HIV, AIDS, AND THE BRAIN

Research Publications:
Association for Research in Nervous and Mental Disease
Volume 72

HIV, AIDS, and the Brain

Research Publications:
Association for Research in Nervous
and Mental Disease
Volume 72

Editors

Richard W. Price, M.D.
Professor and Head
Department of Neurology
University of Minnesota Medical School
Minneapolis, Minnesota

Samuel W. Perry III, M.D.
Cornell University Medical College
The New York Hospital
New York, New York

Raven Press   New York

Raven Press, Ltd., 1185 Avenue of the Americas, New York, New York 10036

Library of Congress Cataloging-in-Publication Data

HIV, AIDS, and the brain / edited by Richard W. Price, Samuel W.
  Perry.
      p.   cm. — (Research publications / Association for Research
  in Nervous and Mental Disease ; v. 72)
      Papers from the 72nd Annual ARNMD Meeting held in New York in Dec.
  1992.
      Includes bibliographical references and index.
      ISBN 0-7817-0063-9
      1. Brain—Infections—Congresses.   2. AIDS (Disease)—
  Complications—Congresses.   3. AIDS dementia complex—Congresses.
  I. Price, Richard W., 1941–   . II. Perry, Samuel, 1940–
  III. Association for Research in Nervous and Mental Diseases.
  Meeting (72nd : 1992 : New York, N.Y.)   IV. Series: Research
  publications (Association for Research in Nervous and Mental
  Disease) ; v. 72.
      [DNLM: 1. AIDS Dementia Complex—physiopathology—congresses.
  2. AIDS Dementia Complex—pathology—congresses.   3. HIV-1—
  pathogenicity—congresses.   W1 RE233P v. 72   1993 / WM 220 H676
  1992]
  RC359.5.H58—1994
  616.97'92—dc20
  DNLM/DLC
  for Library of Congress   93-36006
                                                                      CIP

RESEARCH PUBLICATIONS: ASSOCIATION FOR RESEARCH IN NERVOUS AND MENTAL DISEASE

Titles marked with an (*) are out of print.

Contents

Contributing Authors

Cristian L. Achim, M.D. *Departments of Neurosciences and Pathology, University of California at San Diego, School of Medicine, 9500 Gilman Drive, La Jolla, CA 92093*

M. A. Anderson, Ph.D. *Department of Chemistry, University of Colorado, Boulder, CO 80309*

Helena Bacellar, M.A. *Johns Hopkins School of Hygiene and Public Health, 624 North Broadway, Baltimore, MD 21205*

Anita L. Belman, M.D. *Department of Neurology, SUNY at Stony Brook School of Medicine, Stony Brook, NY 11794*

Etty N. Benveniste, M.D. *Department of Cell Biology, University of Alabama, 1052 Tinsley Harrison Towers, Birmingham, AL 35294*

Celia F. Brosnan, Ph.D. *Department of Pathology (Neuropathology) and the Rose F. Kennedy Center for Research in Mental Retardation and Human Development, Albert Einstein College of Medicine, 1300 Morris Park Avenue, Bronx, NY 10461*

Janice E. Clements, Ph.D. *Department of Neurology, Johns Hopkins University School of Medicine, 720 Rutland Avenue, Baltimore, MD 21205*

Anna da Cunha, D.Phil. *Laboratory of Cell Biology, National Institute of Mental Health, National Institutes of Health, 5600 Fishers Lane, Rockville, MD 20857*

Richard DeTeresa, B.S. *Departments of Neurosciences and Pathology, University of California at San Diego, School of Medicine, 9500 Gilman Drive, La Jolla, CA 92093*

Dennis W. Dickson, M.D. *Department of Pathology (Neuropathology) and the Rose F. Kennedy Center for Research in Mental Retardation and Human Development, Albert Einstein College of Medicine, 1300 Morris Park Avenue, Bronx, NY 10461*

Marc Fishman, M.D. *Department of Psychiatry and Behavioral Science, Johns Hopkins University School of Medicine, Johns Hopkins Hospital, 600 North Wolfe Street, Baltimore, MD 21287*

Nianfeng Ge, M.D.   *Departments of Neurosciences and Pathology, University of California at San Diego, School of Medicine, 9500 Gilman Drive, La Jolla, CA 92093*

Jonathan D. Glass, M.D.   *Department of Neurology, Johns Hopkins University School of Medicine, Johns Hopkins Hospital, 600 North Wolfe Street, Baltimore, MD 21287*

Diane E. Griffin, M.D., Ph.D.   *Department of Neurology, Johns Hopkins University School of Medicine, Johns Hopkins Hospital, 600 North Wolfe Street, Baltimore, MD 21287*

John W. Griffin, M.D.   *Department of Neurology, Johns Hopkins University School of Medicine, Johns Hopkins Hospital, 600 North Wolfe Street, Baltimore, MD 21287*

William Hatch, Ph.D.   *Department of Pathology (Neuropathology) and the Rose F. Kennedy Center for Research in Mental Retardation and Human Development, Albert Einstein College of Medicine, 1300 Morris Park Avenue, Bronx, NY 10461*

Donald R. Hoover, Ph.D., M.P.H.   *Johns Hopkins School of Hygiene and Public Health, 624 North Broadway, Baltimore, MD 21205*

S. V. Joag, M.D., Ph.D.   *Department of Microbiology, Molecular Genetics, and Immunology, University of Kansas Medical Center, 3901 Rainbow Boulevard, Kansas City, KS 66160*

Richard T. Johnson, M.D.   *Department of Neurology, Johns Hopkins University School of Medicine, Johns Hopkins Hospital, 600 North Wolfe Street, Baltimore, MD 21287*

Sunhee C. Lee, M.D.   *Department of Pathology (Neuropathology) and the Rose F. Kennedy Center for Research in Mental Retardation and Human Development, Albert Einstein College of Medicine, 1300 Morris Park Avenue, Bronx, NY 10461*

Stuart A. Lipton, M.D., Ph.D.   *Laboratory of Cellular and Molecular Neuroscience, Department of Neurology, Children's Hospital, Boston, MA 02115; Department of Neurology, Beth Israel Hospital, Brigham and Women's Hospital, and Massachusetts General Hospital, Boston, MA 02115; and Program in Neuroscience, Harvard Medical School, 300 Longwood Avenue, Boston, MA 02115*

Constantine Lyketsos, M.D.   *Department of Psychiatry and Behavioral Science, Johns Hopkins University School of Medicine, Johns Hopkins Hospital, 600 North Wolfe Street, Baltimore, MD 21287*

William D. Lyman, Ph.D.   *Department of Pathology (Neuropathology) and the Rose F. Kennedy Center for Research in Mental Retardation and Human Development, Albert Einstein College of Medicine, 1300 Morris Park Avenue, Bronx, NY 10461*

Eliezer Masliah, M.D. *Departments of Neurosciences and Pathology, University of California at San Diego, School of Medicine, 9500 Gilman Drive, La Jolla, CA 92093*

Linda A. Mattiace, Ph.D. *Department of Pathology (Neuropathology) and the Rose F. Kennedy Center for Research in Mental Retardation and Human Development, Albert Einstein College of Medicine, 1300 Morris Park Avenue, Bronx, NY 10461*

Justin C. McArthur, M.B., B.S., M.P.H. *Department of Neurology, Johns Hopkins University School of Medicine, Johns Hopkins Hospital, 600 North Wolfe Street, Baltimore, MD 21287*

Paul R. McHugh, M.D. *Department of Psychiatry and Behavioral Science, Johns Hopkins University School of Medicine, Johns Hopkins Hospital, 600 North Wolfe Street, Baltimore, MD 21287*

O. Narayan, Ph.D., D.V.M. *Department of Microbiology, Molecular Genetics, and Immunology, University of Kansas Medical Center, 3901 Rainbow Boulevard, Kansas City, KS 66160*

William A. O'Brien, M.D. *Department of Medicine, UCLA School of Medicine, 19833 Le Conte Avenue, Los Angeles, CA 90024*

Michael B. A. Oldstone, M.D. *Head, Viral Immunobiology Laboratory, Division of Virology, Department of Neuropharmacology, The Scripps Research Institute, 10666 North Torrey Pines Road, La Jolla, CA 92037*

Samuel W. Perry III, M.D. *Department of Psychiatry, Cornell University Medical College, The New York Hospital, 525 East 68th Street, New York, NY 10021*

Richard W. Price, M.D. *Professor and Head, Department of Neurology, University of Minnesota Medical School, 420 Delaware Street, SE, Minneapolis, MN 55455*

Ola A. Selnes, Ph.D. *Department of Neurology, Johns Hopkins University School of Medicine, Johns Hopkins Hospital, 600 North Wolfe Street, Baltimore, MD 21287*

Leroy R. Sharer, M.D. *Department of Laboratory Medicine and Pathology, New Jersey Medical School, 185 South Orange Avenue, Newark, NJ 07103*

John J. Sidtis, Ph.D. *Department of Neurology, University of Minnesota Medical School, 420 Delaware Street, SE, Minneapolis, MN 55455*

Glenn Treisman, M.D., Ph.D. *Department of Psychiatry and Behavioral Science, Johns Hopkins University School of Medicine, Johns Hopkins Hospital, 600 North Wolfe Street, Baltimore, MD 21287*

William R. Tyor, M.D. *Department of Neurology, Medical University of South Carolina, Charleston, SC 29425*

Ljubisa Vitkovic, Ph.D. *Division of Neuroscience and Behavioral Science, National Institute of Mental Health, National Institute of Health, 5600 Fishers Lane, Rockville, MD 20857*

Steven L. Wesselingh, M.B.B.S., Ph.D. *Department of Neurology, Johns Hopkins University School of Medicine, Johns Hopkins Hospital, 600 North Wolfe Street, Baltimore, MD 21287*

Clayton A. Wiley, M.D., Ph.D. *Departments of Neurosciences and Pathology, University of California at San Diego, School of Medicine, 9500 Gilman Drive, La Jolla, CA 92093*

M. C. Zink *Department of Neurology, Johns Hopkins University School of Medicine, 720 Rutland Avenue, Baltimore, MD 21205*

Preface

The astonishing and tragic appearance of acquired immunodeficiency syndrome (AIDS) over the last decade made it the "disease of the 1980s." Unfortunately, the continued worldwide explosive growth of the epidemic will also render it the disease of the 1990s and the early 21st century. Among the manifestations of human immunodeficiency virus type 1 (HIV-1) infection and AIDS are an array of clinically important and diverse disorders of the nervous system. While, as with any systemic disease, the major neurological vulnerability relates to profound immunosuppression and consequent opportunistic infections, other disease processes also affect the nervous system; they include autoimmunity, secondary consequences of systemic organ dysfunction (e.g., hypoxic encephalopathy), and toxicities of therapies. The psychological impact of infection and progressive disease is also profound. In addition to these *secondary* effects of HIV-1 on the central nervous system (CNS), the AIDS retrovirus also appears capable of initiating a *primary* neurological disorder variously termed the AIDS dementia complex (ADC), HIV cognitive-motor complex, HIV dementia, and, in children, HIV encephalopathy. This primary effect of HIV on the brain was the subject of the 72nd Annual ARNMD Meeting held in New York in December 1992 and was the basis for the contributions to this volume.

There are several reasons for the circumscribed focus on this single neurological complication. Foremost is its clinical importance. ADC is common, particularly in the late stage of HIV-1 infection in the context of full-blown AIDS, and in severe form it is a source of devastating neurological morbidity. Even when mild, it can importantly interfere with the activities of daily living over a protracted period. A second important reason for detailed attention relates to its pathobiological interest and the evidence that ADC appears to be caused by HIV-1, itself, rather than by a second opportunistic organism. Because of this, its viral pathogenesis is of great interest both with respect to the specifics of the interaction of HIV-1 and the central nervous system and in the more general context as a "model" of viral and immunological diseases of the nervous system that holds broader lessons for CNS disease pathogenesis.

This focus also allows us to deal in considerable depth with various aspects of ADC and CNS HIV-1 infection. The volume begins with a broad introduction by Richard W. Price that highlights the salient observations and considers the general issues of pathogenesis, offering models attempting to reconcile some of the more puzzling observations. This provides a starting point for the more detailed discussion in the chapters that follow.

A background section then deals with basic aspects of the principal pathogenic forces thought to be involved in causing brain dysfunction: the AIDS virus, basic immune system interactions with viruses, and cytokine circuits in the nervous system. William O'Brien's chapter on HIV-1 provides an up-to-date review of the molecular biology of the virus that also focuses particularly on one of the critical issues of neuropathogenesis, namely, the genetic basis of HIV-1 neurotropism. Etty Benveniste reviews the subject of cytokine circuits in the brain, including their cells of origin and effects, and discusses their possible general role in viral regulation and disease pathogenesis and their potential role in ADC. Michael Oldstone emphasizes the potential role of cytotoxic lymphocytes and other immune reactions in protection and neuropathogenesis.

The next section deals in more detail with particular aspects of neuropathology and pathogenesis, presenting evidence from several complementary viewpoints. Dennis Dickson, et al. present a thoughtful review of neuropathology with its major focus on the role of macrophages and microglial cells in pathogenesis based on their studies of patients with AIDS. Eliezer Masliah et al. also review human studies, but with its principal focus on neuronal changes and their relation to immunohistochemically defined infection. These studies of human material are followed by two contributions dealing with an animal model of a related lentivirus, simian immunodeficiency virus (SIV). The first, by Leroy Sharer, reviews the neuropathology of SIV infection in macaque monkeys, including similarities to and differences from HIV-1 in humans. The contribution by Janice Clements, et al. describes a series of experimental studies focusing on the genetic determinants of brain infection and neurotropism.

While peripheral nervous system disease complicating HIV-1 infection was not a primary subject of the conference, John Griffin et al. present results of elegant studies of the common predominantly sensory neuropathy of AIDS with a view to how such studies provide insight into ADC pathogenesis. Their results suggest a possible dysregulation of cytokines with perhaps a deficiency of "inhibiting" cytokines. Stuart Lipton reviews the role of toxins in mediating neuronal injury in ADC emphasizing the final common pathway of amino acid excitotoxicity and the N-methyl-D-aspartate (NMDA) receptor with an eye to its possible therapeutic implications. Ljubisa Vitkovic et al. follow this with a review of their studies of cytokine expression in the brains of AIDS patients and propose a scenario of cytokine-mediated brain injury in ADC.

The next section of the volume is devoted to clinical aspects of HIV-1 infection and its effects on the central nervous system. Two contributions deal with psychiatric disorders. The first, by Samuel Perry, reviews the experience with depression as a complication of HIV-1 infection, including aspects of epidemiology, diagnosis, and treatment. Glenn Treisman, et al. then describe its clinical experience of psychiatric disease in HIV-1-infected subjects. The subject then turns back to "neurological disease" with a review by Justin McArthur, et al. which centers on the epidemiology, natural history, and risk factors of ADC. John Sidtis describes ADC evaluation methodologies and reviews their rationale and the experience with their application to natural history and treatment studies of ADC. Anita Belman reviews the very important pediatric equivalent of ADC—namely, HIV encephalopathy—including its clinical, pathological, pathogenetic, and treatment aspects. Finally, Richard Johnson closes with a historical perspective and an articulation of major questions and future needs.

Altogether the contributions in this book provide a cohesive and provocative picture of a fascinating and important new neurological disease and outline the progress being made in understanding its clinical and pathogenetic aspects. This volume should prove of interest to both clinicians and scientists. For the neurologist, psychiatrist, infectious disease specialist, or other physician as well as for the nonphysician dealing with AIDS patients, there are valuable discussions of both the theory and practice of diagnosis and management of ADC. For the clinical or laboratory scientist engaged in or interested in HIV-1 research or on other issues of viral pathogenesis or neuro-immunology, there are lessons for their own work. This volume should serve as both a milestone in understanding the clinical and pathobiological aspects of ADC and the interactions of HIV-1 and the nervous system, and as a foundation and stimulus for additional study.

Richard W. Price
Samuel W. Perry III

HIV, AIDS, AND THE BRAIN

Research Publications:
Association for Research in Nervous and Mental Disease
Volume 72

HIV, AIDS and the Brain, edited by
R. W. Price and S. W. Perry.
Raven Press, Ltd., New York © 1994.

1

Understanding the AIDS Dementia Complex (ADC)

The Challenge of HIV and Its Effects on the Central Nervous System

Richard W. Price

*Department of Neurology, University of Minnesota Medical School,
Minneapolis, MN 55455*

This chapter provides a selective introduction to some of the central aspects of the AIDS dementia complex (ADC) and its relationship to human immunodeficiency virus type 1 (HIV-1) infection. Its emphasis is on pathogenesis. Despite growing interest and investigation of AIDS and HIV-1 infection, in general, and ADC, in particular, current understanding of the mechanisms involved in this neurological condition remains limited. Yet these pathogenetic issues are both interesting and important, not only with respect to HIV-1 infection, itself, but in relation to other viral and immunological disorders.

BACKGROUND ON SOME PATHOGENETIC ISSUES

Before proceeding to introduce what we *do know* about ADC and central nervous system (CNS) HIV-1 infection, it is useful to consider some of the things we would *like to know*. Table 1 articulates two broad categories of inquiry into pathogenesis of ADC. The first of these relates to understanding the *character of brain dysfunction,* and falls within the traditional purview of the clinical and basic neurobiologist. On a "macro" scale, this includes the questions of how integrated brain function is perturbed, resulting in the characteristic clinical deficits noted in afflicted patients. What is the balance of dysfunction in basal ganglia, cortex, and white matter, and how do these lead to the stereotyped "subcortical" dementia that these patients exhibit? On a "micro" level, questions are directed at the cellular basis for the loss

1

TABLE 1. *Desired levels of understanding of the ADC and CNS HIV-1 infection*

Neuropathophysiology: nature and character of altered brain function
Integrated brain function
What brain structures are disturbed, and how does this disturbance induce the charac-
teristic clinical deficits of ADC?
Individual brain cell function
What brain cells are primarily and secondarily altered, resulting in disturbed integrated
brain function?
Viral pathogenesis: mechanisms of CNS infection and relation to brain dysfunction
Mechanisms of infection bearing on ADC
When and how is the brain infected in the course of systemic infection?
What is the nature of brain infection?
What cells are infected?
What factors determine the course and severity of brain infection?
What factors suppresses and enhance infection?
What host factors?
What viral factors?
Mechanisms of cell dysfunction bearing on ADC
How does infection relate to brain dysfunction?
How does the "viral burden" relate to clinical severity?
What cells are primarily altered by HIV-1, and how?
What causes dysfunction of the important "functional" cells of the CNS?
What cells are secondarily altered by HIV-1, and how?

of integrated brain function. Which cell types and populations are primarily and secondarily injured, and how does this injury result in altered function?

Answers to such neurobiological questions must then be integrated with those relating to the second category, that dealing with *viral and immunological pathogenesis* and the interaction of the virus and its genes with the host organism and particularly its immune system, both within and outside the CNS. When and how does virus reach the CNS, what cells are infected, and what are the consequences of infection? What factors suppress or enhance CNS infection? This is the *principal focus* of this review. While most investigators favor the general hypothesis that ADC relates to a fundamental effect of HIV-1, itself, rather than to an opportunistic infection by another organism, the relation of brain injury to HIV-1 infection and the mechanisms underlying brain injury are not at all well understood (1).

To highlight the questions raised by HIV-1 and ADC, it is instructive to contrast them with the paradigm of CNS infection derived from another era of intense public and investigative attention, namely, poliovirus infection. In the case of this neurotropic picornavirus, there have been for some time reasonably satisfactory and detailed answers to the questions listed in Table 1, although pursuit of a more molecular understanding continues to reveal fascinating detail. The characteristic symptoms and signs of poliomyelitis (i.e., flaccid motor weakness) relate to acute direct infection and consequent death of spinal motor neurons. Neuronal cytolysis results from the action of the poliovirus genome *from within* infected neurons.

By contrast, in the case of HIV-1 and ADC, the view of pathogenesis, and particularly the connection between the virus and cell dysfunction, is much hazier. This is because the relation between HIV-1 and neurological dysfunction is less direct and seemingly more complicated (1,2). HIV-1 infection within the CNS involves cells derived from the bone marrow, recently invading monocyte-derived macrophages or more remotely invading microglia with similar properties, and not the "functional cells" of the brain derived from neuroectoderm—that is, the neurons, oligodendrocytes, or astrocytes (3–15; Dickson et al., *this volume*). How are these functional cells then disturbed *from without?* The underlying pathology is also heterogeneous and, along with the number and distribution of infected cells, does not immediately explain the clinical state. To deal with these observations, most investigations now focus on *indirect* mechanisms of cell injury, rather than direct cytolytic activity of the virus as in polio.

TABLE 2. *Sources of information pertaining to the pathogenesis of ADC and CNS HIV-1 infection*

Data source	Derived concepts
Experimental laboratory-based studies	
In vitro models	Cell and molecular biology of viral replication and gene expression: general and relevant cell-specific
	Assessment of viral effects (signals, toxicity) on relevant cells
In vivo (animal) models	Assessment of pathogenetic mechanisms
	Assessment of viral gene determinants of infection and disease
Patient-based studies	
Clinical studies of systemic disease	Background understanding of interaction of HIV-1 with human host, including immune system
Neurological characterization	Character of "subcortical" brain dysfunction
Neurological history	
Neurological examination	
Neuropsychological testing	
Epidemiology/natural history	Relation of ADC to systemic immunosuppression and virus load
Neuroimaging	
Anatomical (CT/MRI)	Presence and correlations of brain atrophy
	Focal increased water, blood–brain barrier disruption
Physiological (PET/SPECT)	Disturbed diencephalic–cortical relations
	Reduced cortical metabolism and blood flow
Cerebrospinal fluid analysis	
Virology	Early viral invasion
Host responses	Late immune activation associated with ADC
Pathology	
Microscopic histopathology	Heterogeneous pathologies and correlates
	Individual cell changes
Virus identification/localization	Identity and correlation of virus detection
Human virology	
Isolation, cloning	Identification of "neurotropic" strains

The overall understanding of pathogenesis is also complicated by the protracted course and important systemic effects of HIV-1 infection, in contrast to the acute course of polio affecting only the gastrointestinal tract in addition to brain. ADC occurs in the setting of a complex and evolving relation of HIV-1 with the host immune system and a resultant background of progressive immunodeficiency (for review, see ref. 16). To address the pathogenetic challenge of ADC, it is important to integrate observations from both the clinic and the laboratory. Patient-based studies are the touchstone of pathogenic formulations, and hypotheses must always return to the patient for testing. These are complemented by experimental studies which provide a proving ground, particularly for probing mechanisms at the cellular and molecular levels. Patient and experimental studies each profit from continuous cross-checking and cross-fertilization. Table 2 outlines some of the principal sources underlying current understanding, dividing them into experimental laboratory-based and patient-based studies.

This chapter approaches these issues in three major sections: The *first* briefly considers selected general aspects of HIV-1 infection which appear particularly relevant to CNS infection and ADC, the *second* reviews some of the major patient-based observations which provide the foundation for understanding, and the *third* attempts a synthesis in the form of models of pathogenesis. The chapter then closes with brief consideration of some general implications for neurology.

SOME GENERAL ASPECTS OF HIV-1 INFECTION

While it is well beyond the scope of this introductory chapter to discuss the molecular and general biology of HIV-1, it may be useful to briefly underscore some selected aspects of HIV-1 in order to provide a context for considering certain aspects of neuropathogenesis.

Viral Glycoproteins

HIV-1 is a member of the lentivirus group of retroviruses; like other members of this group, it has a complex genome with several regulatory genes in addition to the major *env, pol,* and *gag* genes and the long terminal repeat (LTR) shared across the retroviruses (for reviews, see refs. 17–19 and O'Brien, *this volume*). Its genome is efficiently packaged in a membrane-bound virion, and its *life cycle* begins with interaction of the virion surface glycoprotein, gp120, with the major cell receptor, CD4, on a subset of lymphocytes and macrophages. Binding, penetration, and uncoating appear to also involve secondary interactions of these and other molecules. Gp120 is also secreted by infected cells and may have intercellular signal activities in addition to its binding function (O'Brien, *this volume*).

One of the important properties of HIV-1 is its *genetic variability*. In fact, individual patients are infected by what has been termed a "quasispecies," a population of related viruses derived from the original infecting inoculum (20). This genetic heterogeneity translates into variability in both antigenic and biologic properties. Among the latter, differences in cell tropism relate largely to differences in the sequences coding gp120 that determine, for example, the relative ability to infect macrophages compared to lymphocyte cell lines as discussed in detail elsewhere (21; O'Brien, *this volume*). A second glycoprotein, the transmembrane glycoprotein, gp41, is involved in penetration and also mediates cell–cell fusion and hence the characteristic cytopathology of multinucleated-cell syncytia. Both gp120 and gp41 are coded from the *env* region of the genome and are, in fact, cleavage products of a single precursor.

Reverse Transcriptase

The viral reverse transcriptase (RT), which is coded by the *pol* region of the genome and catalyzes the production of proviral DNA copies of the viral (single-stranded RNA) genome, is critical to both latency and productive infection. This viral enzyme is brought into the cell as part of the virion. As a result of its differences from cellular DNA polymerase, this enzyme can be targeted by antiviral therapy and serves as the basis of the selective action of zidovudine and the other nucleoside anti-retrovirals (22). With the help of another viral gene derived from the *pol* gene, the proviral DNA usually integrates into the cellular genome and thus becomes a part of the host DNA complement, replicating as these cells divide. It is this integration property which assures the long-term survival of the viral genome in the host until death. The poor fidelity of RT also underlies the variability of HIV-1 and the generation of quasispecies.

Replication

Subsequent to integration, the initiation and course of gene expression and replication is regulated in a highly complex manner which can be considered to involve two major phases: The first is directed to production of regulatory gene products, and the second is directed to structural gene products and progeny virus. The initiation and regulation of replication is "focused" through the LTR portion of the genome which contains sequences that respond to intracellular signals—including, for example, NFκB and SP1, which normally regulate cellular genes. Indeed, it is part of the "genius" of HIV-1 that its regulation shares mechanisms with cellular regulatory processes; this allows physiological cell stimuli to up- or down-regulate viral gene expression and replication. Among these are signals from cells of the immune system, and in this way regulation of HIV-1 expression becomes intimately involved in networks of immune cell regulation. These mechanisms appear important in determining the slow tempo of systemic infection and disease, assuring that latent virus is expressed, but not all at once. Products of two of the regulatory genes, *tat* and *nef,* have been hypothesized to act as neurotoxins mediating brain dysfunction (23,24).

Development of Immunosuppression and AIDS

These genes and their packaging in the HIV-1 virion are ultimately responsible for AIDS. While the disease process is complicated, it is mediated principally by the capacity of the virus to infect and, eventually destroy, $CD4^+$ T lymphocytes, a population of cells critical to defending the host against a range of intracellular microbes. While the mechanisms of T-cell attrition remain somewhat controversial, recent evidence showing more active replication and a higher percentage of infected cells in lymph nodes than previously suspected from analysis of peripheral blood is consistent with the basic concept that HIV-1 infection slowly, but directly, kills these cells (8,16,25). This may involve apoptosis or other killing mechanisms. Infection of monocyte-derived macrophages and related cells may also contribute to the profile of immunosuppression. These cells can differ from lymphocytes in the profile of infection, supporting chronic productive infection without cytolysis rather than simple phasic, cytolytic infection, which is characteristic of lymphocyte infection once replication is triggered (26).

While lethal immunosuppression is the ultimate outcome, it is useful to consider HIV-1 infection as a syndrome of immune *dysregulation* in which abnormal immune activation, including frank autoimmunity, may also occur (Oldstone, *this volume*). HIV-1 infection can not only lead to simple cell death, but also to abnormal regulation of immune responses, either as sequelae of the effects on $CD4^+$ T-cell-related regulation of immunity or perhaps as a result of effects of secreted viral gene products on uninfected cells. In this sense the issues to be discussed below regarding "indirect" pathogenetic mechanisms for CNS disease may apply to some aspects of systemic disease as well.

The most important clinical complications defining AIDS are secondary to the virus-induced immunosuppression, and the threshold for their appearance is near 200 $CD4^+$ cells/mm^3, with lower counts increasing their likelihood. At these levels the host has increasing difficulty dealing with a number of intracellular pathogens, including particular parasites, fungi, bacteria, and viruses. Progressive disease is also accompanied by evidence of systemic up-regulation of cytokines. This derives from elevated concentrations in the blood of certain "surrogate markers," including beta-2-microglobulin (β_2M) and neopterin, which rise with disease severity and carry prognostic implications similar to that of falling $CD4^+$ T-cell counts (27a,28).

PATIENT-BASED STUDIES OF ADC AND CNS HIV-1 INFECTION

Patient studies using a variety of tools, both those available routinely to the clinician and those more specialized and restricted to the clinical investigator or the laboratory scientist, have provided important and challenging insight into the interaction of HIV-1 infection and neurological dysfunction. These include clinical observation, epidemiological and natural history studies, anatomic and functional neuroimaging, analysis of cerebrospinal fluid (CSF), and studies of brain, itself, usually obtained at autopsy.

Neurological Dysfunction: Character and Terminology

In considering terminology, it is important to begin by emphasizing an essential distinction between HIV-1 infection, on the one hand, and ADC, on the other. HIV-1 infection of the CNS refers to a *pathobiological process* involving the virus and its interaction with the host. This infection is a complicated process which begins early in the course of systemic infection and pursues a variable evolution over a time frame of several years. ADC, by contrast, refers only to a *clinical syndrome* identified on the basis of characteristic symptoms and signs, time course, and laboratory test profile (29–32). Most contributions to this volume are predicated, either explicitly or implicitly, upon the belief that these two are interrelated and that, indeed, the ADC syndrome relates, at least in part, to CNS retroviral infection. However, at present the nature of such a relationship is not well understood; indeed, cause and effect are by no means established with certainty. For this reason, it is important to continue to keep CNS infection and the clinical ADC syndrome separate, both in our minds and in our vocabularies.

Terminology and ADC Staging

While what we now call ADC was recognized early in the epidemic under a variety of appellations (33–37), the designation of this tripartite term in 1985 (29,38) crystallized certain important concepts that remain relevant today. *AIDS* was included in the term because the morbidity and prognosis of this condition can parallel that of other AIDS-defining illnesses. Subsequently, this recognition was incorporated into the Centers for Disease Control (CDC) definition of AIDS (39), although with further experience it is reasonable to restrict this clinical AIDS definition to patients suffering a degree of severity defined by Stage 2 ADC or greater (see below). *Dementia* was part of the term because cognitive dysfunction is the most common presenting problem and the principal source of morbidity. However, *complex* was incorporated because these patients suffer a constellation of abnormalities which importantly include motor and behavioral components and not simply an isolated dementia such as early Alzheimer's disease.

It was also recognized early that this syndrome fit best within the group of so-called "subcortical dementias" based upon patients' characteristic psychomotor slowing and difficulty with attention and concentration, similar to other diseases within this classification, such as Parkinson's disease, Huntington's disease, and hydrocephalus (40,41). This is in distinction from the "cortical dementias" characterized by difficulties with memory, language, or other focal cortical syndromes. Unfortunately, inclusion of the word *dementia* has led to some confusion since in recent years this term has improperly evolved to be synonymous with dementia of the Alzheimer's type in some circles, rather than retaining its broader generic meaning. Nonetheless, we still favor the ADC nomenclature at this phase of our understanding (32,42).

In order to provide a common vocabulary for the severity of ADC for clinicians as well as for correlative studies linking clinical observations with various laboratory results, including pathological and virological findings, we empirically derived a simple ADC staging scheme based on functional status in the cognitive and motor domains, denoting patients as unaffected (Stage 0), subclinically or equivocally affected (Stage 0.5), or suffering mild (Stage 1), moderate (Stage 2), severe (Stage 3), and end-stage disease (Stage 4) using simple criteria (30,153; also see Sidtis, *this volume*).

More recently, a derivative classification was proposed by the World Health Organization (WHO) and the American Academy of Neurology (AAN) (44,45a) using the term *HIV-1 associated cognitive/motor complex* to encompass the full constellation of ADC and adding subcategories to refer to patients with predominantly cognitive (*HIV-1-associated dementia*) or myelopathic (*HIV-1-associated myelopathy*) presentations of sufficient severity to interfere with work or activities of daily living (a severity equivalent to ADC Stages 2–4). The term *HIV-1-associated minor cognitive/motor disorder* was introduced to designate patients with mild but definite symptoms and signs and only minimal functional impairment of work or activities of daily living (equivalent to Stage 1 ADC).

We have discussed elsewhere how the WHO/AAN terminologies can be "translated" (32). The WHO/AAN terminology tends to "split" what the ADC term "lumps." Thus, the former attempts to separate patients with predominant myelopathy (and, as described below, likely to exhibit vacuolar spinal cord pathology) from those with cognitive changes. While this may eventually have implications for prognosis and therapy, unfortunately many patients will have elements of both cognitive impairment and myelopathy, and the findings may be difficult to accurately separate. The WHO/AAN terminology restricts the term *dementia* to patients with a level of cognitive impairment consistent with that used in other formal definitions, whereas ADC includes this term in the entire spectrum, but always qualified by the inclusion of "complex" indicating referral to the broader syndrome. The WHO/AAN classification also does not convey an implicit assumption that the disorder is a single disease entity differing only in severity, but allows for the possibility that milder and more severe disease could be discontinuous processes; as discussed below, this is an important, but unsettled, pathogenetic issue. It might also simplify reporting this condition as a clinical AIDS-defining disorder if one restricts this designation to patients with sufficient functional severity to be termed *HIV-1 associated dementia* or *HIV-1 associated myelopathy*. Requirement for this level of severity (equivalent to ADC Stage 2 or greater ADC) is likely both biologically and prognostically consistent with other AIDS-defining conditions and simplifies thinking of AIDS versus non-AIDS, although this consideration may be largely superseded by the recent revision of the CDC definition which uses $CD4^+$ T-lymphocyte counts of <200 cells/mm^3 to define AIDS (39,40a). On the other hand, the WHO/AAN terminology was derived not only from ADC staging, but also from other disease definitions, and suffers from the artificiality of consolidating some features of other dementias in an effort to be "consistent." In contrast, the ADC classification was empirically derived from clinical experience and analysis of the condition (Sidtis, *this volume*). ADC classification also admits that what is considered "minor" disease in the WHO/AAN classification is not always minor to patients and friends of those afflicted. Additionally, we have found the ADC Stage 0.5 very useful for both clinical and investigative characterization of patients, allowing a needed middle ground between normal and abnormal. For these reasons we have continued to adhere to the ADC terminology until a more advanced classification can be based on clearer understanding of disease etiology and pathogenesis.

Epidemiology and Natural History

In addition to its utility in guiding diagnostic probabilities and prognosis, definition of the epidemiology and natural history, and particularly the relation of ADC onset and severity to the state of systemic viral infection and immunosuppression, is important to understanding pathogenesis. The systemic and neurological complications of HIV-1 infection are *stage-related;* that is, specific clinical conditions characteristically arise in the context of particular levels of immunosuppression (10,16,46). This is also true for ADC, making it useful to examine this disorder in the context of other complications of HIV-1 (Table 3). As a general rule, severe ADC (Stage 2 or greater) occurs in the same setting as the major opportunistic infections, when $CD4^+$ cells are severely depressed to below 200 cells/mm^3 and usually lower. Hence it

TABLE 3. *Stages of systemic and CNS HIV-1 infection and disease[a]*

Systemic infection/disease	CNS infection/ADC
Acute infection	
Viremia	
Immune-mediated virus suppression	
Clinical latency	*Neurologically asymptomatic*
Early immunodominant (CD4$^+$ >500 cells/mm^3)	Immunodominant.
	Silent infection, CNS entry and ?
Silent infection: virus persists and replicates in lymph organs	persistence
Transition, pre-AIDS	*Mild ADC (Stages 0.5–1)*
Waning immunity (CD4$^+$ 200–500)	
Minor opportunistic infections	
Virus escape, increased viral burden	
Cytokine up-regulation	Cytokine up-regulation: gliosis-pallor
AIDS	*More severe ADC (Stages 2–4)*
Severe immunosuppression (CD4$^+$ < 200).	
Major opportunistic infections	
Virus dominant, increased viremia	Virus-dominant: multinucleated-cell, HIV-1, encephalitis
Cytokine up-regulation	Cytokine up-regulation: gliosis-pallor
Viral CNS entry	
Immune-mediated virus suppression	

[a] The listing includes speculations regarding possible parallels between systemic and CNS events and relations between both the virus and immune reactions and clinical brain dysfunction.

occurs in the setting of immunosuppression and a high viral burden. This association suggests that severe ADC is also an opportunistic complication, but one in which the same organism, HIV-1, both "creates" the opportunity by systemic infection and then "exploits" it in causing CNS infection and disease.

However, within a given range of CD4$^+$ cells, the incidence of ADC varies greatly. At the one extreme are patients who suffer repeated episodes of life-threatening opportunistic infection but continue to work normally between hospitalizations, and at the other extreme are patients who develop ADC as the sole and prevailing complication of HIV-1 infection without other major complications (47). Also, while most Stage 2–4 ADC patients show laboratory evidence of major immunosuppression, a rare patient has more preserved T-cell counts. This is not unlike the case with some of the opportunistic infections in which a group probability can be based on serological evidence of previous exposure to the opportunistic organism and CD4$^+$ counts (48), but predicting whether or when an individual patient will develop active infection is difficult. Individual variability in reactivation of dormant infections may relate to differences in the general and organism-specific functional severity of immunosuppression at given CD4$^+$ counts and to differences in the previous experience with the organism, as well as other undefined host susceptibility factors. Individual ADC incidence is similarly difficult to predict. These patients generally harbor a high virus load, with detectable viremia or p24 antigenemia, but so do many patients without ADC. These considerations allow the conclusion that immunosuppression has a *permissive* effect on development of more advanced ADC but is insufficient in itself. Other factors clearly are also involved.

The case of milder ADC, both Stage 1 and the subclinical fraction of Stage 0.5, is less clear (153). Certainly, the incidence of this form of ADC also increases with depression of CD4$^+$ counts, and, indeed, before zidovudine treatment, it was our impression based on a highly selected experience that the majority of late AIDS patients showed evidence of neurological abnormality (29,38). Additionally, an appreciable number of patients with intermediate level CD4$^+$ levels (200–500 cells/mm^3) could be classified in these milder categories. Whereas Stage 2 or greater ADC is generally a progressive condition, the lower-stage syndrome is therefore more variable and can pursue a benign course. In some of these, both the patients' histories and follow-up examinations suggest a static course without progression for a period of years. Does this mean that the mild and severe ADC are, in fact, different disorders with differing pathogeneses despite their phenotypic similarity, or are differences merely quantitative, reflecting varying severity of the underlying processes?

Neuroimaging: A Dynamic View of Gross Brain Morphology and Physiology

Anatomical and functional neuroimaging studies have provided important insight but have also raised fundamental questions regarding ADC pathogenesis. They have given a general picture of loss of brain substance, increase in water within white and subcortical gray matter, and altered metabolic activity of certain brain regions. These abnormalities generally correlate with clinical onset and severity and can be reversed, at least in part, by antiretroviral therapy.

Brain atrophy is foremost among the anatomical changes revealed by computed tomography (CT) and magnetic resonance imaging (MRI) in ADC patients (29,49–51,51a). In fact, imaging studies of the brain in life have been more sensitive to the presence and degree of brain substance loss than has gross inspection at autopsy. While the presence of brain atrophy has limited specificity and should not be used to diagnose ADC independent of the clinical findings, reduced brain volume and concomitant increase in CSF volume within enlarged cerebral ventricles and subarachnoid space is nearly universal in ADC and generally increases with severity. A number of studies are now more rigorously examining the quantitative relation between brain atrophy to brain dysfunction. Among the fundamental question provoked by observations of atrophy are: What is the anatomical basis of the brain volume loss? What component(s) are reduced: neurons, white matter, neuropil? Perhaps all are affected, but better quantitative evaluation of both neuroimaging studies and pathological materials will be needed to answer this question.

MRI scanning has also shown that there may be conspicuous changes in brain water content in some ADC patients, best seen on T2-weighted images. The most common pattern is a "diffuse" increase signal in involving the deeper white matter with sparing the "U" fibers immediately adjacent to the cortex. In other cases, increased signal is detected in a multifocal or patchy distribution. Similar changes in water are sometimes also evident in the basal ganglia. These abnormalities are presumably *in vivo* counterparts of defined pathological changes considered below and signify disruption of the blood–brain barrier. Thus, diffuse signal in the white matter is likely the imaging counterpart of white matter pallor and gliosis, whereas patchy focal changes in the white matter or diencephalon may relate to foci of multinucleated-cell (HIV-1) encephalitis, although these correlations have not been established directly by rigorous radiographical–pathological correlation studies. Anecdotally arguing in favor of at least some of the focal white matter changes relating to HIV-1 encephalitis is their improvement following zidovudine therapy (52; BJ Brew and RW Price, *unpublished observations*).

Metabolic imaging has shown altered regional glucose utilization using positron emission tomography (PET) in conjunction with fluorodeoxyglucose (FDG) as a metabolic tracer (53). Several types of abnormality have been reported, including global metabolic defect and heterogeneity of cortical metabolism. These abnormalities have been noted to normalize with zidovudine treatment (54). Perhaps most intriguing from the standpoint of understanding the nature of altered brain physiology in the ADC are the FDG–PET findings which show a pattern of disturbed metabolic relationships between cortical and diencephalic nuclei, with relative cortical hypometabolism and diencephalic hypermetabolism (53). This change in pattern may correlate with early difficulties with attention-concentration and reaction time and may eventually help to understand the nature of a dementia in which cortical skills are slowed well before they are lost.

Single-photon-emission computed tomography (SPECT) using a cerebral blood-flow tracer has shown heterogeneity of brain blood flow in some ADC patients (55). While not as readily quantitated as PET, SPECT is more widely available and might prove useful in some cases, particularly where differentiation from psychiatric disease is needed. However, further study is needed to prove the clinical utility and cost-effectiveness of this modality.

CSF Analysis

Studies of the CSF have also provided a view of the dynamic aspects of CNS HIV-1 infection and ADC. Indeed, sampling of this fluid that surrounds the brain and spinal cord has provided unique and provocative information regarding exposure of the CNS to HIV-1 early in the course of systemic infection and immune activation later accompanying the onset of neurological dysfunction. Before briefly describing some of these findings, it is worthwhile to pause and raise the important caveat that findings in CSF do not always reflect processes occurring within the brain. While CSF sampled by simple lumbar puncture can provide a unique window into the CNS, the composition of CSF compartment is not identical to brain interstitial fluid, and processes affecting the two compartments may be either parallel or divergent. Therefore, any extrapolation from CSF to brain must eventually be tested more directly. With this caution, it is fair to say that CSF analysis has provided a view of HIV-1 infection unavailable by any other means, particularly with respect to analyzing early infection and registering serial observation on individual patients.

Early Infection

Studies of subjects early in HIV-1 infection give evidence of both early entry of HIV-1 into the CSF and local host responses (56–65). A number of studies of seropositive, systemically and neurologically asymptomatic subjects studied early in the course of infection, including patients in proximity to seroconversion as well as later in the course of clinical latency, have shown evidence of the virus's presence. This includes the indirect evidence afforded by intrathecal synthesis of antibody directed against viral antigens as well as direct detection of both viral nucleic acid by polymerase chain reaction (PCR) and infectious virus by culture isolation. Careful assessment of these "virus-positive" subjects indicates that they are usually neurologically normal, not only by history and bedside examination but by formal and sensitive quantitative neuropsychological testing. Additionally, they may remain clinically normal in follow-up evaluation over a period of years. Indeed, there is no clear proof that such abnormalities, including virus detection, predict later ADC.

The most reasonable interpretation of these observations is that HIV-1 reaches the CSF compartment early and either persists locally or is continually reseeded throughout the course of infection. How the virus enters, whether as free virus or within cells, and whether it persists locally—and, if so, in what form—all remain to be addressed. However, if access is in the form of intracellular virus involving a "Trojan Horse" mechanism (66,67), high-level exposure may relate to the nonspecific enhancement in the traffic of lymphocytes or even monocytes into the CNS which follows immune cell activation (68). That early entry might involve the brain parenchyma in a fashion similar to that of CSF is supported anecdotally by the case reported by Davis et al. (69) of an unfortunate individual who was mistakenly injected with HIV-1-infected white blood cells and in whom infected cells were later identified in postmortem brain days later.

While these CSF observations provide evidence of the early and, perhaps, chronic nature of HIV-1 infection, they do not further clarify the activity of viral replication or viral gene expression, including whether infection is locally propagated and persistent. Replication is presumably, at best, very indolent because p24 antigen is not usually detected in CSF at this stage, nor are high titers of cell-free virus. It is challenging to try to integrate these observations with recent reports of more active systemic viremia and lymph node infection during the phase of clinical latency than recognized earlier (8,25). The large load of viral particles contacting lymph-node follicular dendritic cells indicates that virions are actively circulating and raises the question of whether these particles may access the CSF through the choroid plexus, either as free virions or complexed with antibody. Likewise, the large number of latently infected CD4$^+$ T lymphocytes and macrophages could explain cell-associated entry. In any event, it seems apparent from CSF studies that this compartment and, by extrapolation, possibly the brain parenchyma as well participates in this protracted infection in the absence of symptoms or signs of organ dysfunction.

One explanation for the absence of symptoms during this phase might be that immune defenses are able to confine local replication to a level that precludes cytopathology. Circumstantial support for this comes from evidence that CSF virus is "detected" by the host. Not only are there nonspecific local responses, including increased immunoglobulin, protein, and cell counts, but, as mentioned, there is also local (intrathecal) synthesis of antibody against viral antigens. Anti-HIV-1 cytotoxic T cells (CD8$^+$) can also be identified in CSF (71). These reactions, if echoed in the brain as well, could account for the very limited replication of entering or persistent virus and explain why, despite the "opportunity" for CNS HIV-1 infection very early in the course of systemic infection, it does not take place. Local defenses derived from systemic protective mechanisms seem able to reach the brain and suppress replications as they do elsewhere in the body.

Late Infection

Certain observations of CSF sampled late in infection, and particularly in association with ADC, have also been informative and provocative. These include studies providing the initial support for the suggestion that brain injury might result from immune activation and cytokine-directed cytotoxicity. Important in this regard are observations that concentrations of certain "surrogate markers" of immune activation are increased in the CSF of ADC patients. Among the markers initially studied were $\beta_2 M$, neopterin, and quinolinic acid (72–76). While diagnostically nonspecific (because similar elevation accompanies a variety of inflammatory conditions), in the absence of confounding conditions the elevation of these markers appear to reflect immune activation provoked by HIV-1 itself. In this regard, CSF elevations parallel those that can be detected in blood, although their concentration in CSF generally reflects a separate compartment in the absence of major blood–brain barrier disruption (73,74). As noted earlier, blood concentrations of $\beta_2 M$ and neopterin have been shown to be predictive markers of prognosis, although the mechanisms underlying the increased concentrations have not been established. $\beta_2 M$ is the light-chain, noncovalently bound component of the major histocompatibility class 1 (MHC-1) surface molecule and is up-regulated by a variety of cytokines, including interferon gamma (IFN-γ). Neopterin is a product of pteridine metabolism, and its production is increased when macrophages are "activated" by IFN-γ and other cytokines. Neither of these molecules is known to directly mediate altered cell function, although neopterin is speculated to have some influence over certain biochemical pathways (77).

Quinolinic acid appears to be activated in parallel; indeed, the three markers are generally highly intercorrelated. However, this product of tryptophan metabolism is known to be biologically active as a neurotoxin, acting as an endogenous excitotoxin at the N-methyl-D-aspartate (NMDA) receptor. Heyes, in particular, has been a champion of the role of quinolinic acid as an important toxin in ADC and other inflammatory conditions (78). He and his co-workers have shown that quinolinic acid may be present in CSF, and, more recently, in brain at concentrations which can kill neurons in cell culture.

The mechanisms underlying the induction of these "markers" are discussed in speculative terms later. Neither their cell source, mechanisms of induction, nor pathogenic role are established with certainty. While macrophages are the suspected candidates for the principal cell source and IFN-γ is suspected as being the major inciting cytokine, this has not been directly shown and probably is a simplification of the complex pleiotropic and redundant system of cytokine activation and action.

Studies of HIV-1 in the CSF late in infection have been less informative. While ADC, particularly in its severe forms, may be accompanied by more active CSF infection in the form of detectable p24 HIV-1 core antigen, this is not regularly the case (58,61,79). As a result, detection of p24 in CSF is generally too insensitive to be of practical clinical use. Perhaps of more interest pathogenetically, comparison of viral isolates from CSF and brain may reveal differences, indicating that infection of these two compartments may differ with respect to virus traffic, persistence, or replication. While this has not been studied systematically, it is illustrated by the studies of Chen and colleagues (80; see also O'Brien, *this volume*), who isolated two prototype HIV-1 variants from one ADC patient: *JR-FL* from the frontal lobe of brain and *JR-CSF* from the CSF. Only the first of these has the strong properties of macrophage tropism. This brings us back to the earlier caution regarding extrapolating findings in CSF to brain.

Studies of Autopsied Brain: Pathology and Identification
of the Virus in Brain

While the autopsy is a fading institution, its findings are a principal foundation for our understanding of CNS infection and ADC. It is the critical source of tissue for direct analysis of virological, immunological, and biochemical data. Fortunately, early in the epidemic, autopsy rates for AIDS patients surged as the tide of curiosity swept patients' relatives along with the medical community, who together sought answers to the questions surrounding this novel disease. Dickson (*this volume;* see also ref. 81) provides a splendid and thoughtful review of the pathology of ADC and CNS HIV-1 infection, so consideration here will be brief and emphasize only a few points: the heterogeneity of pathologies, the character and localization of CNS infection, the correlations of pathology with both clinical state and virological findings, and the character of viral isolates from brain.

Spectrum of Brain Pathologies and their Virological and Clinical Correlates

Pathological analysis provides yet another viewpoint from which to approach the interaction of HIV-1 and the CNS and the clinical sequelae. Indeed, such analysis has provided an additional set of terms to be reconciled and correlated with clinical manifestations and virological findings (82). The power of pathological analysis is such that it should provide the "glue" to reconcile these various approaches, particularly when coupled with current methods of analyzing viral and cellular gene expression in conjunction with morphology.

One of the impediments to any simple formulation of the pathogenesis of ADC is the heterogeneity of the pathological findings (83). In an effort to analyze clinical–pathological correlates, we segregated the common pathologies into three major categories: (i) white matter pallor and gliosis, the most common yet least pathologically specific; (ii) multinucleated-cell encephalitis, the next most common and, as discussed below, related to productive HIV-1 infection; and (iii) vacuolar myelopathy overlapping both (Fig. 1) (1,38). Other pathologies occur less commonly, including vacuolation or spongiform change within brain as well as microfocal areas of necrosis. These pathologies have in common their preferential involvement of subcortical structures compared to cortex. Table 4 outlines some general correlations among the clinical, pathological and virological findings.

Gliosis-pallor characteristically affects the deeper white matter, sparing the subcortical "U" fibers and extends into the deep gray matter as well.

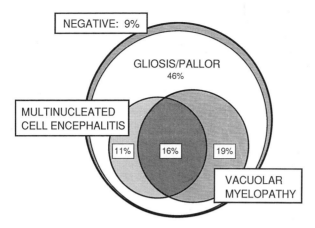

FIG. 1. Major neuropathologies of ADC. The figure diagrams the findings of Navia et al. (38) analyzing the overlapping incidence of the three major pathologies noted at autopsy in AIDS patients in which opportunistic infections and other unrelated pathologies were excluded.

The substrate of myelin pallor is unclear, but it should not be misconstrued as true demeylination, since the integrity of the myelin sheath appears to be preserved. Pale staining of white matter may relate chiefly to increased interstitial water concentration. This would fit with the higher water content noted in the white matter by MRI discussed earlier. Both astrocytes and microglia are also increased in the background. This is the most common finding and can be the sole abnormality in patients dying with milder ADC. In our hands, "conventional" tools for virus detection, including immunohistochemistry and *in situ* hybridization, fail to detect evidence of virus in most of these cases (84; BJ Brew, M Rosenblum, K Cronin, and RW Price, *unpublished observations*). This may relate to the relative insensitivity of these methods which require active transcription and translation, likely in the process of productive infection, to detect the viral signal. More recent studies using PCR have shown that proviral DNA can be found more frequently in such cases (27,85a,150), but even with this ultrasensitive methodology,

TABLE 4. *Clinical correlations with neuropathology and virology*

Clinical	Pathology	Virology
Mild ADC (ADC Stage 0.5–1)	Gliosis-pallor	Negative or minimal productive infection
Severe ADC (ADC Stage 2–4)	Multinucleated-cell encephalitis	Productive infection
Myelopathic ADC (ADC Stage 1–4: spastic/ataxic paraparesis)	Vacuolar myelopathy	Negative for productive infection

proviral DNA is not ubiquitous and the signal is likely small, consistent with a low viral burden in these brains.

Multinucleated-cell encephalitis is marked by the presence of multinucleated cells derived from macrophages and microglia, often in clusters around blood vessels. Additional infected and uninfected macrophages and microglia may be conspicuous in the parenchyma (81; Dickson et al., *this volume*). The clusters of multinucleated cells may be accompanied by surrounding microfocal tissue rarefaction and, occasionally, true demyelination (38). These changes are superimposed on a background of diffuse gliosis and pallor. All methods of virus detection usually readily detect viral signal in multinucleated-cell encephalitis (3–7,9–15,84,87,87a; Dickson et al., *this volume*). Indeed, this pathology can be legitimately called HIV-1 encephalitis. The multinucleated cells are HIV-1-infected cells that have undergone virus-induced cell fusion. Some patients will have a similar encephalitis with few or no multinucleated cells, perhaps because the viral strain is less fusogenic. These encephalitic patients usually have moderate-to-severe ADC occurring in the setting of marked immunosuppression. The systemic viral burden is also usually high. While it is presumed that their clinical condition relates to this pathology, they all have underlying gliosis-pallor as well (38).

While vacuolar myelopathy may involve the entire spinal cord, it is often more severe in the cervical and high thoracic segments (88). It usually more severely affects the lateral and posterior columns in a funicular rather than a systemic distribution, but all zones of the cord white matter may be involved in the most marked cases. Vacuolation may also extend into the white matter of the medulla and pons in some cases. Pathologically, it is indistinguishable from the myelopathy of subacute combined degeneration secondary to vitamin B_{12} deficiency, although these patients usually have normal serum levels of this cofactor. Vacuolar myelopathy is perhaps the most puzzling of the pathologies. Clinically, it correlates with spastic–ataxic paraparesis of varying degree and generally occurs in late systemic disease. Although not universally agreed upon, our own studies indicate that vacuolar myelopathy is not related to productive infection, at least not in the same way as multinucleated-cell encephalitis or its spinal cord extension, multinucleated-cell myelitis (89). Whether vacuolar myelopathy relates fundamentally to HIV-1 infection at all, or to a metabolic disorder only indirectly related to HIV-1, is wholly a matter of speculation at this point. Because there is now little clue regarding this issue, vacuolar myelopathy is largely omitted from considerations of pathogenesis below.

Cellular and Regional Localization of Infection

Definition of infected brain cells at present pertains only to those productively infected and hence only to cases with multinucleated-cell encephalitis or its mononuclear variant, since these are the only cases in which current techniques allow localization of viral signal in tissue sections. While there was considerable controversy in early studies regarding the identity of infected cells, this has diminished as near consensus has been approached (6,14,84,90). It is now generally agreed that productive infection is confined principally or nearly exclusively to macrophages and related microglial cells of bone marrow origin (15,81,91–93,93a; Dickson et al., *this volume*). Oligo-dendrocytes may occasionally be infected (94), and vascular endothelial cell infection is still advocated by some (15). The *absence* of convincing evidence of productive neuronal or astrocytic infection *in vivo* underlies the major question of what causes neuronal or other neuroectodermal cell dysfunction.

Of course, due to their limited sensitivity, results of immunocytochemical and *in situ* hybridization studies do not preclude infection of neuroectodermal cells in which the proviral genome is latent or in which there is only very limited gene expression—that is, below the limits of detection. Supporting this possibility are experimental laboratory studies of cultured glial and neuronal cells or cell lines in which infection yields only very limited progeny virus which may be difficult to detect without sensitive rescue techniques (95–97). Whether this type of infection has an *in vivo* counterpart should soon be addressed by emerging combined PCR–*in situ* technology combining nucleic acid sequence amplification with tissue localization (25). However, the low signal by conventional PCR in brains with gliosis-pallor may predict that such infection will be rare in this setting (27). Additionally, even if proviral DNA is detected in occasional neurons or astroglial cells, this does not ensure their important role in disease pathogenesis.

The restriction of major productive infection to macrophages and microglia likely simply reflects the principal role of the CD4 receptor in infection (93,98,99) and suggests that alternative receptors which are involved in *in vitro* infections of neural cells may not mediate infection *in vivo*. These alternative receptors, identified in some studies as either galactocerebroside or a surface glycoprotein (99a,99b), if not mediating infection, might however be involved in reception of signals involved in toxicity to uninfected cells.

In addition to being restricted to bone marrow-derived cells, productive HIV-1 infection also exhibits a relatively selective predilection for certain brain regions. Our own analysis (BJ Brew, M Rosenblum, K Cronin, and RW Price, *unpublished observations*) parallels that of Dickson and colleagues (7,81) showing a propensity for infection to involve diencephalic and mesencephalic structures along with deep white matter but with relative cortical sparing. The reason for this selective vulnerability is not known. One hypothesis is that it might reflect the predominant *route of viral entry* through the choroid plexus and ventricular CSF in proximity to these structures. While this may be partially explanatory, it does not account for the highest infection rate in the globus pallidus rather than in the caudate nucleus or hypothalamus, both of which are closer to the ventricular wall. Another explanation speculates that the *properties of capillary endothelial cells* may differ in these structures, allowing greater access to virus-infected cells. A third explanation centers on the idea that these structures may be *more vulnerable to virus- or immune-induced cytotoxicity,* which then causes a secondary activation of macrophages and, in turn, greater permissiveness for local HIV-1 replication; in this case, regional predominance of infection would result from conditions favoring local amplification rather than entry per se.

While active HIV-1 has thus been identified in brain, the connection between local infection and brain injury and consequent clinical dysfunction remains problematic. Not only is the clinical–pathological subset of mild ADC and gliosis-pallor usually negative for productive infection, but the relationship of the viral burden to more severe ADC is also variable. Analysis of our own material for p24 antigen by immunohistochemistry suggests that the extent of infection is often less than might be anticipated by the clinical ADC severity (BJ Brew, M Rosenblum, K Cronin, and RW Price, *unpublished observations*). This includes not only ADC Stage 1 patients without detectable infection, but also some Stage 2, 3, and 4 patients with anatomically circumscribed infection and, occasionally, no detectable infection. Vazeux et al. (100) have reported similar findings in children with AIDS. This type of observation drives the search for additional mechanisms that might cause, or at least amplify, neurological dysfunction in the face of limited direct CNS infection. However, Masliah et al. (*this volume;* see also ref. 101) have shown a good correlation between the cortical viral burden and local dendritic and synaptic changes in their pathological series.

Character of Virus and Cytokine Responses in the CNS

As reviewed in detail by O'Brien (*this volume*), a principal finding to emerge from studies of virus strains identified in the CNS is that they have the common property of *macrophage tropism*. Thus, viruses isolated by cell culture and cloned directly from brain without culture selection have the property of readily infecting macrophages but generally not infecting lymphocyte-derived cell lines. Hence, what was first sought as "neurotropism" is now identified as the capacity to infect macrophages rather than neuroectodermal cells as first suggested (102,103). This property is, of course, consistent with the observation that macrophages and microglia, which share in this same tropism, are productively infected *in vivo;* it has been genetically mapped to changes in sequences in the V3 region of HIV-1 gp120, the external glycoprotein (21,98,104–111). A second intriguing observation is that viruses identified in brain exhibit reduced genetic heterogeneity in comparison to those from other organs such as spleen (112–114). This suggests that not only are brain viruses derived from an individual's quasispecies and selected on the basis of the general property of macrophage tropism, but that such selection involves a very limited subset of the population of circulating virus.

How important are these properties of cell tropism and selection in determining whether or not productive brain infection occurs? Do they *drive* the development of encephalitis or are they simply the necessary substrate needed to express other determining factors? The character of virus in brains of asymptomatic or mild ADC patients, whether latent or in transit, has not yet been analyzed with respect to macrophage tropism, so one cannot be certain if macrophage-tropic strains reside in the brain chronically to emerge later, or if they only enter the brain and replicate in temporal proximity to clinical disease manifestation. Analysis of blood-derived isolates indicates that macrophage-tropic variants might be available early and throughout the course of infection (45,115,116). However, it is possible that there may be something different about strains that replicate rapidly in brain macrophages compared to macrophages elsewhere in the body. If so, then development of such variants would be more likely to occur later in infection when active replication generates more mutants and the immune system permits escape of these mutants. In such a scenario, development of these mutants might be the limiting factor in the development of true HIV-1 encephalitis, although the permissive effect of immune system compromise would also be needed to allow such escape and rapid amplification of virus in susceptible macrophages. During late-stage infection, these would also be the dominant susceptible cell, with the number of T lymphocytes having been severely reduced in number. In this way, early viruses entering the brain in CD4$^+$ T cells as a result of nonspecific activation might not be suitable to cause later encephalitis because they would have difficulty amplifying in resident microglia or blood-derived macrophages.

Following the lead of CSF studies, recent efforts have begun to directly analyze cytokine activation in brain parenchyma using both immunohistochemical and PCR technologies to detect products and mRNA transcripts (117–119). These have, in general, conceptually confirmed the CSF findings. Studies have shown enhanced expression of tumor necrosis factor alpha (TNF-α) and several other cytokines or indicators of cytokine activity, including up-regulation of MHC antigens. Some of these results are reviewed by Vitkovic et al. (*this volume*).

PATHOGENETIC SYNTHESIS

Having reviewed the background material and pointed out some of the major questions, I will now describe pathogenetic models which attempt to both simplify principal concepts and serve as an organizing framework for future studies. In doing this, I will take a two-step approach. The first step attempts to isolate the major *elements* of pathogenesis and outline the essen-

TABLE 5. *Some observations supporting a primary pathogenic role of HIV-1 in causing ADC*

ADC is clinically and pathologically unique to HIV-1 infection.
Not described in other immunosuppressed patients
The CNS is exposed early and probably continuously to HIV-1.
Other lentiviruses cause CNS infection and disease.
Visna
Simian immunodeficiency virus (SIV)
ADC correlates (to some extent) with the magnitude of brain infection (viral load).
Principally in more severe forms
Infection has a predilection for subcortical structures.
Compatible as a substrate for the clinical symptoms and signs
CNS infection involves viral variants.
Macrophage-tropic strains
With restricted heterogeneity

tial features of their interactions. The second step presents a simple model of cellular interactions.

These modeling approaches begin with an overall assumption that HIV-1 is intimately involved in ADC pathogenesis and that the pathologies discussed earlier are indeed the substrate of neurological dysfunction. They attempt to reconcile clinical ADC, on the one hand, and CNS HIV-1 infection, on the other, the two processes that I cautioned earlier should be considered separately. Before starting, let us first reconsider the justification for this starting point. Table 5 summarizes some of the observations that support a connection between HIV-1 infection of the CNS and ADC, while Table 6 lists several points challenging a simple relationship between virus infection and brain dysfunction. The models try to reconcile these conflicts.

The Elements of Pathogenesis

The pathogenesis of ADC can be considered to involve three essential elements: the *virus*, the *immune system*, and the *CNS* (2). The relationship

TABLE 6. *Some observations challenging a primary pathogenic role of HIV-1 in causing ADC*

ADC does not always correlate with viral load.
Particularly in milder forms in which productive infection is sparse or absent
Productive infection is anatomically circumscribed
Productive infection is confined almost exclusively to bone-marrow-derived cells.
Macrophages and microglia
Neuroectodermal cells are spared from direct infection.
Immune activation in CSF correlates better with ADC severity than with identified viral burden.

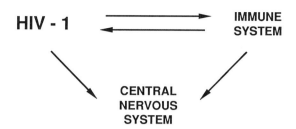

FIG. 2. The essential elements of ADC pathogenesis and their interrelations.

among these three is a dynamic one (Fig. 2) that evolves over the course of infection, and hence one can add a fourth element, *time* (Table 7). HIV-1 is the primary agonist that initiates the process. The immune system is both defender and secondary agonist by virtue of its capacity to initiate immuno-pathology. The CNS is the target and can be altered by both of these.

The Virus

This model views HIV-1 infection, or rather more specifically viral ge-nome, as the *prime mover* in pathogenesis. The genome persists and repli-cates and is the primary agonist that initiates and perpetuates events. Its systemic actions on the immune system determine immunosuppression and

TABLE 7. *Some interactions of the "elements" of ADC pathogenesis*

Effects of HIV-1 (the primary agonist) on the immune system
Immunosuppression
    Attrition of $CD4^+$ T lymphocytes
    Altered function of $CD4^+$ T lymphocytes, macrophages, and other immune defenses
Immune activation
    Primary effects (immune dysregulation): B-cell activation
    Secondary effects (reactive immune activation): macrophage activation
Effects of the immune system (a secondary agonist) on HIV-1 infection
Control of HIV-1 replication
    Surveillance of infected cells and virus: $CD4^+$, $CD8^+$, natural killer, B (antibody) cells
    Direct (up or down) modulation of viral replication: IFN-γ, other cytokines acting
        through transcription factors at LTR
Selection of virus variants
Effects of HIV-1 and immune system on CNS
Infection of cells in CNS
Elaboration of virus-coded neurotoxins
Stimulation of cell-coded neurotoxins
Element of time: factors underlying development of virus predominance
Loss of immune control of replication
    Sequela of loss of global T-cell defenses
Emergence of virus variants
    Altered cell tropism
    Altered virulence
    Immune escape

clearly influence subsequent processes in the CNS. The arrows drawn in Fig. 2 between HIV-1 and the immune system are bidirectional, since these two elements are interactive, joined in a relationship that evolves over time with each of the elements altering the other. In simple terms, the virus causes immune dysregulation with gradual immunosuppression evolving over the course of years. This slow evolution is, itself, remarkable and indicates an element of stability, particularly if measured in a time frame of months. It is thus an evolving, *unstable equilibrium.*

Immune responses are not only involved in globally suppressing viral replication, but also in monitoring viral variants (45). The constant generation of mutants related to the limited fidelity of viral RT results in emergence of immunologically distinct variants. During early infection, these are presumably suppressed as they emerge, and the immune system recognizes them as distinct. However, as the immune system is damaged, its response repertoire is reduced, and eventually it can no longer be able to respond to novel viral antigens. Thus, there is a constant interplay between virus and immunity with the eventual effect of increased viral burden and suppressed immunity against both HIV-1, itself, and other pathogens. After initial viremia is suppressed, HIV-1 infection gradually evolves from an ''immune-dominant'' state to a ''virus-dominant'' state as a result of this complex interaction setting the stage for productive infection in the CNS.

The virus and its gene products may also have effects on the CNS. As reviewed above, there is little to suggest that neurons or astrocytes are productively infected *in vivo,* but brain macrophages and microglia are infected. Additionally, viral gene products, including gp120 and perhaps *tat* and *nef,* may be toxic to neurons or other neural cells in culture (see Lipton, *this volume*).

The Immune System

The immune system plays multiple roles in AIDS and in ADC pathogenesis. Not only are its cells the primary targets of HIV-1 infection, it has further actions as both protector and pathogenic agonist (Table 7). While the relative importance of different mechanisms is uncertain, specific immune responses suppress primary viremia and exert a controlling effect on HIV-1 replication. As discussed earlier, it is only when certain defenses fail that viral replication accelerates into the final stages. Likely, CD4$^+$ T cells, perhaps of the Th1 phenotype, are involved in these defenses, along with cytotoxic CD8$^+$ T cells and perhaps antibody (16,120–122). While these defenses suppress replication, they clearly cannot eliminate the HIV-1 genome. Nor are they fully effective against active infection which continues during the period of clinical latency, albeit in sequestered fashion at a low level.

While true autoimmune phenomena may occur in the early or intermediate stages of HIV-1 infection, there is limited data to support specific responses against self-antigens in the pathogenesis of ADC (see *Oldstone, this volume*). However, as discussed earlier, evidence regarding immune activation late in disease is more substantial and comes from observations of increased concentrations of surrogate markers in both blood and CSF and, more directly, of cytokine up-regulation in brain. To what extent increased cytokines and markers of their activation derive directly from infected cells or secondarily from indirect effects on uninfected cells is uncertain, but this activation clearly indicates that, seemingly paradoxically, immunosuppression is accompanied by a type of immune activation. We have previously suggested that this may result from increased stimulation of "ineffective" immune responses, as if resulting from a defective feedback loop (123). Whatever the mechanism, this immune activation has the potential to result in immuno-pathology when toxic cytokines are released. Quinolinic acid is one example of a toxic molecule which can be released in the course of such activation, but TNF-α, nitric oxide (NO), and other toxic substances might be released in these circumstances (78,124–129). In this way, immune cells become pathological agonists releasing substances capable of damaging cells in the brain.

The CNS

The CNS is the target organ, vulnerable to injury related to the two pathogenic agonists. While the spectrum of gross and light microscopic pathology has been described, the important perturbations of different cell types remain poorly understood and the contributions of each to clinical dysfunction is likewise uncertain. While neurons and perhaps oligodendrocytes are the obvious major foci of interest regarding the ultimate target, it is possible that injury to astrocytes and vascular endothelial cells might be important participants in the process of brain injury. Each of these various cell types is considered below.

Cell Models of ADC Pathogenesis

Given these general considerations of the principal elements of pathogenesis, we can now proceed to examine the cellular interactions responsible for these interactions. To help in this, it is useful to begin very simply and then to build added complexity, starting with consideration of a one-cell model and proceeding to two-, three- and four-cell models. Since the precise roles of individual cells remain uncertain, I have chosen to think primarily in terms of cell *functions* and *types of interactions* in the model and secondarily deal with candidate cells and specific mechanisms which might fulfill these functions.

Direct Injury: 1 Cell Model   **Indirect Injury: 2 Cell Model**

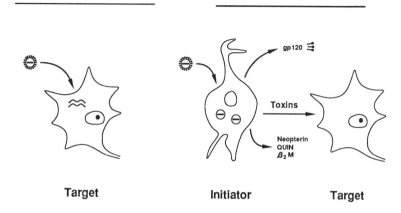

Target   Initiator   Target

Indirect Injury: 3+ Cell Model

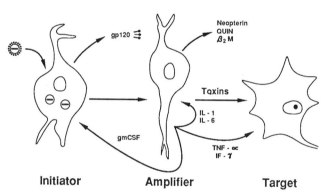

Initiator   Amplifier   Target

FIG. 3. Cell models of ADC pathogenesis involving HIV-1. The one-cell model entails *direct* infection of the functional target cell, whereas the two- and three-cell models involve *indirect* mechanisms of target cell injury (see text).

One-Cell Model

For comparative purposes it is instructive to first view a simple one-cell model (Fig. 3) in which a virus directly infects the target cell and the subsequent action of the viral genome results in dysfunction or death of that cell. This brings us back to the poliovirus paradigm discussed earlier of *cytolysis from within* in which the anterior horn cell is destroyed by direct infection. However, on the basis of available evidence, this model does not appear tenable in HIV-1 infection of the CNS, particularly with respect to neurons.

As discussed earlier, these "functional" targets of neuroectodermal origin are not productively infected. Hence, widespread brain dysfunction cannot be attributed to a direct action of the HIV-1 genome within these cells. For this reason, we turn to models of *indirect* injury that involve more than one cell and in which infection actually occurs in a cell other than the functional target.

Two-Cell Model

The simplest model of indirect injury involves two cells (Fig. 3), namely, an infected *initiator cell* and an uninfected *target cell*. In this model infection of the initiator results in the release of toxic molecules that alter the function of the target. These toxins might be of two types: (i) *virus-coded* gene products related to the expression of the HIV-1 genome, or (ii) *cell-coded* products induced in the infected cell as a result of alterations in the profile of cell gene expression. These two types of toxins might then be released in the course of infection.

Three-Cell Model

This extension of the indirect model involves an intervening *amplifier cell* between the initiator and target. In this model, the initiator cell releases or expresses products on its surface which signal the amplifier cell. These signals again may be virus- or cell-coded, although the former are hypothetically more attractive. These signals then, in turn, change the synthetic profile of the amplifier cell so that it subsequently releases cell-coded signals which alter the target cell. The signal molecules would fall into the broad category of cytokines. This model could be expanded to involve additional cells and cytokine circuits before the eventual effect on the target. The attractiveness of including the amplifier cell is that it could explain more widespread pathology and cell dysfunction in the face of limited presence and distribution of infected cells.

Four-Cell Model

While the three-cell model includes the essential elements needed to consider the mechanisms of brain dysfunction, a fourth element is needed to adequately deal with the element of time and the role of the immune system in determining the course of infection and disease. Figure 4 incorporates this fourth element in a *modulator cell* which exerts control on the profile of viral replication in the initiator cell. The capacity of this modulator cell to down-

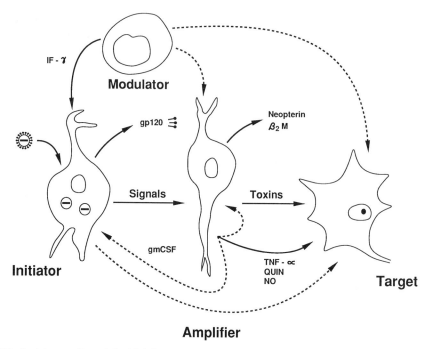

FIG. 4. A four-cell model which incorporates a modulator cell to account for the element of time (see text).

regulate HIV-1 replication varies over time, diminishing as infection progresses.

Functions of the Cells in the Model

Having sequentially built this four-cell model, one can now begin to consider the identity of each of the cellular elements and their interactions (Table 8).

Modulator Cell

The role of the putative modulator cell is that of exerting control on the level of viral replication and gene expression. This might be effected in two general ways. The *first* of these is the elimination or neutralization of virus-infected cells and free virions. CD4$^+$ T lymphocytes are likely involved in this defense, at the least in their helper capacity; the TH1 phenotype might be most effective in this regard. CD8$^+$ T lymphocytes are also likely involved in direct cytotoxicity whereas B lymphocytes are likely involved in produc-

TABLE 8. *Candidate identity and functions of the cells of the four-cell model of ADC pathogenesis*

Cell class	Candidate cells	Role in model
Modulator	CD4$^+$ (TH1), CD8$^+$ T lymphocytes	Modulate level of HIV-1 gene expression and replication in initiator cell
Initiator	Monocyte/microglia, CD4$^+$ T lymphocyte	Support HIV-1 replication and gene expression, including secretion of virus-coded and virus-induced cell-coded signals
Amplifier	Monocyte/microglia, astrocyte	Receive signals from initiator cell; secrete cell-coded signals, including cytokines
Target	Neuron, oligodendrocyte, endothelium	Undergo functional alteration in response to signals from amplifier and initiator cells

tion of antiviral antibodies, both neutralizing and participating in antibody-dependent cellular cytotoxicity (ADCC) (16,120–122).

The *second* mechanism involves some of the same cell types, including CD4$^+$ and CD8$^+$ lymphocytes, in more direct modulation of viral gene expression within the infected cell by altering the profile of cell transcriptional factors and their subsequent effects on the viral LTR. These might be involved in direct up- or down-regulation of replication. A number of cytokines have been shown to exhibit these properties (16,26,97). In the case of down-regulation, IFN–γ might be particularly important, but several of the interleukins, colony-stimulating factors, and other cytokines might act alone or together to decrease or increase viral gene expression.

As discussed above, the balance of these influences changes over time. Systemically, following acute infection, host defenses are able to suppress viremia, clearly demonstrating effectiveness in curtailing replication. However, they do not eliminate latent virus and, indeed, cannot fully inhibit viral replication, and eventually their power erodes and the end stage of AIDS is characterized by escape of HIV-1 with active viral replication and a high viral burden. The defenses within the CNS derive from the circulation and therefore are likely largely the same as in the body, but with perhaps some differences in relative profiles and importance.

The Initiator Cell

The ultimate prime mover is the HIV-1 genome. Its ability to insert itself into the host genome and to remain latent or to "turn on" full productive infection confers enormous power to survive and propagate in the infected host. The cell that harbors this genome is the initiator cell. In our model, this cell not only is the source of virus, but also has the principal function of signaling the amplifier cell or, alternatively, short-circuiting the latter by more directly signaling the target (two-cell toxicity). While effective replication of HIV-1 is not required for this function, neurotoxicity likely occurs in the course of replication and can be considered a "byproduct" of full-blown infection.

Over the long course of infection, the $CD4^+$ T lymphocyte is the predominant initiator cell. Lymphocyte infection is important in disseminating virus throughout the body, including into the CNS. Trafficking activated lymphocytes probably move in and out of the brain and might initiate local reactions and, conceivably, local replication. However, macrophages and microglia appear to be more important for ADC and carry the major burden of replication in the brain later in infection when $CD4^+$ cells are depleted. The limited genetic variation, the well-mapped tropism, and the histologic identification of infected cells as macrophages all indicate this role in HIV-1 multinucleated-cell encephalitis.

The signals might be released during the course of replication, either phasically (lymphocyte infection) or chronically (macrophage infection), or might derive from cell lysis. Most attractive as putative signals are viral gene products, either by virtue of intrinsic biological signal properties or as antigens triggering recognition and subsequent immune responses. As noted above, among the candidate viral products receiving attention are gp120 and the regulatory gene products of *tat* and *nef* (23,24,85,126,128,129,131–134; Lipton, *this volume*). Cell-coded signals induced by viral gene expression in the infected cell represent a variant of the model in which the infected cell plays a dual role of both inducer and amplifier, with signals being *intra-* rather than *inter*cellularly mediated. However, there is limited experimental evidence that HIV-1 can directly up-regulate cytokine production within infected cells.

Amplifier Cell

The amplifier cell (a) receives signals from the initiator, (b) transduces these signals in the course of responding by altering its own synthetic profile, and (c) releases toxic cytokines acting on the target. The amplifying function involves increasing both the intensity and volume of effect. Two principal cell types are major candidates for this role: macrophages/microgliocytes and astrocytes. Both are cytokine producers and responders (see Benveniste, *this volume*), and both are increased in number and morphologically altered in HIV-1 infection. They are therefore clearly responding to external signals, although whether or not they are, in turn, the source of important toxins is less clear (135). However, as examples of stimulated cell-coded toxins, evidence of increased TNF-α expression by uninfected macrophages has been cited earlier, and Heyes and colleagues (78) have provided a schema whereby quinolinic acid might be released by uninfected cells.

A variety of additional cell-coded toxic signals have been identified or proposed, either from *in vivo* observations or from cell culture studies. In addition to quinolinic acid and TNF-α, they include a glutamate agonist, NO, interleukin 1 (IL-1), arachidonic acid metabolites, and a low-molecular-weight product of infected macrophages (43,73,124–126,128,129,133,136). Which of these are truly active in ADC and their relative importance awaits further work. However, the accumulating data identifying and providing support for these processes should provide a firmer understanding and perhaps a basis for therapeutic intervention (see below) in the future. Investigation of this issue comes at a time of growing recognition and understanding of the role of cytokines in infections and immune responses and their interactions with the nervous system (Benveniste, *this volume*).

Target Cells

The target cells are functionally altered by the toxins emanating from the amplifier (or initiator) cells. The targets may be killed or undergo disturbance in their "luxury" functions. Principal candidate cells are the neurons and oligodendrocytes. Vascular endothelial cells might also be considered, although alteration of these cells might be conceptually considered a hybrid of amplifier and target cell roles.

Several studies have now documented loss of neurons in cerebral cortex (137,138) and, more recently, in basal ganglia and cerebellum (70,139) and have shown alteration of dendritic morphology and synaptic density in cortex (101,140; Masliah et al., *this volume*). Further work is clearly needed on the neurobiology of cytokines and mechanisms whereby neuronal survival, trophic function, reception, modulation, and transmission of signals might be modified.

Evidence that oligodendrocytes are importantly functionally altered is less secure. Esiri and colleagues (94,141) demonstrated hyperplasia with oligodendrocytes expressing cell proliferation markers. However, whether these changes importantly relate to major ADC functional alterations or are simple epiphenomena needs further study. Likewise, a role for myelin dysfunction needs to be defined because common white matter pallor is not true demyelination and also because the latter is noted only in areas of microscopic rarefaction accompanying multinucleated-cell encephalitis or leukoencephalitis. In general, the molecular pathogenesis of white matter disease has received less experimental study than have neuronal abnormalities, but *in vitro* observations have shown TNF-α to be toxic to myelin (43,85,136).

Vascular endothelium might have a number of important roles in ADC and CNS HIV-1 infection. Altered adhesion molecule expression may be critical in initiation and amplification of CNS HIV-1 infection. In a putative role as a target, the vascular endothelium might be altered by cytokines from either the luminal (systemic circulation) or abluminal (brain) side. Altered function might not only then impact on the earlier events in the model (initiation and modulation), but also on secondary disturbed neuronal function because a damaged blood–brain barrier results in altered ionic and biochemical composition of the brain interstitial fluid. In this regard, astrocytes might also be considered primary targets rather than amplifiers, given their critical function in maintaining the brain extracellular environment.

Some Additional Considerations

This four-cell model presents a very simplified picture, and one can easily develop variations and further layers of complexity to incorporate additional hypotheses and observations. However, its simplicity allows a potentially clearer vision or framework for comprehending fundamental principles. Most importantly, it is a framework for further study because as one defines the cells along with the signals and toxins represented by the connecting arrows, a deeper level of understanding, the molecular level, will come into focus. This will, in turn, allow refinement of the cell interaction model.

Having completed this description, it is worthwhile to emphasize a few points. The model defines ADC and its relation to HIV-1 infection as a *cytokine disease,* at least with respect to cytokines being the likely final common pathway leading to brain dysfunction. But it is a cytokine disease *driven by the virus.* If the virus is eliminated or contained, the stimulus to cytokine excess is removed and pathological processes halted or reversed. While these same processes are likely involved in many infections, their importance is exaggerated in ADC because: (a) unlike most organisms causing CNS infection, HIV-1 is not directly cytopathic for neuroectodermal cells; (b) infection is extremely protracted, allowing even mild effects to cause accumulating damage; and (c) these effects occur in the setting of dysimmunity in which inflammation is inconspicuous yet there is activation of cytokines, perhaps with disturbance in the normal regulatory circuits.

Finally, in describing this model, it was assumed that the cell interactions all occur within the CNS. However, one can easily extend these considerations to envision a series of parallel processes occurring primarily outside of brain, yet with CNS sequelae. If systemic infection produces excessive and toxic cytokines, they might impact on the CNS through effects on endothelial cells or on neurons and glia. Indeed, parallel processes developing both systemically and within the brain could be invoked to deal with the issue of whether mild ADC with gliosis and pallor and more severe ADC with multinucleated-cell encephalitis are, in fact, continuous and related processes. As emphasized earlier, while sharing these apparent pathological and virological differences, the clinical pictures are "phenotypically" similar; that is, the character of the patients' symptoms and signs are parallel, seeming to differ in severity but not in type. One way to reconcile these differences and similarities is to consider that early-mild disease relates principally to systemic infection and circulating cytokines whereas late-severe disease results from these same processes extending directly into the brain. Severe disease involves "metastatic" infection which brings these same toxic processes directly into the brain. If this is the case, clinical phenocopy might relate to selective vulnerabilities impacting on both events. In the case of systemic toxicity, selective vulnerability might relate to differences in endothelial sensitivities in different brain regions or to differential vulnerabilities of cell populations to toxins. Late disease might then relate to these same vulnerabilities; additionally, sites of infection might secondarily involve brain regions where the systemic toxicities have been at work. Thus, when cells are injured, secondary alterations of endothelial adhesion and entry of infected or permissive macrophages may occur in these regions, feeding a vicious cycle of local infection.

Therapeutic Implications of the Cell Model

One test of a disease model is whether it can be helpful in preventing or treating the disease. While this has not yet been tested in the case of our ADC models, they are helpful in organizing a logical approach to different therapy modalities. As outlined in Table 9, one can consider targeting treatment to each of the cells of the four-cell model.

Treatment of the Modulator Cell

Augmenting the antiviral efficacy of the modulator cell can be considered *immunomodulatory therapy*. The objective is to increase the antiviral efficacy of existing host systems. This strategy has historically been attempted in a number of settings, both infectious and neoplastic. Unfortunately, direct attempts at such efforts in AIDS have not yet shown efficacy. The use of IFN-γ might be considered to follow this rationale as a supplement to its

TABLE 9. *Applying the four-cell model of ADC pathogenesis to therapy*

Cell class	Treatment objectives
Modulator	*Immunomodulatory therapy:* Preserve and augment host antiviral defenses.
Initiator	*Antiviral Therapy:* Reduce systemic viral burden; reduce entry of virus replication and spread in CNS.
Amplifier	*Adjunctive therapy:* Interfere with signal reception, transduction, toxin secretion, and toxin action.
Target	*Symptomatic/neuroprotective therapy:* Block reception of, and response to, toxic signals; compensate neurochemical perturbation.

more direct antiviral effect. At present the most effective way to prevent progressive immunosuppression is to lessen the systemic viral burden with antiviral nucleoside therapy and thereby, secondarily, reduce the virus-induced decline in immune function.

Treatment of the Initiator Cell

Attacking this cell is the principal therapeutic approach now being taken in the clinic and is the one likely to be most selective and specific. These *antiviral therapy* measures are aimed at combatting the virus, which is the prime mover of the disease. Theoretically, several objectives of therapy can be targeted, including reduction of the systemic viral burden, inhibition of entry of the virus into the nervous system, suppression of local replication within the CNS, and elimination or inactivation of latent virus. With the exception of the last, these are the main aims of current prevention and treatment methods. Available antiviral drugs are directed against the viral RT and include the zidovudine and the other nucleosides. Non-nucleoside RT inhibitors are also being tried, and intensive efforts are underway to develop and test agents which interfere with other steps in the replicative cycle, including binding and penetration of the virus, regulatory gene function, and other late processing steps (22).

Treatment of the Amplifier Cell

This strategy can be considered *adjunctive therapy* and aims to interfere with (a) the effect of signals to amplifier cells and their subsequent transduction, (b) production of cell-coded toxins by these cells, and (c) the effects of these toxins on targets. While such approaches, in attempting to interfere with "normal" host responses to a pathogen, lack specificity and may not yield powerful effects without concomitant side effects altering other favorable sequelae of these responses, they might still contribute importantly to reducing neural cell dysfunction and death and, hence, alleviate symptoms and signs of ADC. In fact, there are now several efforts in varying stages of clinical trial pursuing this general approach. These include (a) the use of pentoxifylline to inhibit production and effects of TNF-α and (b) the use of memantine to block the action of a putative toxin acting at the NMDA receptor. As we begin to learn more about the relevant intermediaries produced by amplifier cells, additional variations of this strategy will undoubtedly be introduced.

Treating the Target Cell

The final approach aims to "normalize" or compensate for perturbations in luxury functions of target cells (*symptomatic therapy*) or to prevent disturbance of constitutive cell function and cell viability (*neuroprotective therapy*). A number of symptomatic therapies are already in use in certain clinical settings. These include the use of (a) neuroleptic or anticonvulsants in patients with secondary movement disorders or seizures, (b) lithium or neuroleptic for mania, and (c) amphetamines and related compounds for psychomotor retardation. The proposed use of calcium channel blockers to protect neurons from death (142) could be considered a neuroprotective approach as could peptide-T acting as a vasointestinal peptide agonist with trophic function (143–145). Thus, this approach includes (a) current therapies used by psychiatry and neurology for management of symptoms in other disease settings and (b) more novel approaches aimed at stabilizing the vulnerable cell. Because the latter parallels similar efforts in stroke and other neurodegenerative diseases, there will likely be further development in this area in the coming years.

Lessons from the Treatment Experience

Just as the model of pathogenesis may instruct development of therapy, so the experience with treatment may hold lessons for or test the theories of pathogenesis. Table 10 outlines some lessons and possible interpretations derived from the experience with antiviral therapy in ADC. Several studies have now shown that zidovudine can not only arrest progression, but even reverse the severity of ADC (146–152). Most AIDS clinicians have witnessed dramatic examples of improvement in some patients. While this may partially relate to neural plasticity and compensation by uninjured brain cells, particularly in children, the degree of reversal in some patients suggests not only that HIV-1 is the driver of ADC, but that the latter likely results from an *active process* in which functional change precedes cell death. Such a reversible metabolic insult is fully compatible with the model outlined, particularly with the intercellular signaling and toxin production and reception. The observation that treatment of ADC with zidovudine is accompanied by reduction in concentrations of surrogate markers of cytokine activation in the CSF also supports the role of *HIV-1 as the driver* of cytokine activation.

TABLE 10. *Pathogenic lessons for ADC from the treatment experience with zidovudine*

HIV-1 is the driver (cause) of ADC.
  Symptoms and signs respond to treatment and prevention.
There is a "metabolic component" to ADC.
  ADC is partially reversible with treatment.
Cytokine activation is driven by HIV-1.
  Treatment results in reduction of CSF cytokine activation markers.
A CNS "reservoir" of HIV-1 may not be rate-limiting to treatment, and major emphasis may appropriately rest with systemic treatment.
  ADC is prevented by antiretroviral treatment, even at modest doses.

A more controversial interpretation of some of the studies relates to the primacy of systemic treatment in preventing ADC. Available evidence suggests that zidovudine reduces the incidence of ADC among infected subjects, even at current doses of 500–600 mg/day (86,148,149). This might suggest that a putative reservoir of latent HIV-1 in the CNS and subsequent escape and replication from this reservoir is not a rate-limiting step in ADC development. This is also consistent with speculation that ADC develops as a result of late, active systemic infection, either from effects of systemically released toxins or from hematogenous infection developing in temporal proximate to the onset of symptoms. Restricted heterogeneity of macrophage-tropic strains in brain then derives from the systemic circulation of variants of the patient's quasispecies which have adapted to replication in brain macrophages. Treating systemic infection may therefore be the critical and essential step in preventing this from happening. If so, analogy with childhood leukemia, in which the brain serves as a sequestered reservoir of malignant cells protected from systemic chemotherapy, may not be apt for HIV-1.

SOME BROADER IMPLICATIONS FOR NEUROLOGY

While there are those in neurobiology as in other scientific fields, as well as among the lay public, who argue that the "excessive" attention to HIV-1 and AIDS diverts funding and more generally detracts from work on other issues and diseases, it is also possible to argue to the contrary, that the intensive work on the neurology and neurobiology of HIV-1 infection, with rapid deployment of the most advanced tools available, will importantly help advance these other areas as well. Table 11 lists some of the lessons for clinical neuroscience that one can cite among these advances. Outside of its immediate clinical implications, work on AIDS has and will continue to have scientific, practical, and sociopolitical implications for other fields.

ADC has now become a paradigm of subcortical dementia, and studies focusing on cortical–diencephalic relations using a variety of approaches to evaluation and pathophysiological study, including functional neuroimaging, should stimulate new understanding of this type of CNS dysfunction. Similarly, the issues raised and the advances made in understanding the pathogenesis of CNS dysfunction related to noncytopathic infection and cytokine-related immunopathology surely will have important lessons for other infectious and immunological nervous system diseases with regard to understanding pathogenesis and approaches to treatment.

The study of AIDS has clearly accelerated a number of general biomedical advances. Rapid development and practical clinical application of PCR technology is one such example. In the case of CNS disease, PCR–*in situ* techniques are being pioneered by investigations of HIV-1 (25). The application of CSF surrogate markers and cytokines is also being advanced by studies

TABLE 11. *Some lessons for neurobiology from ADC and HIV-1 infection of the CNS*

Definition of pattern of brain dysfunction: subcortical dementia
   Evaluation methodology
   Pathophysiological understanding
Viral and immune neuropathogenesis
   Cellular and cytokine mechanisms
   Approaches to symptom control
New diagnostic and monitoring tools
   Accelerated application of PCR, combined with *in situ* detection
   Use of CSF cytokine markers for diagnosis and disease/therapy monitoring
Management of opportunistic neurological disorders
   Diagnosis
   Treatment
Extending paradigm of antiviral therapy
Alteration of drug testing and approval process
   Development of the "parallel track"
Role of constituent group advocacy/militancy
   Determining clinical trials
   Influencing funding
   Patient education

of ADC and should have application to other conditions. The intensive experience with certain opportunistic infections has similarly led to improved diagnosis and management applicable to other settings with parallel susceptibilities. For example, whereas diagnosis and treatment of cerebral toxoplasmosis was sufficiently uncommon that diagnosis might be delayed and treatment regimens uncertain, this disorder is now routinely recognized and effectively managed. Progressive multifocal leukoencephalopathy (PML) was an orphan disease with no prospect for therapeutic study, but soon a program to test treatment efficacy will begin. The example of AIDS is another important step in accepting antiviral therapy as a practical therapeutic objective and follows the lead of acyclovir in treating herpes simplex virus. Patients with other disorders thus profit both now and in the future from advances in AIDS.

AIDS has also clearly had an important impact on certain social and political aspects of medicine. It has seen the emergence of fervid interest groups who have served as (a) consumer advocates, (b) sources of information for patients, (c) lobbyists, and (d) a powerful force for change in physician–patient relations and, on a larger scale, in policies regarding the testing and approval of new drugs. These changes will certainly spill over into other areas, including neurology and psychiatry. We have already seen an example in the approval process of a drug for Alzheimer's disease which followed precedent set by experience with didanosine, one of the antiviral nucleosides. We will also likely see it in a more militant stance of some disease advocacy groups. If these changes continue to follow the lead of AIDS, physicians and scientists may become frustrated and annoyed on occasion, but in the long run the net result will likely be more rapid progress in both basic understanding and the development and implementation of new treatments.

CONCLUSIONS

Table 12 summarizes some of the major issues and hypothetical formulations discussed in this chapter in an attempt to reconcile the observations regarding ADC and HIV-1 which both favor (Table 5) and challenge (Table 6) a link between this neurological syndrome and the AIDS retrovirus. Interpretation of observations from a variety of sources leads to a picture of brain disease driven by systemic and CNS HIV-1 infection but involving cytokine-related immunopathology as a principal mechanism of cell injury. The condition involves complex interactions of HIV-1 and the immune system as a foundation for eventual selective damage of the CNS mediated by virus- and cell-coded signals and toxins. While these mechanisms stand out because of their predominating role in ADC, they are likely also involved in many other CNS diseases caused by other organisms or involving immunopathological processes. For this reason, further study to test and extend the models pre-

TABLE 12. *Reconciling a primary pathogenic role of HIV-1 infection in ADC: pieces of a unifying hypothesis*

HIV-1 likely initiates and sustains pathogenic processes leading to brain dysfunction.
    The pathologies parallel topography of infection.
    The distribution of infection and pathology are a compatible substrate for the clinical symptoms and signs.
But immune reactions play an important pathogenic role.
    In defense, by controlling viral replication.
    As an agonist, causing brain dysfunction.
Brain injury is not the result of direct virus-induced cytolysis of neuroectodermal cells.
    Neuroectodermal cells are only rarely productively infected.
    Rather productive brain infection involves macrophages and microglia.
Brain injury results from "indirect" neurotoxic processes.
    Involves cytokine signals and toxins.
    Involves viral gene product signals or toxins.
The combination of HIV-1 as the driver and cytokine circuits as amplifiers reconciles the limited correlation of brain infection with clinical dysfunction.
    Low virus load and gliosis in ADC Stage 0.5–1; may relate to systemic infection and cytokine generation.
    Higher virus loads and local replication in ADC Stages 2–4; may reflect metastatic infection.
The temporal profile of development and progression of ADC in relation to systemic disease is determined by interrelated changes in both the immune system and the virus.
    Immunosuppression has a permissive effect on HIV-1 replication and escape of mutants.
    Brain infection involves development of neurotropic strains which replicate preferentially in macrophages and microglia.
Selective vulnerability to toxicity or viral entry and viral amplification explains common anatomic distribution and phenotypic similarity of mild and severe disease.
    Involves diencephalic nuclei and deep white matter.

sented here has important implications for both HIV-1-infected people and patients suffering other neurological diseases.

REFERENCES

1. Price RW, Sidtis JJ, Brew BJ. AIDS dementia complex and HIV-1 infection: a view from the clinic. *Brain Pathol* 1991;1:155–162.
2. Spencer DC, Price RW. Human immunodeficiency virus and the central nervous system. *Annu Rev Microbiol* 1983;46:655–693.
3. Budka H. Human immunodeficiency virus (HIV) envelope and core porteins in CNS tissues of patients with the acquired immune deficiency syndrome (AIDS). *Acta Neuropathol* 1990;79:611–619.
4. Gabuzda DH, Ho DD, DeLaMonte SM, Hirsch MS, Rota TR, Sobel RA. Immunohistochemical identification of HTLV-III antigen in brains of patients with AIDS. *Ann Neurol* 1986;20:289–295.
5. Koenig S, Gendelman HE, Orenstein JM, et al. Detection of AIDS virus in macrophages in brain tissue from AIDS patients with encephalopathy. *Science* 1986;233:1089–1093.
6. Kure K, Lyman WD, Weidenheim KM, Dickson DW. Cellular localization of an HIV-1 antigen in subacute AIDS encephalitis using an improved double-labeling immunohistochemical method. *Am J Pathol* 1990;136(5):1085–1092.
7. Kure K, Weidenheim KM, Lyman WD, Dickson DW. Morphology and distribution of HIV-1 gp41-positive microglia in subacute AIDS encephalitis. *Acta Neuropathol* 1990;80: 393–400.
8. Pantaleo G, Graziosi C, Demarest JF, et al. HIV infection is active and progressive in lymphoid tissue during the clinically latent stage of disease. *Nature* 1993;362:355–358.
9. Peudenier S, Hery C, Montagnier L, Tardieu M. Human microglial cells: characterization in cerebral tissue and in primary culture, and study of their susceptibility to HIV-1 infection. *Ann Neurol* 1991;29:152–161.
10. Price RW, Brew BJ, Sidtis J, Rosenblum M, Scheck AC, Cleary P. The brain in AIDS: central nervous system HIV-1 infection and AIDS dementia complex. *Science* 1988;239: 586–592.
11. Pumarole-Sune T, Navia BA, Cordon-Cardo C, Cho E-S, Price RW. HIV antigen in the brains of patients with the AIDS dementia complex. *Ann Neurol* 1987;21:490–496.
12. Sharer LR, Prineas JW. Human immunodeficiency virus in glial cells, continued. *J Infect Dis* 1988;157:204.
13. Stoler MH, Eskin TA, Benn S, Angerer RC, Angerer LM. Human T-cell lymphotropic virus type III infection of the central nervous system. A preliminary *in situ* analysis. *JAMA* 1986;256:2360–2364.
14. Vazeux R, Brousse N, Jarry A, et al. AIDS subacute encephalitis: identification of HIV-infected cells. *Am J Pathol* 1987;126:403–410.
15. Wiley CA, Schrier RD, Nelson JA, Lampert PW, Oldstone MBA. Cellular localization of human immunodeficiency virus infection within the brains of acquired immune deficiency patients. *Proc Natl Acad Sci USA* 1986;83:7089–7093.
16. Pantaleo G, Graziosi C, Fauci AS. The immunopathogenesis of human immunodeficiency virus infection. *N Engl J Med* 1993;328:327–335.
17. Coffin JM. Retroviridae and their replication. In: Fields B, Knipe D, Chanock R, eds. *Virology,* 2nd ed. New York: Raven Press, 1990;1437–1500.
18. Cullen BR. Regulation of HIV-1 gene expression. *FASEB J* 1991;5:2361–2368.
19. Haseltine WA. The molecular biology of HIV-1. In: DeVita VT Jr, Hellman S, Rosenberg SA, eds. *AIDS: etiology, diagnosis, treatment and prevention.* Philadelphia: JB Lippincott, 1992;3:39–59.
20. Wain-Hobson S. HIV genome variability *in vivo. AIDS* 1989;3(suppl 1):S13–S18.
21. O'Brien WA, Koyanagi Y, Namazie A, et al. HIV-1 tropism for mononuclear phagocytes can be determined by regions of gp120 outside the CD4-binding domain. *Nature* 1990;348: 69–73.

22. Hirsch MS, D'Aquila RT. Therapy for human immunodeficiency virus infection. *N Engl J Med* 1993;328:1686–1695.
23. Sabatier J-M, Vives E, Marbrouk K, et al. Evidence for neurotoxic activity of tat from human immunodeficiency virus type 1. *J Virol* 1991;65(2):961–967.
24. Werner T, Ferroni S, Saermark T, et al. HIV-1 nef protein exhibits structural and functional similarity to scorpion peptides interacting with K^+ channels. *AIDS* 1991;5:1301–1308.
25. Embertson J, Zupancic M, Ribas JL, et al. Massive covert infection of helper T lymphocytes and macrophages by HIV during the incubation period of AIDS. *Nature* 1993;362:359–362.
26. Epstein LG, Gendelman HE. Human immunodeficiency virus type 1 infection of the nervous system: pathogenetic mechanisms. *Ann Neurol* 1993;33:429–436.
27. Gadler H, Hahn BH, Shaw GM, Brew BJ, Rosenblum M, Price RW. Analysis of brain from AIDS patients for HIV-1 DNA sequences using the polymerase chain reaction. In: *Proceedings of the V international conference on AIDS,* Montreal, 1989; abstract WCP 84.
27a. Kramer A, Wiktor SZ, Fuchs D, et al. Neopterin: a predictive marker of acquired deficiency syndrome in human immunodeficiency virus infection. *J AIDS* 1989;2:291–296.
28. Lifson AR, Hessol NA, Buchbinder SP, O'Malley PM, Barnhart L, Segal M, et al. Serum β_2-microglobulin and prediction of progression to AIDS in HIV infection. *Lancet* 1992;339:1436–1440.
29. Navia BA, Jordan BD, Price RW. The AIDS dementia complex. I. Clinical features. *Ann Neurol* 1986;19:517–524.
30. Price RW, Brew BJ. The AIDS dementia complex. *J Infect Dis* 1988;158:1079–1083.
31. Price RW, Sidtis JJ. The AIDS dementia complex. In: Wormser GP, ed. *AIDS and other manifestations of HIV infection.* New York: Raven Press, 1992;373–382.
32. Worley J, Price RW. Management of neurologic complications of HIV-1 infection and AIDS. In: Sande MA, Volberding PA, eds. *The medical management of AIDS, 4th ed.* Philadelphia: WB Saunders 1992;13:193–217.
33. Belman AL, Ultmann MH, Horoupian D, et al. Neurological complications in infants and children with acquired immune deficiency syndrome. *Ann Neurol* 1985;18:560–566.
34. Epstein LG, Sharer LR, Joshi VV, Fojas MM, Koenigsberger MR, Oleske JM. Progressive encephalopathy in children with acquired immune deficiency syndrome. *Ann Neurol* 1985;17:488–496.
35. Gopinathan G, Laubenstein LJ, Mondale B, Krigel RG. Central nervous system manifestations of the acquired immunodeficiency syndrome in homosexual men. *Neurology* 1983;33(suppl 2):105.
36. Horowitz SL, Benson DF, Gottlieb MS, Davos I, Bentson JR. Neurological complications of gay-related immunodeficiency disorder. *Ann Neurol* 1982;12:80.
37. Snider WD, Simpson DM, Neilsen S, Gold JW, Metroka CE, Posner JB. Neurological complications of acquired immune deficiency syndrome: analysis of 50 patients. *Ann Neurol* 1983;14:403–418.
38. Navia BA, Cho E-W, Petito CK, Price RW. The AIDS dementia complex. II. Neuropathology. *Ann Neurol* 1986;19:525–535.
39. Centers for Disease Control: Revision of the CDC surveillance case definition for acquired immunodeficiency syndrome. *MMWR* 1992;36:3S–14S.
40. Benson DF. The spectrum of dementia: a comparison of the clinical features of AIDS dementia and dementia of the Alzheimer's type. *Alzheimer Dis Assoc Dis* 1987;1(4):217–220.
40a. CDC. 1993 Revised classification system for HIV infection and expanded surveillance case definition for AIDS among adolescents and adults. *MMWR* 1993;41(RR-17).
41. Cummings JL, Benson DF. Subcortical dementia: review of an emerging concept. *Arch Neurol* 1984;41:874–879.
42. Brew BJ, Perdices M. HIV nomenclature. *Neurology* 1992;42:265.
43. Robbins DS, Shirzai Y, Drysdale B, et al. Production of cytoxic factor for oligodendrocytes by stimulated astrocytes. *J Immunol* 1987;139:2593–2597.
44. Report of a working group of the American Academy of Neurology AIDS task force, 1991: Nomenclature and research case definitions for neurologic manifestations of human immunodeficiency virus-type 1 (HIV-1) infection. *Neurology* 41:778–785.

45. Wolfs TFW, De Jong J-J, Van Den Berg H, Tunagel JM, Krone WJA, Goudsmit J. Evolution of sequences encoding the principal neutralization epitope of HIV-1 is host-dependent, rapid, and continuous. *Proc Natl Acad Sci USA* 1990;87(24):9928–9942.
45a. World Health Organization consultation on the neuropsychiatric aspects of HIV-1 infection. *AIDS* 1990;4(9):935–936.
46. Brew B, Sidtis J, Petito CK, Price RW. The neurological complications of AIDS and human immunodeficiency virus infection. In: Plum F, ed. *Advances in contemporary neurology*. Philadelphia: FA Davis Co, 1988;1–49.
47. Navia BA, Price RW. The acquired immunodeficiency syndrome dementia complex as the presenting or sole manifestation of human immunodeficiency virus infection. *Arch Neurol* 1987;44:65–69.
48. Grant IH, Gold JWM, Rosenblum M, et al. *Toxoplasma gondii* serology in HIV-infected patients: the development of central nervous system toxoplasmosis in AIDS. *AIDS* 1991; 4:519–523.
49. Gelman BB, Guinto FC. Morphometry, histopathology and tomography of cerebral atrophy in the acquired immunodeficiency syndrome. *Ann Neurol* 1992;32(1):31–40.
50. Jakobsen J, Gyldensted C, Brun B, Bruhn P, Helweg-Larsen S, Arlien Soborg P. Cerebral ventricular enlargement relates to neuropsychological measures in unselected AIDS patients. *Acta Neurol Scand* 1989;79:59–62.
51. Post MJ, Tate LG, Quencer RM, et al. CT, MR, and pathology in HIV encephalitis and meningitis. *AJR* 1988;151:373–380.
51a. Jarvik JG, Hesselink JR, Kennedy C, et al. Acquired immunodeficiency syndrome. Magnetic resonance patterns of brain involvement with pathologic correlation. *Arch Neurol* 1988;45(7):731–736.
52. Tozzi V, Narciso P, Galgani S, et al. Effects of zidovudine in 30 patients with mild to end-stage AIDS dementia complex. *AIDS* 1993;7:683–692.
53. Rottenberg DA, Moeller JR, Strother SC, et al. The metabolic pathology of the AIDS dementia complex. *Ann Neurol* 1987;22:700–706.
54. Pizzo PA, Eddy J, Falloon J, et al. Effect of continuous intravenous infusion of zidovudine (AZT) in children with symptomatic HIV infection. *N Engl J Med* 1988;319:889–896.
55. Pohl P, Vogl G, Fill H, Rossler H, Zangerle R, Gerstenbrand F. Single photon emission computed tomography in AIDS dementia complex. *J Nucl Med* 1988;29(8):1382–1386.
56. Appleman ME, Marshall DW, Brey RL, et al. Cerebrospinal fluid abnormalities in patients without AIDS who are seropositive for the human immunodeficiency virus. *J Infect Dis* 1989;158:193–199.
57. Buffet R, Agut H, Chieze R, et al. Virological markers in the cerebrospinal fluid from HIV-1 infected individuals. *AIDS* 1991;5:1419–1424.
58. Chiodi F, Norkrans G, Hagberg L, et al. Human immunodeficiency virus infection of the brain. II. Detection of intrathecally synthesized antibodies by enzyme linked immunosorbent assay and imprint immunofixation. *J Neurol Sci* 1988;87:37–48.
59. Elovaara I, Iivanainen M, Valle SL, Suni J, Tervo T, Lahdevirta J. CSF protein and cellular profiles in various stages of HIV infection related to neurological manifestations. *J Neurol Sci* 1987;78:331–342.
60. Goswami KK, Miller RF, Harrison MJ, Hamel DJ, Daniels RS, Tedder RS. Expression of HIV-1 in the cerebrospinal fluid detected by the polymerase chain reaction and its correlation with central nervous system disease. *AIDS* 1991;5:797–803.
61. Goudsmit J, DeWolf F, Paul DA, et al. Expression of human immunodeficiency virus antigen (HIV-Ag) in serum and cerebrospinal fluid during acute and chronic infection. *Lancet* 1986;2(8500):177–180.
62. Ho DD, Rota TR, Schooley RT, et al. Isolation of HTLV-III from cerebrospinal fluid and neural tissues of patients with neurologic syndromes related to the acquired immunodeficiency syndrome. *N Engl J Med* 1985;313:1493–1497.
63. McArthur JC, Cohen BA, Farzadegan H, et al. Cerebrospinal fluid abnormalities in homosexual men with and without neuropsychiatric findings. *Ann Neurol* 1988;23(suppl): S34–S37.
64. Marshall DW, Brey RL, Cahill WT, Houk RW, Zajac RA, Boswell RN. Spectrum of cerebrospinal fluid findings in various stages of human immunodeficiency virus infection. *Arch Neurol* 1988;45:954–958.

65. Resnick L, Berger JR, Shapshak P, Tourtellotte WW. Early penetration of the blood–brain barrier by HIV. *Neurology* 1988;38:9–14.
66. Haase AT. Pathogenesis of lentivirus infections. *Nature* 1986;322:130–136.
67. Peluso R, Haase A, Stowring L, Edwards M, Ventura P. A Trojan Horse mechanism for the spread of visna virus in monocytes. *Virology* 1985;147:231–236.
68. Hickey WF. Migration of hematogenous cells through the blood–brain barrier and the initiation of CNS inflammation. *Brain Pathol* 1991;1:97–105.
69. Davis LE, Hjelle BL, Miller VE, et al. Early viral brain invasion in iatrogenic human immunodeficiency virus infection. *Neurology* 1992;42:1736–1739.
70. Everall I, Bames H, Spargo E, Lantos P. Evidence for selective neuronal loss in the putamen in HIV infected patients using spatial analysis. *Clin Neuropathol* 1993;12:S10.
71. Walker BD, Harrer T, Rosenthal TW, et al. HIV-1 specific cytotoxic lymphocytes release inflammatory cytokines when they encounter their target antigens. *Neurology* 1992;43(4S): A370.
72. Brew BJ, Bhalla RB, Fleisher M, et al. Cerebrospinal fluid B$_2$-microglobulin in patients infected with human immunodeficiency virus. *Neurology* 1989;39:830–834.
73. Brew BJ, Bhalla RB, Paul M, et al. Cerebrospinal fluid neopterin in human immunodeficiency virus type 1 infection. *Ann Neurol* 1990;28:556–560.
74. Brew BJ, Bhalla R, Paul M, et al. Cerebrospinal fluid B$_2$-microglobulin in patients with AIDS dementia complex: an expanded series including response to zidovudine treatment. *AIDS* 1992;6:461–465.
75. Heyes MP, Brew BJ, Martin A. Quinolinic acid in cerebrospinal fluid and serum in HIV-1 infection: relationship to clinical and neurologic status. *Ann Neurol* 1991;29:202–209.
76. Heyes MP, Brew B, Martin A, et al. Cerebrospinal fluid quinolinic acid concentrations are increased in acquired immune deficiency syndrome. *Adv Exp Med Biol* 1991;294:687–690.
77. Fuchs D, Weiss G, Semenitz E, Dierich MP, Wachter H. Increased neopterin concentrations in CSF of HIV infected patients may contribute to brain tissue damage. *Clin Neuropathol* 1993;12:S2.
78. Heyes MP, Saito K, Crowley JS, et al. Quinolinic acid and kynurenine pathway metabolism in inflammatory and non-inflammatory neurological disease. *Brain* 1992;115:1249–1274.
79. Paul MO, Brew BJ, Khan A, Gallardo M, Price RW. Detection of HIV-1 in cerebrospinal fluid (CSF): correlation with presence and severity of the AIDS dementia complex. *V Intl Conf AIDS Abst* 1989:238.
80. Koyangi Y, Miles S, Mitsuyasu RT, Merrill JE, Vinters HV, Chen ISY. Dual infection of the central nervous system by AIDS viruses with distinct cellular tropism. *Science* 1987;236:819–822.
81. Dickson DW, Mattiace LA, Kure K, Hutchins K, Lyman WD, Brosnan CF. Biology of disease: microglia in human disease, with an emphasis on acquired immune deficiency syndrome. *Lab Invest* 1991;64:136–156.
82. Budka H, Wiley CA, Kleihues P, et al. HIV-associated disease of the nervous system: review of nomenclature and proposal for neuropathology-based terminology. *Brain Pathol* 1991;1:143–212.
83. Rosenblum MK. Infection of the central nervous system by the human immunodeficiency virus type 1: morphology and relation to syndrome of progressive encephalopathy and myelopathy in patients with AIDS. *Pathol Ann* 1990;25:117–169.
84. Michaels J, Price RW, Rosenblum MK. Microglia in the human immunodeficiency virus encephalitis of acquired immunodeficiency syndrome: proliferation, infection, and fusion. *Acta Neuropathol* 1988;76:373–379.
85. Kimura-Kuroda J, Nagashima K, Yasui K. HIV-1 gp 120 causes demyelination in a primary culture of rat cerebral cortex. *Clin Neuropathol* 1993;12:S3.
85a. Kleihues P, Boni J, Emmerich BS, Schupbach J. PCR identification of HIV-1 DNA in the CNS of patients with HIV encephalopathy. *Clin Neuropathol* 1993;12:S3.
86. Schmitt FA, Bigley JW, McKinnis R, Logue PE, Evans RW, Drucker JL. AZT Collaborative Working Group, 1988. Neuropsychological outcome of zidovudine (AZT) treatment of patients with AIDS and AIDs-related complex. *N Engl J Med* 319:1573–1578.
87. Shaw GM, Harper ME, Hahn BH, et al. HTLV-III infection in brains of children and adults with AIDS encephalopathy. *Science* 1985;227:177–182.
87a. Budka H, Costanzi G, Cristina S, et al. Brain pathology induced by infection with the

human immunodeficiency virus (HIV). A histological, immunocytochemical and electron microscopical study of 100 autopsy cases. *Acta Neuropathol (Berl)* 1987;75:185–198.

88. Petito CK, Navia BA, Cho E-S, Jordan BD, George DC, Price RW. Vacuolar myelopathy pathologically resembling subacute combined degeneration in patients with acquired immune deficiency syndrome (AIDS). *N Engl J Med* 1985;312:874–879.

89. Rosenblum M, Scheck AC, Cronin K, et al. Dissociation of AIDS-related vacuolar myelopathy and productive human immunodeficiency virus type 1 (HIV-1) infection of the spinal cord. *Neurology* 1989;39:892–896.

90. Budka H. Neuropathology of HIV encephalitis. *Brain Pathol* 1991;1:163–175.

91. Chiodi F, Wilt S, Dubois-Dalcq M. The capacity to replicate in microglial cells is a common property of primary HIV isolates. *Clin Neuropathol* 1993;12:S2.

92. Graeber MB, Streit WJ. Microglia: immune network in the CNS. *Brain Pathol* 1990;1: 2–5.

93. Watkins BA, Dorn HH, Kelly WB, et al. Specific tropism of HIV-1 for microglial cells in primary human brain cultures. *Science* 1990;249:549–553.

93a. Gartner S, Markovits P, Markovits DM, Betts RF, Popovic M. Virus isolation from and identification of HTLV-III/LAV producing cells in brain tissue from a patient with AIDS. *JAMA* 1986;256:2365–2371.

94. Esiri MM, Morris CS, Millard PR. Fate of oligodendrocytes in HIV-1 infection. *AIDS* 1991;5:1081–1088.

95. Dewhurst S, Sakai D, Bresser J, Stevenson M, Evinger-Hodges MJ, Volsky DJ. Persistent productive infection of human glial cells by human immunodeficiency virus (HIV) and by infectious molecular clones of HIV. *J Virol* 1987;61:3774–3782.

96. Dewhurst S, Sakai K, Zhang XH, Wasiak A, Volsky DJ. Establishment of human glial cell lines chronically infected with the human immunodeficiency virus. *Virology* 1988; 162(1):151–159.

97. Tornatore C, Nath A, Amemiya K, Major EO. Persistent human immunodeficiency virus type 1 infection in human fetal glial cells reactivated by T-cell factor(s) or by the cytokines tumor necrosis factor alpha and interleukin-1 beta. *J Virol* 1991;65(11):6094–6100.

98. Chesebro B, Nishio J, Perryman S, et al. Identification of human immunodeficiency virus envelope gene sequences influencing viral entry into CD4-positive HeLa cells, T-leukemia cells, and macrophages. *J Virol* 1991;65(11):5782–5789.

99. Jordan CA, Watkins BA, Kufta C, Dubois-Dalcq M. Infection of brain microglial cells by human immunodeficiency virus type 1 is CD4 dependent. *J Virol* 1991;65(2):736–742.

99a. Harouse JM, Bhat S, Spitalnik SL, et al. Inhibition of entry of HIV-1 in neural cell lines by antibodies against galactosyl ceramide. *Science* 1991;253:320–322.

99b. McAlarney T, Apostolski S, Latov N. Antibodies to galactocerebroside (GalC) inhibit the binding of gp120 to a glycoprotein receptor in neurons. *Clin Neuropathol* 1993;12:S4.

100. Vazeux R, Lacroix-Ciaudo C, Blanche S, et al. Low levels of human immunodeficiency virus replication in the brain tissue of children with severe acquired immunodeficiency syndrome encephalopathy. *Am J Pathol* 1992;140:137–144.

101. Masliah E, Achim CL, Ge N, DeTeresa R, Terry RD, Wiley CA. Spectrum of human immunodeficiency virus-associated neocortical damage. *Ann Neurol* 1992;32:321–329.

102. Castro BA, Cheng-Mayer C, Evans LA, Levy JA. HIV heterogeneity and viral pathogenesis. *AIDS* 1988;2(suppl 1):S17–S27.

103. Cheng-Mayer C. Biological and molecular features of HIV-1 related to tissue tropism. *AIDS* 1990;4(suppl 1):S49–S56.

104. Cann AJ, Churcher MJ, Boyd M, et al. The region of the envelope gene of human immunodeficiency virus type 1 responsible for determination of cell tropism. *J Virol* 1992;66(1): 305–309.

105. Hwang SS, Boyle TJ, Lyerly HK, Cullen BR. Identification of the envelope V3 loop as the primary determinant of cell tropism in HIV-1. *Science* 1991;253:71–74.

106. Liu Z-Q, Wood C, Levy JA, Cheng-Meyer C. The viral envelope gene is involved in macrophage tropism of a HIV-1 strain isolated from brain tissue. *J Virol* 1990;64(12): 6148–6153.

107. Page KA, Stearns SM, Littman DR. Analysis of mutations in the V3 domain of gp160 that affect fusion and infectivity. *J Virol* 1992;66(1):524–533.

108. Shioda T, Levy JA, Cheng-Mayer C. Macrophage and T cell-line tropisms of HIV-1 are determined by specific regions of the envelope gp120 gene. *Nature* 1991;349:167–169.

109. Takeuchi Y, Akutsu M, Murayama K, Shimizu N, Hoshino H. Host range mutant of human immunodeficiency virus type 1: modification of cell tropism by a single point mutation at the neutralization epitope in the env gene. *J Virol* 1991;65(4):1710–1718.
110. Westervelt P, Gendelman HE, Ratner L. Identification of a determinant within the human immunodeficiency virus 1 surface envelope glycoprotein critical for productive infection of primary monocytes. *Proc Natl Acad Sci USA* 1991;88:3097–3101.
111. Westervelt P, Trowbridge DB, Epstein LG, et al. Macrophage tropism determinants of human immunodeficiency virus type 1 *in vivo*. *J Virol* 1992;66:2577–2582.
112. Epstein LG, Kuiken C, Blumberg BM, et al. HIV-1 V3 domain variation in brain and spleen of children with AIDS: tissue specific evolution within host-determined quasispecies. *Virology* 1991;180:583–590.
113. Li Y, Kappes JC, Conway JA, Price RW, Shaw GM, Hahn BH. Molecular characterization of human immunodeficiency virus type 1 cloned directly from uncultured brain tissue: identification of replication-competent and -defective viral genomes. *J Virol* 1991;65(8): 3973–3985.
114. Pang S, Vinters HV, Akashi T, O'Brien WA, Chen ISY. HIV-1 env sequence variation in brain tissue of patients with AIDS-related neurological disease. *J AIDS* 1991;4:1082–1092.
115. Keyes B, Albert J, Kvamees J, Chiodi F. Brain-derived cells can be infected with HIV isolates derived from both blood and brain. *Virology* 1991;183:834–839.
116. Schuitemaker H, Koot M, Kootstra NA, et al. Biological phenotype of human immunodeficiency virus type 1 clones at different stages of infection: progression of disease is associated with a shift from monocytotropic to T-cell tropic virus populations. *J Virol* 1992; 66(3):1354–1360.
117. Tyor WR, Glass JD, Griffin JW, et al. Cytokine expression in the brain during the acquired immunodeficiency syndrome. *Ann Neurol* 1992;31:349–360.
118. Tyor JW, Glass JD, Baumrind N, et al. Cytokine expression of macrophages in HIV-1-associated vacuolar myelopathy. *Neurology* 1993;43:1002–1009.
119. Wesselingh SL, Power C, Glass JD, et al. Intracerebral cytokine mRNA expression in AIDS. *Ann Neurol* 1993;33(6):576–582.
120. Autran B, Plata F, Debre P. MHC-restricted cytotoxicity against HIV. *J AIDS* 1991;4: 361–367.
121. Ljungrenn K, Biberfeld G, Jondal M, Fenyo EM. Antibody dependent cellular cytotoxicity detects type and strain specific antigens among HIV types 1 and 2 and SIV mac isolates. *J Virol* 1989;63:3376–3380.
122. Nixon DF, McMichael AJ. Cytotoxic T-cell recognition of HIV proteins and peptides. *AIDS* 1991;5:1049–1059.
123. Price RW, Brew BJ, Rosenblum M. The AIDS dementia complex and HIV-1 brain infection: a pathogenetic model of virus-immune interaction. In: Waksman BH, ed. *Immunologic mechanisms in neurologic and psychiatric disease*. New York: Raven Press, 1990; 269–290.
124. Dawson VL, Dawson TM, Uhl GB, Snyder SH. HIV coat protein neurotoxicity mediated by nitric oxide in primary cortical cultures. *Proc Natl Acad Sci USA* 1992 *(in press)*.
125. Giulian D, Vaca K, Noonan CA. Secretion of neurotoxins by mononuclear phagocytes infected with HIV-1. *Science* 1990;250:1593–1596.
126. Lipton SA. Requirement for macrophages in neuronal injury induced by HIV envelope protein gp120. *Neuro Report* 1992;3:913–915.
127. Pulliam L, Herndler BG, Tanf NM, McGrath MS. Human immunodeficiency virus-infected macrophages produce soluble factors that cause histological and neurochemical alterations in cultured human brains. *J Clin Invest* 1991;87:503–512.
128. Tardieu M, Hery C, Peudenier S, et al. Human immunodeficiency virus type 1-infected monocytic cells can destroy human neural cells after cell-to-cell adhesion. *Ann Neurol* 1992;32:11–17.
129. Wahl LM, Corcoran ML, Pyle SW, et al. Human immunodeficiency virus glycoprotein (gp120) induction of monocyte arachidonic acid metabolites and interleukin 1. *Proc Natl Acad Sci USA* 1989;86:621–625.
130. Kaiser PK, Offerman JT, Lipton SA. Neuronal injury due to HIV-1 envelope protein is blocked by anti-gp-120 antibodies but not by anti-CD4 antibodies. *Neurology* 1990;40: 1757–1761.

131. Lipton SA. Human immunodeficiency virus-infected macrophages, gp120 and N-methyl-D-aspartate neurotoxicity. *Ann Neurol* 1993;33:227–228.
132. Lipton SA, Sucher NJ, Kaiser PK, Dreyer EB. Synergistic effects of the HIV coat protein and NMDA receptor-mediated neurotoxicity. *Neuron* 1991;7:111–118.
133. Merrill JE, Koyanagi Y, Zack J, et al. Induction of interleukin-1 and tumor necrosis factor alpha in brain cultures by human immunodeficiency virus type 1. *J Virol* 1992;66:2217–2221.
134. Toggas S, Masliah E, Rockenstein E, Mueke L. Neurotoxicity of viral proteins-HIV-1 gp 120 effects in transgenic models. *Clin Neuropathol* 1993;12:S4.
135. Bernton E, Bryant D, Decoster M, et al. No direct neuronotoxicity by HIV-1 virions or culture fluids from HIV-1 infected T-cells or monocytes. *AIDS Res Hum Retroviruses* 1992;8:495–501.
136. Selma KW, Raines CS. Tumor necrosis factor mediates myelin and oligodendrocyte damage *in vitro*. *Ann Neurol* 1988;23:339–346.
137. Everall IP, Luthert PJ, Lantos PL. Neuronal loss in the frontal cortex in HIV infection. *Lancet* 1991;337:1119–1121.
138. Ketzler S, Weis S, Haug H, Budka H. Loss of neurons in the frontal cortex in AIDS brains. *Acta Neuropathol* 1990;80:92–94.
139. Abe H, Weis S, Mehraein P. Degeneration of the cerebellar dentate nucleus and the inferior olivary nucleus in HIV-1 infection: a morphometric study. *Clin Neuropathol* 1993;12:S7.
140. Wiley CA, Masliah E, Morey M, et al. Neocortical damage during HIV infection. *Ann Neurol* 1991;29:651–657.
141. Esiri MM, Morris CS. Markers of cell proliferation in the brain in HIV-1 infection. *Clin Neuropathol* 1993;12:S10.
142. Dreyer EB, Kaiser PK, Offermann JT, Lipton SA. HIV-1 coat protein neurotoxicity prevented by calcium channel antagonists. *Science* 1990;248:364–367.
143. Brenneman DE, Westbrook GL, Fitzgerald SP, et al. Neuronal cell killing by the envelope glycoprotein of HIV and its prevention by vasoactive intestinal peptide. *Nature* 1988;335:639–642.
144. Bridge TP, Heseltine PNR, Parker ES, et al. Results of extended peptide T administration in AIDS and ARC patients. *Psychopharmacol Bull* 1991;27(3):237–245.
145. Panlilio LV, Hill JM, Brenneman DE. Gp120 and VIP receptor antagonists impair Morris water maze performance in rats. *Soc Neurosci Abstr* 1990;16:1330.
146. Brouwers P, Moss H, Wolters P, Eddy J, Balis F, Poplack DG. Effects of continuous-infusion zidovudine therapy on neuropsychologic functioning in children with symptomatic human immunodeficiency virus infection. *J Pediatr* 1990;116:980–985.
147. Gray F, Geny C, Dournon E, Fenelon G, Lionnet F, Gherardi R. Neuropathological evidence that zidovudine reduces the incidence of HIV infection of brain. *Lancet* 1991;337:852–853.
148. Portegies P, de Gans J, Lange JM, et al. Declining incidence of AIDS dementia complex after introduction of zidovudine treatment. *Br Med J* 1989;299:819–821.
149. Portegies P, Enting RH, de Gans J, et al. Presentation and course of AIDS dementia complex: 10 years of follow-up in Amsterdam, the Netherlands. *AIDS* 1993;7:669–675.
150. Scaravilli F, Sinclair E, Gray F, Ciardi A. PCR detection of HIV proviral DNA in the brain of asymptomatic HIV-positive patients; correlation with morphological changes. *Clin Neuropathol* 1993;12:S13.
151. Sidtis JJ, Gatsonis C, Price RW, et al. Zidovudine treatment of the AIDS dementia complex: results of a placebo controlled trial. *Ann Neurol* 1992;33:343–349.
152. Yarchoan R, Berg G, Brouwers P, et al. Response of human immunodeficiency virus associated neurological disease to 3′-azido-3′-deoxythymidine. *Lancet* 1987;1:132–135.
153. Price RW, Sidtis JJ. Early HIV infection and the AIDS dementia complex. *Neurology* 1990;40:323–326.

HIV, AIDS and the Brain, edited by
R. W. Price and S. W. Perry.
Raven Press, Ltd., New York © 1994.

2

Genetic and Biologic Basis of HIV-1 Neurotropism

William A. O'Brien

Department of Medicine, UCLA School of Medicine, Los Angeles, CA 90024

Human immunodeficiency virus type 1 (HIV-1) infection is frequently complicated by a variety of disease processes affecting the central nervous system (CNS). Although many opportunistic infections and neoplasms can occur, the most common CNS complication is the AIDS dementia complex (ADC), now also termed HIV-associated cognitive/motor complex. ADC is characterized by a progressive disease that may include cognitive, motor, and/or behavioral symptoms (1). Although ADC may be the first or sole manifestation of HIV-1 infection, the prevalence of neurologic symptoms increases in later clinical stages. This dementia appears to be a consequence of HIV-1 infection in the brain. HIV-1 has been recovered from neural tissues (2–4), but productive HIV-1 brain infection is confined nearly exclusively to mononuclear phagocytes, which include macrophages, microglia, and derivative multinucleated cells that are formed by virus-induced cell fusion (5–8). HIV-1 infection of macrophages thus appears to be critical for HIV-1 entry and replication in the CNS. However, factors important for development of neurologic disease are poorly defined, and are likely to be complex. In this review, we will focus on virologic aspects of HIV-related neurologic disease. HIV-1 replication in primary cells will be reviewed, and genetic determinants for efficient HIV-1 infection of mononuclear phagocytes will be described.

GENERAL RETROVIROLOGY

HIV-1 and HIV-2 are members of the Retroviridae virus family. These viruses are characterized by a single-stranded RNA genome and an RNA-dependent DNA polymerase (reverse transcriptase) carried in infectious virions. HIV-1 is more prevalent in the United States, whereas HIV-2 infection is seen primarily in parts of Africa, South America, and Europe. Simian immunodeficiency virus (SIV) is related to HIV-1 and HIV-2 and can cause an AIDS-like syndrome in certain nonhuman primates. Stable retroviral infection of a cell is usually associated with formation of a double-stranded DNA copy of the retroviral genome and covalent integration into chromosomal DNA of host cells. The HIV genome is approximately 9 kilobases (kb) in size; it exists in the virion as a dimer with two identical RNA subunits, designated as plus (+) strands since they are in the same orientation as messenger RNA (mRNA). Proteins are translated from RNA of this polarity.

Structural Genes

Retroviral particles consist of RNA genomes associated with core nucleoproteins encapsulated by an outer lipid envelope. There are three structural genes present in all retroviruses which are required for production of fully infectious progeny viruses. The *gag* gene encodes a precursor protein of 70–80 kilodaltons (kD), which is cleaved post-translationally to form the nucleocapsid products. The principal *gag* protein in HIV-1 is 24 kD (p24). The *pol* gene encodes protease, reverse transcriptase, integrase, and RNase H activities. These sequences are highly conserved among related strains of viruses. The *env* gene encodes membrane-associated glycoproteins. Surface glycoproteins are encoded by the virus project through the lipid membrane, and are seen by electron microscopy as spikes attached to the viral core. In HIV-1, a glycosylated precursor polypeptide (gp160) is cleaved to (a) a larger external polypeptide (gp120) which is involved in recognition and binding to receptors on the surface of target cells and (b) a smaller hydrophobic transmembrane polypeptide (gp41).

Long Terminal Repeat (LTR)

All retroviruses have functional regions at the terminal ends of the genome that contain regulatory elements required in *cis* for replication. Reverse transcription is initiated at the primer binding site (PBS) near the 5' terminal region. Sequence redundancy of the R region of the RNA genome at the 5' and 3' ends allows DNA strand transfer during reverse transcription. There is also a second binding site near the 3' terminal region for initiation of synthesis of plus strand DNA at the polypurine tract (PPT). Between these binding sites and R at each end are two other regions, U5 and U3, which are duplicated during reverse transcription to form two copies of the LTR. Regions in the LTR direct initiation of transcription and replication, and are the regions where integration into the host chromosome occurs during formation of the provirus.

HIV-1 LIFE CYCLE

An overview of the HIV-1 life cycle is schematically shown in Fig. 1. Successful retrovirus infection of a cell requires entry of viral genes into the cell and synthesis of a full-length double-stranded DNA copy of the RNA genome. The first step in the life cycle is adsorption of the virion to the surface of the host cell. This event involves attachment of the virus to a cell surface receptor; and in most cases for HIV-1, this is the cell surface molecule CD4. Although there appear to be other mechanisms for HIV entry that do not involve CD4, only cells expressing CD4 are infected with high efficiency (virus binding and entry are discussed below in the section entitled "HIV-1 Macrophage Tropism").

Formation of the Provirus

Following virus binding to target cells, the core nucleoprotein complex containing the viral RNA genome enters the cellular cytoplasmic space following a fusion event. There, virion-associated reverse transcriptase synthesizes a linear, double-stranded DNA copy of the viral genome. Virion-associated $tRNA_{lys}$ primer initiates synthesis of the first strand of viral DNA, and RNase H degrades the RNA component of the viral RNA-DNA dimer. Retroviral reverse transcription is complex, and involves at least two initiation events and two template switches. Reverse transcription is completed in 4–6 hours in activated T lymphocytes (9,10) but is incomplete in quiescent, nondividing T cells, which do not produce virus following *in vitro* infection (11). In mononuclear phagocytes, a third pattern of reverse transcription is seen, where 36–48 hours are required for formation of full-length viral DNA (11a). Reverse transcription in mononuclear phagocytes can be accelerated by addition of high concentrations of exogenous nucleosides, which indicates that nonviral factors are also important for efficient HIV-1 reverse transcription. However, addition of exogenous nucleosides apparently does not allow completion of reverse transcription in quiescent PBL, suggesting that other cell factors may be involved in this process (JA Zack, *personal communication*).

Some of the full-length reverse transcribed viral DNA migrates to the nucleus where integration can occur by collinear insertion of the ends of the viral LTRs into chromosomal DNA. This integrated DNA copy of the retrovirus genome is called a *provirus*. Viral genes are replicated along with host chromosomal DNA, and can thus persist for the life of the cell. For most retroviruses, integration is associated with cell division and is accomplished by the viral integrase protein, which is encoded by the *pol* gene. However, macrophages generally do not divide, and it is not certain whether chromosomal integration in these nondividing cells is required for productive

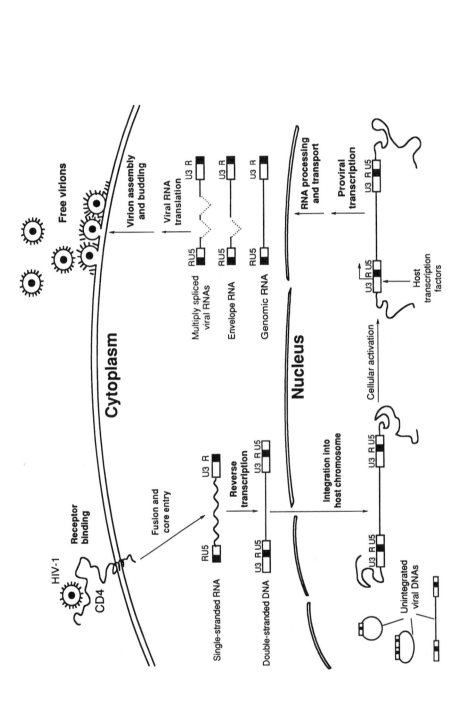

infection. Although most of the HIV-1-specific DNA in productively infected macrophages is associated with the high-molecular-weight fraction (12), covalent integration of viral DNA sequences with chromosomal sequences in mononuclear phagocytes has not been demonstrated.

Expression of the HIV-1 Genome

The next phase of infection involves expression of integrated retroviral genes leading to the formation of progeny virus. This is predominantly performed by host cell mechanisms. Host factors perform synthesis and processing of viral RNA, and translate viral mRNA on host ribosomes to synthesize viral proteins. Signals for initiation of transcription of viral genes are located in the viral LTR. There are enhancer sequences that are present in the LTR which can increase the level of transcription following binding of host regulatory proteins to these sequences. These include the cellular transcription factors Sp1 and NF-κB. Following translation of the processed viral mRNA on host ribosomes and protease cleavage of peptide precursors, viral proteins are assembled. This occurs near the plasma membrane of the infected cell. Retrovirus core particles containing reverse transcriptase and the RNA genome bud through the membrane in regions that are enriched for the Env protein complex. Intact infectious progeny virions are released by budding through the cell membrane, and can infect other permissive host cells.

NOVEL HIV GENES

There are complex regulatory systems in HIV and other primate lentiviruses, such as SIV, that are not found in other retroviruses. In addition to the three genes *(gag, pol,* and *env)* required for replication in all animal retroviruses, there are six additional overlapping open reading frames (ORFs) identified that encode viral gene products (13). These auxiliary genes are generally well conserved within each primate lentivirus group, suggesting that they play an important role in the viral life cycle. The proviral organiza-

FIG. 1. Retrovirus life cycle. Viral RNA enters the cell after binding to the surface of the host cell and viral-cell fusion. A double-stranded DNA copy is synthesized from genomic RNA by virion-associated reverse transcriptase. The LTRs are formed by duplication of U3 and U5 at the terminal regions. Some of the double-stranded DNA enters the nucleus, and the provirus is formed by collinear integration into the host genome. Viral RNA can be expressed from provirus, and viral proteins are synthesized on host ribosomes. Progeny virions are formed by budding through the membrane of infected cells.

tion of the human immunodeficiency viruses is shown in Fig. 2. SIV organization is similar to that of HIV-2.

The *tat* Gene

The *tat* (*trans*-activator of transcription) gene encodes a 14-kD protein in two distinct regions of the HIV genome that is essential for HIV replication. The Tat protein is an early gene product, and is synthesized from a multiply spliced, subgenomic mRNA. The Tat protein enhances HIV gene expression by (a) interacting with cellular factors and (b) binding to *trans*-activation-responsive (TAR) RNA sequences located in the R region. These sequences are present at the 5' end of all HIV-1 transcripts. Tat may increase HIV gene expression by stabilizing mRNA transcripts and facilitating elongation (14,15).

The *rev* Gene

Rev (regulator of expression of virion proteins) is also formed from a multiply-spliced RNA, and is required for HIV replication (16,17). The Rev protein localizes to the nucleus of transfected cells and binds to HIV-1 RNAs through sequences located within the *env* gene, termed the Rev-responsive element (RRE) (18–20). Rev is found associated with the RRE-containing RNAs in the cytoplasm of infected cells (21). Rev acts at the post-transcriptional level to increase the nuclear export and translation of the RRE-containing RNAs (22,23). As a result, Rev is required for the expression of Gag and Env structural proteins and indirectly down-regulates its own expression as well as that of *tat* and *nef*.

The *nef* Gene

The *nef* gene is present in all primate lentiviruses, the protein is highly immunogenic (24), and like the other two multiply-spliced HIV-1 proteins, Tat and Rev, Nef appears to be an early gene product. This gene is apparently not required for HIV-1 replication in culture because many strains, including the prototypic HTLV-III strain, are replication-competent despite having defective *nef* genes. In early studies (25,26), *nef*-expressing strains were found to exhibit a modest decrease in efficiency of viral spread in culture when compared with *nef*-deficient viruses, and the gene was therefore named "negative factor" (*nef*). Action as a specific repressor of HIV-1 transcription was proposed (27), although this effect was not reproduced by other groups, and currently the function of Nef is not clear (28,29). Nef is myristilated, is associated with cytoplasmic membrane structures, and may down-regulate

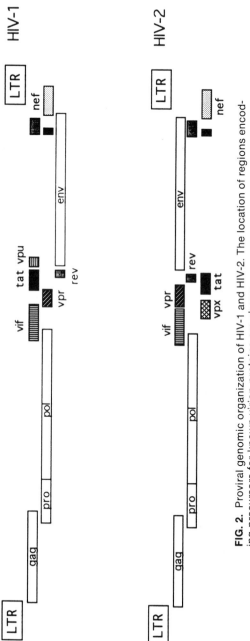

FIG. 2. Proviral genomic organization of HIV-1 and HIV-2. The location of regions encoding precursors for known virion proteins are shown.

surface expression of CD4 (13,30). Thus, Nef may be involved with either protein transport or membrane signaling. Importantly, *in vitro* studies may not reveal the function of Nef in clinical disease. Studies to determine the role of Nef *in vivo* have been performed in the SIV system using modified forms of the infectious clone, SIV_{max239}/*nef*-closed, which has a premature in-frame stop signal in the *nef* gene (31). Although no difference was observed in the replicative ability between *nef*-mutant and wild-type *nef* strains in cultured cells, mutant strains with large deletions in *nef* did not replicate to high titer in rhesus monkeys and did not cause clinical disease after 2 years. In contrast, monkeys infected with SIV_{max239}/*nef*-open, which encoded a full-length Nef protein, had much higher levels of virus replication and exhibited dramatic clinical progression. In animals infected with SIV_{max239}/*nef*-closed, viral strains that overcame the stop signal by spontaneous point mutation appeared quickly, and became predominant in infected animals. Therefore, in SIV, Nef appears to be required for vigorous virus replication *in vivo,* as well as for pathogenic effects. Based on these results, *nef* mutant strains have been proposed for testing as an experimental vaccine (13).

The *vpr* Gene

The virion protein R *(vpr)* gene, located between *pol* and *env,* encodes a 15-kD protein that is associated with the virion (32). Nonetheless, Vpr is not required for virion assembly, and is not required for virus replication in cell culture. Mutations in *vpr* do not appear to affect the replication or cytopathic effect of HIV-1 in $CD4^+$ T-cell lines. Vpr appears to act in *trans* to modestly increase expression of heterologous genes driven by the HIV-1 LTR (32).

The *vif* Gene

The viral infectivity factor *(vif)* gene is a late gene product encoded by an ORF overlapping the 3' end of *pol* and the 5' end of *vpr*. Mutations in the *vif* gene product have been shown to drastically decrease infectivity of HIV-1 particles as much as 1000-fold (33,34), but this effect is dependent on the cell type used. In some cell lines, Vif can be dispensable for viral replication. Vif may be involved in viral protein processing by a protease function (35).

The *vpu* Gene

The virion protein U *(vpu)* gene encodes a 15-kD protein in HIV-1; this gene is not present in HIV-2 or SIV. Vpu is required for efficient virus replication, but deletion mutants in *vpu* are not fatal (36). Vpu is phosphorylated and appears to be involved in virus release. *vpu* has also been implicated in HIV-1 envelope processing (37). Strain-dependent differences in *vpu* may affect the cell-surface expression of gp160 and, subsequently, the budding of progeny virions. In the absence of *vpu,* virions appear to congregate in chains attached to the infected cell membrane.

The *vpx* Gene

The virion protein X *(vpx)* gene is not present in HIV-1, but is located in the central portion of the genome between *pol* and *env* in HIV-2 and SIV. This gene encodes a 14-kD protein that is produced in large amounts; however, based on mutational analysis, this gene product appears to be dispensable for virus replication (38). Because of close sequence homology, it has been suggested that *vpx* is a duplicated *vpr* gene (39).

HIV-1 GENETIC VARIATION

There is variability of the molecular sequence between isolates of HIV-1 recovered from different individuals with AIDS, and from HIV-1 isolates recovered from the same patient (4,40,41). Each HIV-1 strain should be considered to be unique. Variability is generated during reverse transcription, because there is no proofreading function associated with retroviral reverse transcriptase. This leads to nucleotide changes at a rate of one per ten thousand base pairs, or about one change for each genome for each replication. However, observed sustainable genetic variation is not distributed evenly throughout the genome. Although some regions are well conserved between HIV-1 isolates, other regions show marked differences, particularly the *env* region (42). This suggests that selective pressures influence development of HIV-1 genetic diversity. As discussed below, variation in the *env* regions appears to be important to viral pathogenesis and persistence.

A number of investigators have examined HIV-1 sequence heterogeneity present in one patient at one time for specific HIV-1 genetic regions. Using the polymerase chain reaction (PCR), a DNA amplification technique, highly related but distinct sequences have been identified in patient blood, and termed "quasispecies" (41,43). The pattern of viral heterogeneity differs in different stages of disease. During acute infection, where there are high levels of viral replication, the sequences are homogeneous, because one virus strain tends to predominate (44,45). Levels of detectable virus typically fall after 4–8 weeks, following development of anti-HIV-1 antibodies. Early isolates, obtained from asymptomatic individuals, usually display slow replication kinetics, are non-syncytium-inducing (NSI), and, consequently, are less efficient at killing infected cells. HIV-1 sequence diversity emerges in patients within several months. Over time, viral load, or copy number of HIV-1 DNA and RNA sequences, gradually increases, as does sequence diversity (45,46).

Virus variants are selected as a result of pressure to escape from antibody neutralization, cell tropism, or other replicative properties. In late stages of AIDS, viral phenotypes are more diverse, include HIV-1 strains which are syncytium-inducing (SI), and replicate to higher titer and with greater cytopathic effect (47,48).

The presence of more "virulent" strains of HIV-1 may correlate with clinical progression from asymptomatic disease to AIDS. It has been hypothesized that SI strains may be present during acute infection but are suppressed by the competent anti-HIV immune response of the host, whereas NSI strains escape host immune surveillance and establish a persistent infection throughout the asymptomatic period of the disease (49). At later disease stages, as a result of CD4 lymphocyte depletion, the weakened immune system is no longer able to prevent the emergence of the SI HIV-1 strains. The emergence of these strains may further hasten clinical decline.

HIV-1 strains isolated from different tissues of an HIV-infected individual display biologic phenotypes that may enable them to propagate better in particular body compartments. For example, HIV-1 strains isolated from brain tissue tend to replicate efficiently in mononuclear phagocytes, whereas blood-derived HIV-1 strains may or may not be capable of replication in mononuclear phagocytes (50). Infection of these cells in body tissues is associated with disease. In addition, *in vitro* culture conditions will select for HIV-1 variants with certain phenotypes, including the ability to replicate in certain cell types. *In vitro* passage of virus can result in preferential growth of what may be a minor subset of virus strains, which subsequently become the predominant strain (41,43). Therefore, results of experiments using bulk virus cultures, particularly those passaged through transformed cell lines, should be interpreted with caution. We will focus our discussion on HIV-1 replication of primary strains that have not been disturbed by prolonged *in vitro* culture.

HIV-1 MACROPHAGE TROPISM

Blood mononuclear cells expressing CD4, which include the T-helper cell subset of peripheral blood lymphocytes (PBLs) and mononuclear phagocytes, are the predominant targets for HIV-1 infection. Most HIV-1 in circulating blood is associated with PBL (51), whereas HIV-1 in extravascular tissues (except lymph nodes) is associated with mononuclear phagocytes. Nearly all HIV-1 strains replicate in lectin-stimulated PBLs, whether the virus was obtained directly from infected tissues, or following passage in PBLs, transformed cell lines, mononuclear phagocytes, or infected tissues. However, different HIV-1 strains vary markedly in their ability to productively infect mononuclear phagocytes. Distinct differences in target cell tropism have been identified for different HIV-1 isolates obtained from the same individual (4). HIV-1$_{JR-CSF}$ was isolated from cell-free cerebrospinal fluid (CSF) of a patient who died with severe AIDS encephalopathy. This strain replicates efficiently in phytohemagglutinin (PHA)-stimulated PBLs, but does not replicate as well in blood mononuclear phagocytes from most donors. In contrast, the strain HIV-1$_{JR-FL}$, recovered from frontal lobe brain tissue of the same patient, replicates efficiently and to high titer in stimulated PBLs and blood mononuclear phagocytes from all donors tested (over 250); HIV-1$_{JR-FL}$ also replicates in brain microglial cells that are resident macrophages of the brain (52), as well as in alveolar macrophages (53). Although these strains are genetically distinct, they are more closely related to each other than to strains isolated from different individuals (42). Thus, differences in macrophage tropism appear to be related to viral genetic variation.

Viral Determinants for Macrophage Tropism

Phenotypic differences between HIV-1 strains can be mapped by recombinant virus studies. HIV-1$_{HXB2}$ and HIV-1$_{NL4-3}$, which were obtained following serial passage in transformed T-cell lines, replicate very inefficiently in peripheral blood mononuclear phagocytes. Apparently, prolonged culture in transformed cell lines exerts a negative selection for determinants important for macrophage tropism. These laboratory strains are also unable to replicate in primary brain microglial cells (54), but these cells can be productively infected by virus strains that replicate in blood mononuclear phagocytes. Because of the marked differences in the ability of HIV-1$_{JR-FL}$ and HIV-1$_{NL4-3}$ to productively infect mononuclear phagocytes, molecular clones of these strains were used to generate molecular recombinant viruses in order to identify viral regions involved in determining macrophage tropism.

For recombinant virus studies, chimeric proviral clones were constructed by substituting purified DNA fragments of the clone of HIV-1$_{JR-FL}$ into the infectious clone pNL4-3 (55). Recombinant viruses were assessed for ability to replicate in purified blood mononuclear phagocytes. A region of 157 amino acids of HIV-1$_{JR-FL}$ gp120 was identified that was capable of fully conferring mononuclear phagocyte tropism. This region of *env* includes the major neutralization domain (variable region 3, or V3) and does not include the originally defined CD4 binding domain (amino acids 404–447) (56). The third variable domain, V3, comprises a loop structure formed by approximately 30 amino acids bordered by a disulfide-linked cysteine bridge. Other recombinant viruses containing larger substitutions of HIV-1$_{JR-FL}$ *env* that did not include V3 replicated poorly in mononuclear phagocytes.

In subsequent recombinant virus studies, mononuclear phagocyte tropism was mapped to the same region of gp120 by substitution of proviral fragments from other macrophage-tropic strains, including HIV-1$_{SF162}$, HIV-1$_{ADA}$, and

HIV-1$_{BaL}$ (57–59). Hwang et al. (58) have defined the minimal region important for macrophage tropism by substitution of a fragment encoding only the 30 amino acids of the V3 loop.

Cell tropism for transformed T-cell lines appears to map to a similar region of gp120; however, viral determinants of tropism for T-cell lines and mononuclear phagocytes appear to be mutually exclusive (57,58,60). In general, recombinant viruses that replicate efficiently in mononuclear phagocytes do not productively infect transformed T-cell lines, and the converse is also true. Thus, the V3 loop appears to be critically involved with HIV-1 replication events in both mononuclear phagocytes and transformed cell lines.

Mechanism of *env*-Mediated Cell Tropism

The studies that map mononuclear cell tropism of diverse HIV-1 isolates to the *env* gene suggest that tropism is determined by early events in the retroviral life cycle. We tested this hypothesis by analyzing viral DNA formation in a quantitative PCR assay 24–48 hours after infection. Viral DNA formation is the earliest assayable event in productive infection. We found over 100-fold less HIV-1-specific DNA following infection with HIV-1$_{NL4-3}$ or other poorly macrophage-tropic strains, compared with the macrophage-tropic strains (e.g., HIV-1$_{JR-FL}$) or the macrophage-tropic recombinant virus strains (55). Similar differences in HIV-1-specific DNA levels are seen in transformed T-cell lines by PCR analysis (60–62). In this case, macrophage-tropic HIV-1 strains did not productively infect the transformed T-cell lines, and there was very little viral DNA formation following infection. Taken together, the mapping of macrophage tropism to gp120 and the low level of viral DNA seen in cells in nonproductive infection suggest that HIV-1 strain differences and the ability to infect mononuclear phagocytes can result from differences in virus entry, at least for strains which have been examined by this assay. Virus entry involves specific binding to receptors on the cell surface, along with subsequent uptake of the bound virus into the cytoplasm. Although initial binding events between gp120 and CD4 have been well-defined, little is known about post-binding events.

V3 Sequence Analysis and Phenotypic Associations

In addition to its role as a crucial determinant of cell tropism, the envelope V3 region has also been implicated in syncytium induction. These syncytia are multinucleated cell complexes comprised of CD4$^+$ cells that have been fused by interactions with envelope. In infection, viral cores are believed to enter the cytoplasmic space following fusion of viral and target cell membranes. V3 appears to play a role in fusion (63), but virus strains differ in ability to induce syncytia. V3 amino acid sequences from several well-characterized virus strains are aligned in Fig. 3. The amino acid sequence Gly-Pro-Gly-Arg (G-P-G-R) located at the tip of the loop is highly conserved among HIV-1 isolates; the flanking amino acids on both sides are highly variable (64). Analysis of the predicted V3 amino acid sequence of macrophage-tropic and -nontropic strains has identified amino acid patterns that may be important for cell tropism. For example, most macrophage-tropic strains have acidic amino acid residues—either Glu (E) or Asp (D)—at position 317 of HIV-1 *env,* just downstream from the conserved tip of the loop. Strains that do not efficiently replicate in mononuclear phagocytes are more likely to have positively charged amino acids, such as Lys (K) at position 317 (59). V3 sequence analysis of HIV-1 isolates recovered over time reveal phenotypic associations with amino acid charge (65–67). In general, strains having more positively charged amino acid residues in V3 are less efficient at replication in mononuclear phagocytes, readily induce syncytia in T cells, and have expanded tropism for a variety of transformed cell lines. Viral isolates obtained during the early stages of disease tend to be NSI, and replicate in macrophages, although several viral subgroups having SI phenotype can also be found. Over time, with disease progression, SI isolates come to predominate.

Changes introduced by site-directed mutagenesis on either side of the V3 loop, or changes of amino acids on both sides of the loop that increase the net positive charge, have been shown to affect SI phenotype (68). Specific amino acid changes in V3 that alone can confer marked changes in HIV-1 macrophage tropism, however, have not been identified. Spontaneous mutations within the highly conserved tip of the V3 loop can occur during prolonged culture *in vitro,* and have been shown to affect cell tropism (69). The clinical relevance of these findings are not clear, since most clinical strains do not contain these amino acid changes. The virus strain HIV-1$_{89.6}$ is able to replicate efficiently in both mononuclear phagocytes and transformed T-cell lines. This is an SI isolate that encodes many positively charged V3 amino acid residues (70). The relationship between the positively charged V3 loop in this strain and the ability to replicate in macrophages is not clear. Both SI and tropism events appear to occur after initial binding to target cells and involve secondary conformational changes. Perhaps other *env* regions in addition to V3 are involved in determining the phenotype of HIV-1$_{89.6}$, and these regions may impact the confirmational changes that occur following envelope binding to CD4. In addition, structural Env conformations related to the charge of the V3 loop may be complex.

Interactions Between HIV-1 Env and CD4

Env is comprised of two distinct proteins, gp120 and gp41, which are not covalently bound. The transmembrane protein, gp41, has a cytoplasmic tail

virus	V3 loop sequence	M-tropic	syncytia	net(+) charge
ZR6	----YK---Q-TP-·-L-Q-L---RGRTKI-G----	no	yes	9
HXB2	------R-R-QR-----V-I-K·--NM-----	no	yes	9
MN	-----Y-K--R---·--------KN---T----	no	yes	8
SF2	--------Y-·-·-----H-----K---	no	no	8
JRCSF	----S----------------	no	no	5
consensus	293 CTRPNNTRKSIHI·GPGRAFYTTGEIIGDIRQAHC 327			
JRFL	--------------·-·------------	yes	no	5
ADA	--------------·-·-------------	yes	no	5
Bal	--------------L----	yes	no	5
YU-2	------N-·-----L----	yes	no	5
SF162	------T-·------A--D----	yes	no	5
89.6	------RRLS-·-------ARRN-----	yes	yes	9

FIG. 3. Comparison of predicted amino acid sequences of the V3 loop. V3 amino acid sequences are aligned with non-macrophage-tropic strains above the consensus sequence [as determined by LaRosa et al. (64)] and are aligned with macrophage-tropic strains below the consensus sequence. Phenotype and net positive charge are shown to the right. Dots indicate gaps; dashes indicate conserved amino acids. [Adapted from Collman et al. (70), with permission.]

at its carboxy terminus, traverses the cell membrane several times at hydrophobic regions, and extends extracellularly where it is associated with the external membrane protein gp120. The amino terminus of gp41 has been shown to be critical for fusion and viral entry. The C4 domain of gp120, just downstream from the V3 domain, was shown to be crucial for binding to CD4 (56), but changes in amino acids throughout Env have also been shown to affect gp120-CD4 binding affinity (71,72). This suggests that there are multiple contact points between gp120 and CD4, or that amino acid changes in distant regions of Env can alter protein conformation of the CD4 binding site.

Soluble CD4 Neutralization

The soluble form of the receptor molecule CD4 (sCD4) was considered for therapeutic use to block infection by binding virus before it could interact with CD4 expressed on target cells. sCD4 was shown to efficiently neutralize infection by cell-line-adapted strains of HIV-1 in PBLs and transformed cell lines *in vitro,* but there was no detectable antiviral effect in treated patients as assessed by serum p24 antigen levels (73,74) and infectious HIV-1 titers in blood (75). The lack of efficacy appears to be related to virus strain differences. Cell-line-adapted strains can be neutralized at low sCD4 concentrations; however, most primary virus strains are at least 100-fold more resistant to neutralization by sCD4 (75).

Viral-strain-dependent differences in binding affinity to CD4 were considered as an explanation for resistance to sCD4 neutralization, yet there was no appreciable difference in binding affinity between recombinant soluble gp120s from the primary strains, HIV-1$_{JR-FL}$ and HIV-1$_{JR-CSF}$, and the cell-line-adapted strain, HIV-1$_{BH10}$, as well as other primary and laboratory strains (76–78). However, intact virions of primary isolates appear to have a 10- to 30-fold lower affinity for sCD4 than do cell-line-adapted strains (78). In addition, mutagenesis studies with *env* constructs from a cell-line-adapted strain efficiently neutralized by sCD4 demonstrated that amino acid substitutions in gp120 that decreased CD4 binding affinity resulted in a relative resistance to neutralization by sCD4 (79). Thus, virus strain differences in CD4 binding may determine resistance to sCD4, but these experimental systems may not accurately represent the interactions between multimeric *env* on virions and CD4 presented in the context of the cell surface. Recombinant studies have shown that both cell tropism and sensitivity to sCD4 neutralization can be determined by specific domains of gp120 which include the V3 loop (60,80). However, mutational analysis has identified other gp120 regions (in C3 and C4) which are more important for gp120 binding to both gp41 and CD4 (79).

gp120 Shedding

During virion binding to CD4, there are noncovalent interactions of gp120 both with gp41 and with CD4. sCD4 can induce shedding of gp120 from virions, which renders the particles noninfectious (81). The efficacy of sCD4-induced shedding varies between different HIV-1 strains. Primary HIV-1 isolates resistant to sCD4 neutralization not only exhibit decreased sCD4 binding affinity, but also undergo less sCD4-induced gp120 shedding than do sCD4-sensitive isolates, suggesting that these properties together may account for the relative resistance of primary isolates to sCD4 neutralization (82).

Antibody Neutralization

Many HIV-1 proteins have highly immunogenic regions, but the predominant type-specific antibody neutralization epitopes are determinants in V3 (83). Antibodies raised to linear peptides based on the V3 sequence of cloned strains are only able to neutralize the same or closely related strains. Antibodies that recognize conformational envelope epitopes may be more relevant for inhibiting infection. Neutralizing monoclonal antibodies have been identified which interact with discontinuous regions of gp120 (84), and which are much less reactive with denatured gp120 protein. These gp120 epitopes are therefore conformational, in contrast to linear epitopes which are comprised of short stretches of continuous sequences. sCD4 binding to virus can induce an increase in binding of V3-specific antibodies, and can expose gp41 fusion epitopes which were cryptic prior to sCD4 binding (85). Although sCD4 binding to most HIV-1 strains will result in neutralization, sCD4 treatment can actually lead to enhancement of virus infection in the SIV system (86). In this case, sCD4 binding apparently generates conformational changes that increase the efficiency of virus fusion and entry.

Interactions between gp120 and CD4 are complex. Binding is initiated by interaction of gp120 with domain 1 of CD4, and can be blocked with monoclonal antibodies reactive with CD4 domain 1. The regions around CDR3 in domain 2 have been proposed to be critical for fusion, possibly independent from gp120 binding to CD4 (87). This is further suggested by the inability of the monoclonal antibody 5A8 (which is reactive with CD4 domain 2) to block sCD4 binding to virions. Instead, 5A8 appears to block HIV-1 fusion by interfering with sCD4-induced conformational changes in gp120/gp41 that are necessary for virus entry (88). Recent studies using a panel of CD4–vaccinia recombinants altered in CDR3, however, did not affect syncytium formation or gp120 release from HIV-1 envelope protein (89). The mechanism of postbinding HIV-1 entry events remains a matter of speculation.

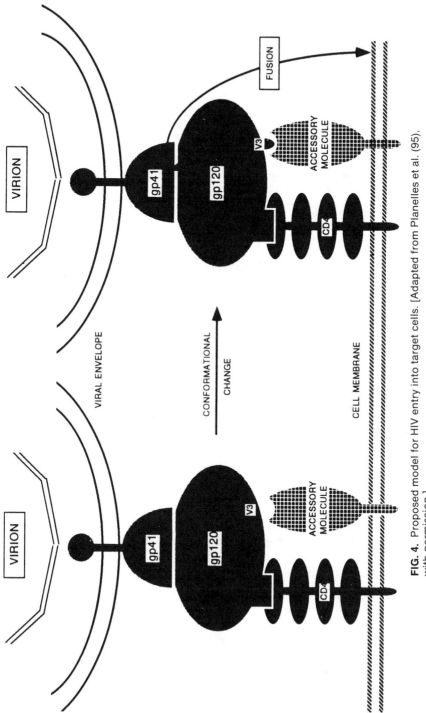

FIG. 4. Proposed model for HIV entry into target cells. [Adapted from Planelles et al. (95), with permission.]

Model of HIV-1 Infection of Mononuclear Phagocytes

Determinants in the gp120 V3 region have been shown to be important for efficient infection of mononuclear phagocytes. CD4 binding plays a crucial role in initiation of infection, based on monoclonal antibody and sCD4 neutralization studies. However, CD4 binding alone is not sufficient for infection of mononuclear phagocytes by all virus strains. In addition, the major gp120 determinants for CD4 binding lie outside V3 (56,71). We propose that conformational changes in gp120 occur following CD4 binding that affect the structure of V3 (see Fig. 4). There appears to be a target cell interaction with V3 in addition to or in conjunction with CD4 binding that is necessary for efficient entry into mononuclear phagocytes. This V3-dependent interaction may involve a second cellular receptor protein, or other domains of CD4 rather than distinct molecules.

Virus internalization is likely to be more complex than the model presented. Although V3 is a critical determinant, studies demonstrating the importance of conformational epitopes suggest the involvement of widely disparate gp120 regions, as well as CD4 regions, in binding and entry of HIV-1 into the cell. Multiple *env* domains may be involved in the virus entry process. In addition, just as each virus strain is different, so too is each individual. Variation in host genetic determinants may affect the efficiency of virus entry into target cells. This is demonstrated by marked differences in susceptibility of mononuclear phagocytes from different donors to infection with the same virus strain (55).

OTHER VIRAL DETERMINANTS FOR MONONUCLEAR PHAGOCYTE TROPISM

Although HIV-1 *env* determinants are implicated in efficient virus entry into mononuclear phagocytes, virus-strain-specific deferences in HIV-1 replication may also be determined by post-entry events. Several viral genetic regions have been identified which appear to affect cell-specific differences in viral replication. Studies with chimeric HIV-1 strains having substitutions in both *env* and *vpr* using sequences from the macrophage-tropic strain HIV-1$_{ADA}$ have shown that efficient viral replication in mononuclear phagocytes can be affected in a two-step process (36). One is determined by envelope at the level of entry, while another yet uncharacterized step is determined by *vpr* sequences in strains with envelope determinants that allow virus entry. *vpr* mutants have also been reported to decrease HIV-2 replication in mononuclear phagocytes (90). The mechanism of these *vpr*-mediated effects is not known.

Murine retroviruses have been shown to exhibit differences in virus expression and cell tropism based on specific alterations in the LTR. However, comparison of expression directed from the LTR of T-cell-tropic strains of HIV-1 with brain-derived or macrophage tropic strain-derived LTRs did not demonstrate any differences in viral gene expression (91). These transient transfection assays may not, however, accurately reflect strain-dependent differences in LTR-directed virus expression that may occur *in vivo*.

The *vpx* gene is found in SIV and HIV-2, but not in HIV-1, and has been shown to be dispensable for virus replication in several different T-cell lines. Mutations in the *vpx* gene of SIV_{mac} diminish levels of replication in primary lymphocytes (92). Decreases in virus replication are even more pronounced in primary macrophages from the same donors, suggested that *vpx* is required for efficient virus replication in both lymphocytes and (particularly) macrophages.

IN VIVO CORRELATES OF NEUROTROPISM

If macrophage tropism truly is important for development of HIV-related neurologic disease, it is expected that HIV-1 sequences present in CNS tissue will have a distribution pattern distinct from that found circulating in blood. Evidence to support this has been shown by examining the HIV-1 sequence distribution from paired brain and blood or spleen samples collected at autopsy from HIV-infected patients. Studies examining V4 *env* sequences in adults (93), as well as studies examining V3 sequences in brain and spleen samples of pediatric patients (94), have shown segregation of viral subtypes in different body compartments. In these studies, the major subtype sequence in the brain was a minor component of the quasispecies in blood or spleen, or was not represented at all. Conversely, the major subtype in blood was much less common in brain tissue. Additional evidence to support independent evolution of variants in different tissues comes from detailed analysis of the genetic variation. The mutations seen were not random, but showed several "hot spot" where changes were clustered. In addition, the rate of silent mutations was lower than expected. Under conditions of no selection pressure, the frequency of silent mutations is approximately 25 percent. In the studies of Pang et al. (93), the silent mutation rates were much lower, generally less than 10 percent. These data suggest that specific genetic changes conferred a selective advantage, either by allowing escape from immune surveillance or by conferring cell tropism which allows replication in CNS.

CONCLUSION

HIV infection of mononuclear phagocytes appears to be important for genesis of HIV-related diseases, particularly in the CNS. The ability to productively infect mononuclear phagocytes can be determined by sequences in the V3 domain of HIV-1 *env*. This region is not only involved in determining cell tropism, but has also been implicated in neutralization by monoclonal antibodies and sCD4. Although this region is critical for efficient entry into mononuclear phagocytes, other *env* domains appear to be involved in complex binding and internalization processes. Studies to more precisely define virus–target-cell interactions, particularly identification of accessory cell proteins, will enhance our understanding of pathogenesis of HIV disease and may lead to development of new therapeutic strategies.

ACKNOWLEDGMENTS

I thank Patricia Page for preparation of the manuscript. I also thank Salvatorre Arrigo, David Camerini, Gerold Feuer, Vicente Plannes, and Jerome Zack for helpful comments and discussions. William O'Brien is supported by a Department of Veteran's Affairs career development award and by PHS grant AI-29894.

REFERENCES

1. Price RW, Brew B, Sidtis J, Rosenblum M, Scheck AC, Cleary P. The brain in AIDS: central nervous system HIV-1 infection and AIDS dementia complex. *Science* 1988;239:586–592.
2. Ho DD, Rota TR, Schooley RT, Kaplan JC, Allan JD, Groopman JE, Resnick L, Felsenstein D, Andrews CA, Hirsch MS. Isolation of HTLV-III from cerebrospinal fluid and neural tissues of patients with neurologic syndromes related to the acquired immunodeficiency syndrome. *N Engl J Med* 1985;313:1494–1497.
3. Levy JA, Shimabukuro J, Hollander H, Mills J, Kaminsky L. Isolation of AIDS-associated retroviruses from cerebrospinal fluid and brain of patients with neurological symptoms. *Lancet* 1985;ii:586–588.
4. Koyanagi Y, Miles S, Mitsuyatsu RT, Merryl JE, Vinters HV, Chen ISY. Dual infection of the central nervous system by AIDS viruses with distinct cellular tropisms. *Science* 1987;236:819–822.
5. Shaw GM, Harper ME, Hahn BH, et al. HTLV-III infection in brains of children and adults with AIDS encephalopathy. *Science* 1985;227:177–181.
6. Gabuzda DH, Hirsch MS. Neurologic manifestations of infection with human immunodeficiency virus. *Ann Neurol* 1986;107:383–391.
7. Koenig S, Gendelman HE, Orenstein JM, et al. Detection of AIDS virus in macrophages in brain tissue from AIDS patients with encephalopathy. *Science* 1986;233:1089–1093.
8. Wiley CA, Schrier RD, Nelson JA, Lampert PW, Oldstone BA. Cellular localization of human immunodeficiency virus infection within the brains of acquired immunodeficiency syndrome patients. *Proc Natl Acad Sci USA* 1986;83:7089–7093.
9. Kim S, Byrn R, Groopman J, Baltimore D. Temporal aspects of DNA and RNA synthesis during human immunodeficiency virus infection: evidence for differential gene expression. *J Virol* 1989;63:3708–3713.
10. Zack JA, Haislip AM, Krogstad P, Chen ISY. Incompletely reverse-transcribed human immunodeficiency virus type 1 genomes in quiescent cells can function as intermediates in the retroviral life cycle. *J Virol* 1992;66:1717–1725.
11. Zack JA, Arrigo SJ, Weitsman SR, Go AS, Haislip A, Chen ISY. HIV-1 entry into quiescent primary lymphocytes: molecular analysis reveals a labile, latent viral structure. *Cell* 1990;61:213–222.
11a. O'Brien WA, Namazi A, Kalhor H, et al. Kinetics of HIV-1 reverse transcription in blood

mononuclear phagocytes is slowed by limitations of nucleotide precursors. Submitted for publication.

12. Weinberg JB, Matthews TJ, Cullen BR, Malim MH. Productive human immunodeficiency virus type 1 (HIV-1) infection of nonproliferating human monocytes. *J Exp Med* 1991;174: 1477–1482.

13. Desrosiers RC. HIV with multiple gene deletions as a live attenuated vaccine for AIDS. *AIDS Res Hum Retroviruses* 1992;8:8411–8421.

14. Feng S, Holland EC. HIV-1 *tat trans*-activation requires the loop sequence within *tar*. *Nature* 1988;334:165–167.

15. Gatignol A, Buckler-White A, Berkhout B, Jeang K-T. Characterization of a human TAR RNA-binding protein that activates the HIV-1 LTR. *Science* 1991;251:1597–1600.

16. Feinberg MB, Jarrett RF, Aldovini A, Gallo RC, Wong SF. HTLV-III expression and production involve complex regulation at the levels of splicing and translation of viral DNA. *Cell* 1986;46:807–817.

17. Sodroski J, Goh WC, Rosen C, Dayton A, Terwillinger E, Haseltine W. A second post-transcriptional *trans*-activator gene required for HTLV-III replication. *Nature* 1986;321: 412–417.

18. Cullen BR, Hauber J, Campbell K, Sodroski JG, Haseltine WA, Rosen CA. Subcellular localization of the human immunodeficiency virus trans-acting art gene product. *J Virol* 1988;62:2498–2501.

19. Daly TJ, Cook KS, Gray GS, Maione TE, Rusche JR. Specific binding of HIV-1 recombinant Rev-responsive element *in vitro*. *Nature* 1989;342:816–819.

20. Zapp ML, Green MR. Sequence-specific RNA binding by the HIV-1 Rev protein. *Nature* 1989;342:714–716.

21. Arrigo SJ, Heaphy S, Haines JK. *In vivo* binding of wild-type and mutant human immunodeficiency virus type 1. *rev* proteins: implications for function. *J Virol* 1992;66:5569–5575.

22. Arrigo SJ, Chen ISY. *Rev* is necessary for translation but not cytoplasmic accumulation of HIV-1 *vif, vpr,* and *env/vpu* 2 RNAs. *Genes Dev* 1991;5:808–819.

23. Malim MH, Hauber J, Fenrick R, Cullen BR. Immunodeficiency virus *rev trans*-activator modulates the expression of the viral regulatory genes. *Nature* 1989;335:181–183.

24. Allan JS, Coligan JE, Lee TH, et al. A new HTLV-III/LAV encoded antigen detected by antibodies from AIDS patients. *Science* 1985;230:810–813.

25. Luciw PA, Cheng-Mayer C, Levy JA. Mutational analysis of the human immunodeficiency virus: the *orf-B* region down-regulates virus replication. *Proc Natl Acad Sci USA* 1987;84: 1434–1438.

26. Cheng-Mayer C, Lannello P, Shaw K, Luciw PA, Levy JA. Differential effects of *nef* on HIV replication: implications for viral pathogenesis in the host. *Science* 1989;246:1629–1632.

27. Ahmed N, Venkatesan S. *nef* protein of HIV-1 is a transcriptional repressor of HIV-1 LTR. *Science* 1988;241:1481–1485.

28. Kim SK, Ikeuchi K, Byrn R, Groopman J, Baltimore D. Lack of a negative influence on viral growth by the *nef* gene of human immunodeficiency virus type 1. *Proc Natl Acad Sci USA* 1989;86:9544–9548.

29. Hammes SR, Dixon EP, Malim MH, Cullen BR, Greene WC. Nef protein of human immunodeficiency virus type 1: evidence against its role as a transcriptional inhibitor. *Proc Natl Acad Sci USA* 1989;86:9549–9553.

30. Guy B, Kieny MP, Rivier Y, Le Peuch C, Dott K, Girard M, Montanier L, LeCocq J-P. HIV F/31 orf encodes a phosphorylated GTP-binding protein resembling an oncogene product. *Nature* 1987;330:266–269.

31. Kestler HW, Ringler DJ, Mori K, Panicall DL, Sehgal PK, Daniel MD, Desrosiers RC. Importance of the *nef* gene for maintenance of high virus loads and for development of AIDS. *Cell* 1991;65:651–662.

32. Cohen EA, Dehni G, Sodroski JG, Haseltine WA. Human immunodeficiency virus *vpr* product is a virion-associated regulatory protein. *J Virol* 1990;64:3097–3099.

33. Fisher AG, Ensoli B, Ivanoff L, et al. The *sor* gene of HIV-1 is required for efficient virus transmission *in vitro*. *Science* 1987;237:888–893.

34. Strebel K, Daugherty D, Clouse K, Cohen D, Folks T, Martin MA. The HIV 'A' *(sor)* gene product is essential for virus infectivity. *Nature* 1987;328:728–730.

35. Guy B, Geist M, Dott K, Spehner D, Kieny M-P, Lecocq JP. A specific inhibitor of cysteine

proteases impairs a Vif-dependent modification of human immunodeficiency virus type 1 Env protein. *J Virol* 1991;65:1325–1331.

36. Westervelt P, Trowbridge DB, Epstein LG, et al. Macrophage tropism determinants of human immunodeficiency virus type 1 *in vivo. J Virol* 1992;66:2577–2582.

37. Willey RL, Maldarelli F, Martin MA, Strebel K. Human immunodeficiency virus type 1 *vpu* protein regulates the formation of intracellular gp160–CD4 complexes. *J Virol* 1992; 66:226–234.

38. Marcon L, Michaels F, Hattori N, Fargnoli K, Gallo RC, Franchini G. Dispensable role of the human immunodeficiency virus type 2 Vpx protein in viral replication. *J Virol* 1991; 65:3938–3942.

39. Tristem M, Marshall C, Karpas A, Petrik J, Hill F. Origin of *vpx* in lentiviruses. *Nature* 1990;347:341–342.

40. Hahn BH, Shaw GM, Taylor ME, et al. Genetic variation in HTLV-III/LAV over time in patients with AIDS or at risk for AIDS. *Science* 1986;232:1548–1553.

41. Goodenow M, Huet T, Saurin W, Kwok S, Sninsky J, Wain-Hobson S. HIV-1 isolates are rapidly evolving quasispecies: evidence for viral mixtures and preferred nucleotide substitutions. *J AIDS* 1989;2:344–352.

42. Myers G, Rabson AB, Bertzofsky JA, Smith TF. *Human retroviruses and AIDS.* Los Alamos, NM: Los Alamos National Laboratory, 1991.

43. Meyerhans A, Cheynier R, Albert J, Seth M, Kwok S, Sninsky J, Morfeldt-Manson L, Asjo B, Wain-Hobson S. Temporal fluctuations in HIV quasispecies *in vivo* are not reflected by sequential HIV isolations. *Cell* 1989;58:901–910.

44. Pang S, Shlesinger Y, Daar ES, Moudgil T, Ho DD, Chen ISY. Rapid generation of sequence variation during primary HIV-1 infection. *AIDS* 1992;6:453–460.

45. McNearney T, Hornickova Z, Markham R, Birdwell A, Arens M, Saah A, Ratner L. Relationship of human immunodeficiency virus type 1 sequence heterogeneity to stage of disease. *Proc Natl Acad Sci USA* 1992;89:10247–10251.

46. Nowak MA, Anderson RM, McLean AR, Wolfs TFW, Goudsmit J, May RM. Antigenic diversity thresholds and the development of AIDS. *Science* 1991;254:963–969.

47. Cheng-Mayer C, Seto D, Tateno M, Levy JA. Biologic features of HIV-1 that correlate with virulence in the host. *Science* 1988;240:80–82.

48. Tersmette M, de Goede REY, Al BJM, Winkel IN, Gruters RA, Cuypers HT, Huisman HG, Miedema F. Differential syncytium inducing capacity of HIV isolates: frequent detection of syncytium inducing isolates in patients with AIDS and ARC. *J Virol* 1988;62:2026–2032.

49. Schuitemaker H, Koot M, Kootstra NA, Dercksen MW, DeGoede REY, Van Steenwijk RP, Lange JMA, Eeftink Schattenkerk JKM, Miedema F, Tersmette M. Biological phenotype of human immunodeficiency virus type 1 clones at different stages of infection: progression of disease is associated with a shift from monocytotropic to T-cell-tropic virus populations. *J Virol* 1992;66:1354–1360.

50. Gartner S, Markovits P, Markovitz DM, Kaplan MH, Gallo RC, Popovic M. The role of mononuclear phagocytes in HTLV-III/LAV infection. *Science* 1986;233:215–219.

51. Schnittman SM, Psallidopoulos MC, Lane HC, Thompson L, Baseler M, Massari F, Fox CH, Salzman NP, Fauci AS. The reservoir for HIV-1 in human peripheral blood is a T cell that maintains expression of CD4. *Science* 1989;245:305–308.

52. Sharpless NE, O'Brien WA, Verdin EM, Kufta CV, Chen ISY, Dubois-Dalcq M. A primary determinant of immunodeficiency virus 1 (HIV-1) neurotropism resides in a region of the *env* glycoprotein that also controls monocyte–macrophage tropism. *J Virol* 1992;66:2588–2593.

53. Rich EA, Chen ISY, Zack JA, Leonard ML, O'Brien WA. Increased susceptibility of differentiated mononuclear phagocytes to productive infection with human immunodeficiency virus type 1 (HIV-1). *J Clin Invest* 1992;89:176–183.

54. Watkins BA, Dorn HH, Kelly WB, Armstrong RC, Potts B, Michaels F, Kufta CV, Dubois-Dalcq M. Specific tropism of HIV-1 for microglial cells in primary human brain cultures. *Science* 1990;249:549–553.

55. O'Brien WA, Koyanagi Y, Namazie A, et al. HIV-1 tropism for mononuclear phagocytes can be determined by regions of gp120 outside the CD4-binding domain. *Nature* 1990;348: 69–73.

56. Lasky LA, Nakamura G, Smith DH, et al. Delineation of a region of the human immunodeficiency virus type 1 gp120 glycoprotein critical for interaction with the CD4 receptor. *Cell* 1987;50:975–985.

57. Shioda T, Levy A, Cheng-Mayer C. Macrophage and T-cell line tropisms of HIV-1 are determined by specific regions of the envelope gp120 gene. *Nature* 1991;349:167–169.
58. Hwang SS, Boyle TJ, Lyerly HK, Cullen BR. Identification of the V3 loop as the primary determinant of cell tropism in HIV-1. *Science* 1991;253:71–74.
59. Westervelt P, Gendelman HE, Ratner L. Identification of a determinant within the HIV-1 surface envelope glycoprotein critical for productive infection of cultured primary monocytes. *Proc Natl Acad Sci USA* 1991;88:3097–3101.
60. O'Brien WA, Daar ES, Ho DD, Chen ISY. HIV-1 resistance to soluble CD4 is conferred by domains of gp120 that determine cell tropism. *J Virol* 1992;66:3125–3130.
61. Cann AJ, Zack JA, Go AS, Arrigo SJ, Koyanagi Y, Green PL, Koyanagi Y, Pang S, Chen ISY. Human immunodeficiency virus type 1 T-cell tropism is determined by events prior to provirus formation. *J Virol* 1990;64:4735–4742.
62. Cann AJ, Churcher MJ, Boyd M, O'Brien WA, Zhao J-Q, Zack JA, Chen ISY. The region of the envelope gene of HIV-1 responsible for determination of cell tropism. *J Virol* 1992; 66:305–309.
63. Freed EO, Myers DJ, Risser R. Identification of the principal neutralizing determinant of human immunodeficiency virus type 1 as a fusion domain. *J Virol* 1991;65:190–194.
64. La Rosa GJ, Davide JP, Weinhold K, Waterbury JA, Profy AT, Lewis JA, Langlois AJ, Dreesman GR, Boswell RN, Shadduck P, Holley LH, Karplus M, Bolognesi DP, Matthews TJ, Emini EA, Putney SD. Conserved sequence and structural elements in the HIV-1 principal neutralizing determinant. *Science* 1990;249:932–935.
65. Groenink J, Fouchier AM, DeGoede REY, DeWolfe F, Gruters RA, Cuypers TM, Huisman HG, Tersmette M. Phenotypic heterogeneity in a panel of infectious molecular human immunodeficiency virus type 1 clones derived from a single individual. *J Virol* 1991;65: 1968–1975.
66. Rouchier RMA, Groenink M, Kootstra NA, Tersmette M, Huisman HG, Miedema F, Schuitemaker H. Phenotype-associated sequence variation in the third variable domain of the human immunodeficiency virus type 1 gp120 molecule. *J Virol* 1992;66:3183–3187.
67. Kuiken CL, de Jong J-J, Baan E, Keulen W, Tersmette M, Goudsmit J. Evolution of the V3 envelope domain in proviral sequences and isolates of human immunodeficiency virus type 1 during transition of the viral biological phenotype. *J Virol* 1992;66:4622–4627.
68. de Jong J-J, Goudsmit J, Keulen W, Klaver B, Krone W, Tersmette M, deRonde A. Human immunodeficiency virus type 1 clones chimeric for the envelope V3 domain differ in syncytium formation and replication capacity. *J Virol* 1992;66:757–765.
69. Takeuchi Y, Akutsu M, Murayama K, Shimizu N, Hoshino H. Host range mutant of human immunodeficiency virus type 1: modification of cell tropism by a single point mutation at the neutralization epitope in the *env* gene. *J Virol* 1991;65:1710–1718.
70. Collman R, Balliet JW, Gregory SA, Friedman H, Kolson DL, Nathanson N, Srinivasan A. An infectious molecular clone of an unusual macrophage-tropic and highly cytopathic strain of human immunodeficiency virus type 1. *J Virol* 1992;66:7517–7521.
71. Olshevsky U, Helseth E, Furman C, Li J, Haseltine W, Sodroski J. Identification of individual human immunodeficiency virus type 1 gp120 amino acids important for CD4 receptor binding. *J Virol* 1990;64:5701–5707.
72. Cordonnier A, Riviere Y, Montagnier L, Emerman M. Effects of mutations in hyperconserved regions of the extracellular glycoprotein of human immunodeficiency virus type 1 on receptor binding. *J Virol* 1989;63:4464–4468.
73. Kahn JO, Allan JD, Hodges TL, Kaplan LD, Arri CJ, Fitch HF, Izu AE, Mordenti J, Sherwin SA, Groopman JE, Volberding PA. The safety and pharmacokinetics of recombinant soluble CD4 (rCD4) in subjects with the acquired immunodeficiency syndrome (AIDS) and AIDS-related complex. *Ann Intern Med* 1990;112:254–261.
74. Schooley RT, Merigan TC, Gaut P, Hirsch MS, Holodniy MH, Flynn T, Liu S, Byington E, Henochowicz S, Gubish E, Spriggs D, Kufe D, Schindler J, Dawson A, Thomas D, Hanson DG, Letwin B, Liu T, Gulinello J, Kennedy S, Fisher R, Ho DD. Recombinant soluble CD4 therapy in patients with the acquired immunodeficiency syndrome (AIDS) and AIDS-related complex. A phase I–II escalating dosage trial. *Ann Intern Med* 1990;112: 247–253.
75. Daar ES, Li XL, Moudgil T, Ho DD. High concentrations of recombinant soluble CD4 are required to neutralize primary HIV-1 isolates. *Proc Natl Acad Sci USA* 1990;87:6574–6578.

76. Ashkenazi A, Smith DH, Marsters SA, Riddle L, Gregory TJ, Ho DD, Capon DJ. Resistance of primary isolates of human immunodeficiency virus type 1 to soluble CD4 is independent of CD4-gp120 binding affinity. *Proc Natl Acad Sci USA* 1991;88:7056–7060.
77. Brighty DW, Chen ISY, Rosenberg M, Ivey-Hoyle M. Neutralization-resistant primary clinical isolates of HIV-1 possess gp120 glycoproteins with high affinity for recombinant sCD4. *Proc Natl Acad Sci USA* 1991;88:7802–7805.
78. Moore JP, McKeating JA, Norton WA, Sattentau QJ. Direct measurement of soluble CD4 binding to human immunodeficiency virus type 1 virions: gp120 dissociation and its implication for virus-cell binding and fusion reactions and their neutralization by soluble CD4. *J Virol* 1991;65:1133–1140.
79. Thali M, Olshevsky U, Furman C, Gabuzda D, Li J, Sodroski J. Effects of changes in gp120-CD4 binding affinity on human immunodeficiency virus type 1 envelope glycoprotein on human immunodeficiency virus type 1 envelope glycoprotein function and soluble CD4 sensitivity. *J Virol* 1991;65:5007–5012.
80. Hwang SS, Boyle T, Lyerly NK, Cullen BR. Identification of envelope V3 loop as the major determinant of CD4 neutralization sensitivity of HIV-1. *Science* 1992;257:535–537.
81. Moore JP, McKeating JA, Weiss RA, Sattentau QJ. Dissociation of gp120 from HIV-1 virions induced by soluble CD4. *Science* 1990;250:1139–1142.
82. Moore JP, McKeating JA, Huang Y, Ashkenazi A, Ho DD. Virions of primary human immunodeficiency virus type 1 isolates resistant to soluble CD4 (sCD4) neutralization differ in sCD4 binding and glycoprotein gp120 retention from sCD4-sensitive isolates. *J Virol* 1992;66:235–243.
83. Rusche JR, Javaherian K, McDanal C, Petro J, Lynn DL, Grimaila R, Langlois AJ, Gallo RC, Arthur LO, Fischinger PJ, Bolognesi DP, Putney SD, Matthews TJ. Antibodies that inhibit fusion of human immunodeficiency virus-infected cells bind a 24-amino acid sequence of the viral envelope, gp120. *Proc Natl Acad Sci USA* 1988;85:3198–3202.
84. Thali M, Furman C, Ho DD, Robinson J, Tilley S, Pinter A, Sodroski J. Discontinuous, conserved neutralization epitopes overlapping the CD4-binding region of human immunodeficiency virus type 1 gp120 envelope glycoprotein. *J Virol* 1992;66:5635–5641.
85. Sattentau QJ, Moore JP. Conformational changes induced in the human immunodeficiency virus envelope glycoprotein by soluble CD4 binding. *J Exp Med* 1991;174:407–415.
86. Allan JS, Strauss J, Buck DW. Enhancement of SIV infection with soluble receptor molecules. *Science* 1990;247:1084–1088.
87. Camerini D, Seed B. A CD4 domain important for HIV-mediated syncytium formation lies outside the principal virus binding site. *Cell* 1990;60:747–754.
88. Moore JP, Sattentau QJ, Klasse PJ, Burkly LC. A monoclonal antibody to CD4 domain 2 blocks soluble CD4-induced conformational changes in the envelope glycoproteins of human immunodeficiency virus type 1 (HIV-1) and HIV-1 infection of CD4+ cells. *J Virol* 1992;66:4784–4793.
89. Broder CC, Berger EA. CD4 molecules with a diversity of mutations encompassing the CDR3 region efficiently support human immunodeficiency virus type 1 envelope glycoprotein-mediated cell fusion. *J Virol* 1993;67:913–926.
90. Hattori N, Michaels F, Fargnoli K, Marcon L, Gallo RC, Franchini G. The human immunodeficiency virus type 2 *vpr* gene is essential for productive infection of human macrophages. *Proc Natl Acad Sci USA* 87:8080–8084.
91. Pomerantz RJ, Feinberg MB, Andino R, Baltimore D. The long terminal repeat is not a major determinant of the cellular tropism of human immunodeficiency virus type 1. *J Virol* 1991;65:1041–1045.
92. Yu X-F, Yu Q-C, Essex M, Lee T-H. The *vpx* gene of simian immunodeficiency virus facilitates efficient viral replication in fresh lymphocytes and macrophages. *J Virol* 1991;65:5088–5091.
93. Pang S, Vinters HV, Akashi T, O'Brien WA, Chen ISY. HIV-1 Env sequence variation in brain tissue of patients with AIDS encephalopathy. *J AIDS* 1991;4:1082–1091.
94. Epstein LG, Kuiken C, Blumberg BM, Hartman S, Sharer LR, Clement M, Goudsmit J. HIV-1 V3 domain variation in brain and spleen of children with AIDS: tissue-specific evolution within host-determined quasispecies. *Virology* 1991;180:583–590.
95. Plannelles V, Li Q-X, Chen ISY. The molecular basis for cell tropism in HIV. In: Cullen BR, ed. *Molecular biology of human retroviruses*. Oxford, England: Oxford University Press, 1993.

HIV, AIDS and the Brain, edited by
R. W. Price and S. W. Perry.
Raven Press, Ltd., New York © 1994.

3

Cytokine Circuits in Brain

Implications for AIDS Dementia Complex

Etty N. Benveniste

Department of Cell Biology, University of Alabama, Birmingham, AL 35294

This chapter on cytokines in the central nervous system (CNS) will emphasize the expression and action of a select group of cytokines, namely, those implicated in contributing to inflammatory and immune responses within the CNS that are associated with the disease of AIDS dementia complex (ADC). These cytokines include interleukin 1 (IL-1), tumor necrosis factor alpha (TNF-α), interleukin 6 (IL-6), granulocyte-macrophage colony-stimulating factor (GM-CsF), and transforming growth factor beta (TGF-β). Specifically, the emphasis will be on the ability of glial cells to both produce and respond to such cytokines.

I will present a brief review on the clinical and pathologic characteristics of ADC. Following this will be an overview of the "traditional" (i.e., immunological) functions of the above cytokines. Finally, the main focus of this chapter is on how glial cells both respond to and synthesize cytokines, and how these changes in gene expression and function may contribute to neurologic disease states such as ADC.

AIDS DEMENTIA COMPLEX

A subacute encephalitis termed ADC afflicts up to 80 percent of adult AIDS patients (1,2). ADC is characterized clinically by cognitive, motor, and behavioral dysfunction. Pathologically, ADC presents with cerebral atrophy and abnormalities of the white matter and deep gray matter structures, including the basal ganglia. These abnormalities include (a) diffuse pallor and vacuolation of the white matter and (b) focal rarefaction accompanied by infiltration of macrophages, multinucleated cells, and lymphocytes. Infiltration of T lymphocytes is limited in degree and is primarily of the CD8[+] phenotype. Discrete areas of demyelination are common and are associated with reactive/hypertrophied astrocytes (astrogliosis) and the presence of microglia, blood-derived macrophages, and multinucleated giant cells.

HIV-1 EXPRESSION IN THE CNS

ADC occurs in the absence of recognized, opportunistic pathogens, and there is strong indication that direct infection of the CNS by human immunodeficiency virus type 1 (HIV-1) is responsible for ADC. HIV-1 DNA and RNA sequences are found in the CNS tissue of individuals with ADC in an abundance greater than that of lymphoid tissues (3). HIV-1 has been directly isolated from both the brain and cerebrospinal fluid (CSF) of AIDS patients (4), and anti-HIV-1 antibodies have been detected in the CSF of AIDS patients in levels indicating intracerebral CNS antibody production (5).

Much attention has been directed at determining which cells in the CNS are infected by HIV-1. A number of laboratories have conclusively determined by *in situ* hybridization coupled with immunocytochemistry that infiltrating monocytes/macrophages, as well as resident microglia, are infected by HIV-1 (6–9). Earlier reports suggested that brain capillary endothelial cells, astrocytes, oligodendrocytes, and neurons could occasionally be infected with HIV-1; however, these examples were quite rare (7,9). The prevailing belief is that macrophages and microglia are the principal (and probably only) cell types productively infected with HIV-1 in the CNS. In support of this theory, Watkins et al. (10) have shown that HIV-1 infection of primary human brain explant cultures resulted in a productive infection of microglial cells whereby astrocytes remained uninfected. While it is clear that macrophages and microglia are the principal targets of HIV-1 infection, there is currently no satisfactory explanation for the extensive neurologic impairment observed clinically in ADC. Because neurons are not directly infected with HIV-1, the severe pathophysiological manifestations of ADC are most likely mediated through *indirect* mechanisms. Because HIV-1-infected macrophages and microglia produce a number of different cytokines (11), it is hypothesized that cytokine production within the CNS may directly damage neurons, or may alter the function of the astrocyte, thereby indirectly compromising the neurons. Cytokines have also been shown to modulate HIV expression in infected cells, and thus are likely to be important in the pathogenesis of ADC.

CYTOKINES

Cytokines play a major role in the initiation, propagation, regulation, and suppression of immune and inflammatory responses. Although cytokines comprise a diverse group of proteins, they share a number of general properties. Cytokines are low-molecular-weight proteins which are produced during the effector phases of immunity, and serve to mediate and regulate immune and inflammatory responses. Most cells do not constitutively produce cytokines; instead, an activation event results in cytokine gene transcription. Cytokines in general are secreted, but can also be expressed on the cell surface. An individual cytokine can be produced by many different cell types, and have multiple effects on different cell types. Cytokines have also been shown to have redundant functions; that is, several cytokines can mediate a common event. Thus, the cytokine system displays pleiotropism and redundancy. Cytokines often influence both the synthesis and function of other cytokines, resulting in complex "cytokine cascades" for immune and inflammatory responses. Cytokines generally act locally, and initiate their action by binding to specific cell-surface receptors on target cells; these receptors generally show high affinities for their ligands, with dissociation constants in the range of 10^{-10}–10^{-12} M. This suggests that very small amounts of a cytokine need to be produced to elicit a biological response. The ultimate response of a particular cell to a particular cytokine is determined by (a) the level of expression of the cytokine receptor, (b) the signal transduction pathways of the target cell that are activated by that cytokine, and (c) the microenvironment of the target cell.

INTERLEUKIN 1

IL-1 is a 17,000-dalton cytokine produced predominantly by activated macrophages, although other cell types such as endothelial cells, B cells, keratinocytes, microglia, and astrocytes can also secrete IL-1 upon stimulation (for reviews see refs. 12 and 13). IL-1 is a cytokine responsible for mediating a variety of processes in the host response to microbial and inflammatory diseases. IL-1 is the major co-stimulator for T-helper cell activation via the augmentation of both IL-2 and IL-2 receptor expression. These effects allow antigen-stimulated T-helper cells to rapidly proliferate and expand in number. IL-1, in cooperation with other cytokines, can also enhance the growth and differentiation of B cells. IL-1 is a principal participant in inflammatory reactions through its induction of other inflammatory metabolites such as prostaglandin, collagenase, and phospholipase A2. IL-1 acts on endothelial cells to promote leukocyte adhesion, and induces the production of various cytokines such as IL-6, TNF-α, CsFs, and IL-1 itself.

TUMOR NECROSIS FACTOR ALPHA

TNF-α is a 17,000-dalton peptide produced primarily by activated macrophages, and is the principal mediator of the host response to gram-negative bacteria (for review see ref. 14). Activated macrophages are the major cellular source for TNF-α, although other cell types such as T cells, mast cells, microglia, and astrocytes can be stimulated to secrete TNF-α. TNF-α is an active participant in inflammatory responses and, in particular, can alter vascular endothelial cell function. Specifically, TNF-α enhances the permeability of endothelial cells (15) and also enhances local adhesion of neutrophils, lymphocytes, and monocytes to the surface of endothelial cells (16), thereby facilitating (a) transendothelial cell migration of polymorphonuclear leukocytes and immune cells and (b) the formation of leukocyte-rich inflammatory infiltrates. TNF-α can modulate immune responses by affecting the expression of class I and class II MHC molecules on a variety of cell types, and can stimulate many cell types to produce numerous cytokines, including IL-1, IL-6, CsFs, and TNF-α itself. TNF-α is produced predominantly as a secreted protein, although a membrane-anchored form of TNF-α has been identified on the surface of macrophages that has lytic activity and may play an important role in intercellular communication (17).

INTERLEUKIN 6

IL-6, similar to IL-1 and TNF-α, is a pleiotropic cytokine involved in the regulation of inflammatory and immunologic responses (for review see ref. 18). IL-6, a 26,000-dalton molecule, is secreted by a wide range of activated cells, including fibroblasts, monocytes, B cells, endothelial cells, T cells, microglia, and astrocytes. The two best-described functions of IL-6 are on hepatocytes and B cells. IL-6 stimulates hepatocytes to synthesize several plasma proteins such as fibrinogen and C-reactive protein, which contribute to the acute-phase response. IL-6 serves as the principal cytokine for inducing terminal differentiation of activated B cells into immunoglobulin-secreting plasma cells. IL-6 can also act as a co-stimulator of T-helper cell activation.

GRANULOCYTE-MACROPHAGE COLONY-STIMULATING FACTOR

The group of cytokines that have potent stimulatory effects on the growth and differentiation of bone marrow progenitor cells are collectively called *colony-stimulating factors* (CsFs). By stimulating the growth and differentiation of bone marrow cells, CsFs act to provide inflammatory leukocytes. We will consider only one of the CsFs in this discussion, namely, granulocyte-macrophage colony-stimulating factor (GM-CsF) (for review see ref. 19).

GM-CsF is a 22,000-dalton glycoprotein produced by a number of activated cells, including T cells, macrophages, endothelial cells, fibroblasts, and astrocytes. GM-CsF acts on bone marrow progenitor cells already committed to differentiate to granulocytes and monocytes. GM-CsF can also interact with various mononuclear phagocytes, including microglia, to induce their activation.

TRANSFORMING GROWTH FACTOR BETA

TGF-β is a dimeric protein of approximately 28,000 daltons that is synthesized by almost all cell types. It is normally secreted in a latent form that must be activated by proteases (for review see ref. 20). The TGF-β family is comprised of several members showing high structural homology. Three closely related TGF-β genes have been identified in mammals; they are TGF-β1, TGF-β2, and TGF-β3. The actions of TGF-β are highly pleiotropic and include: inhibiting the proliferation of many cell types (epithelial, endothelial, lymphoid, and hematopoietic cells), promoting the growth of new blood vessels (angiogenesis), serving as a chemotactic factor for macrophages, and inhibiting immune and inflammatory responses. TGF-β has been demonstrated to inhibit the production of numerous cytokines and is thought to function as a negative regulator of immune responses.

INTERLEUKIN 1 IN THE CENTRAL NERVOUS SYSTEM

Biological Action of IL-1 on Glial Cells

Because one response to brain injury is proliferation of astrocytes, IL-1 was tested for its capacity to induce proliferation of these cells. Purified IL-1 was shown to have a mitogenic effect on astrocyte grown *in vitro* (21), while IL-1 directly injected into the brain can stimulate astrogliosis (22). These results suggest that IL-1, released by inflammatory cells, may contribute to astroglial scarring in damaged mammalian brain, including the disease of ADC. Activated astrocytes, microglia, and oligodendrocytes have been shown to secrete IL-1 *in vitro*, which will be discussed in more detail later. These cells would provide an endogenous brain source of IL-1, which could promote astrogliosis within the CNS.

CNS cells have been shown to produce cytokines in response to IL-1. IL-1 stimulation of primary rat astrocytes primes them for the secretion of TNF-α (23), and induces IL-6 (24–26) and TGF-β (27); primary human astrocytes produce IL-6 and CsFs in response to IL-1 (28); and human astroglial cell lines will produce CsFs (29,30), TNF-α (31), and IL-6 (32) in response to IL-1. With respect to microglia and oligodendrocytes, IL-1 induces TGF-β expression by these cells (33). These are all cytokines involved in mediating immune reactions, inflammatory responses, and modulation of HIV-1 expression; thus, their production by resident brain cells can contribute to the pathology of ADC.

IL-1 Expression by Glial Cells

IL-1 production by glial cells of the CNS was originally suggested by a study in which cultured murine astrocytes, upon stimulation with lipopolysaccharide (LPS), secreted an IL-1-like factor (34). This finding was later confirmed using astrocyte cultures of >95 percent purity, and observing that LPS stimulated astrocytes expressed mRNA for both IL-1α and IL-1β (35). Several human astroglioma cell lines can constitutively secrete IL-1, and both phorbol myristate acetate (PMA) and LPS enhance IL-1 production by these cell lines (36–38). Additionally, primary cultures of human fetal astrocytes produce IL-1 upon stimulation with LPS (38). Both rat and murine microglia produce IL-1 in response to LPS stimulation (35,39–41), and virally transformed microglia clones produce IL-1 (42). The use of double-labeling immunohistochemistry to positively identify cells *in vivo* expressing IL-1 have demonstrated that both astrocytes and microglia express IL-1, but that astrocytes are the more frequent producer of this cytokine in diseased brain (33).

Oligodendrocytes also appear to be capable of producing IL-1 based on the observation that human oligodendroglioma cell lines produce IL-1 *in vitro* (43), and oligodendrocytes in diseased brain stain positively for IL-1 (33). These data indicate that there are three endogenous sources of IL-1 within the CNS: activated astrocytes, microglia, and oligodendrocytes.

INVOLVEMENT OF IL-1 IN ADC

Elevated levels of IL-1 are present in the CSF of ADC patients (44,45), and IL-1-positive cells have been identified in the brains of these patients (45). The IL-1-positive cells appear to be predominantly infiltrating macrophages and resident microglia. IL-1 has been shown to stimulate the HIV-1 enhancer in human T-cell lines via activation of the transcription factor

TABLE 1. *Involvement of IL-1 in ADC*

Evidence
   Elevated levels in CSF
   IL-1 protein in ADC brains
Sources in CNS
   Astrocytes
   Microglia
   Oligodendrocytes
   Infiltrating macrophages
Effects
   Astrocytes
      Induce proliferation → Astrogliosis
      Induce cytokines → IL-6, TNF-α, CsFs, TGF-β
   Microglia
      Enhance HIV-1 replication?
   Oligodendrocytes
      Induce cytokines → TGF-β
   Macrophages
      Enhance HIV-1 replication?

NF-κB (46). Whether IL-1 has any effect on HIV-1 replication in other cells such as macrophages is unknown at this time. A summary of IL-1-mediated effects in the CNS relevant to ADC is shown in Table 1.

TNF-α IN THE CENTRAL NERVOUS SYSTEM

Biological Effects of TNF-α on Glial Cells

TNF-α has a diverse range of functions in the CNS because of its direct effects on astrocytes and oligodendrocytes. Perhaps most relevant to ADC is the ability of TNF-α to mediate myelin and oligodendrocyte damage *in vitro* (47), and its ability to cause cell death of rat oligodendrocytes *in vitro* (48). This aspect of TNF-α activity may contribute directly to myelin damage and/or the demyelination process observed in ADC. TNF-β, the cytokine which is genetically and functionally related to TNF-α, exerts a more potent cytotoxic effect toward oligodendrocytes than does TNF-α, and mediates its effect via apoptosis (49). Thus, both TNF-α and TNF-β can cause death of the oligodendrocyte, the myelin-producing cell of the CNS.

TNF-α has multiple effects on the astrocyte which are noncytotoxic in nature, and it may function in an autocrine fashion because astrocytes (a) express specific high-affinity receptors for TNF-α (50) and (b) secrete TNF-α upon activation by a variety of stimuli (23,31,38,51). TNF-α has been shown to induce proliferation of both primary bovine astrocytes (52) and human astroglioma cell lines (53,54). As mentioned previously, astrocyte proliferation leads to the reactive gliosis associated with ADC, and TNF-α appears to contribute to this process.

TNF-α is a potent inducer of cytokine production in astrocytes. Primary astrocytes and human astroglioma cell lines produce three CsFs upon stimulation with TNF-α: GM-CsF, G-CsF, and M-CsF (28,30,35,55). These cytokines can augment inflammatory responses as a result of their leukocyte chemotactic properties, which would promote migration of granulocytes and macrophages to inflammatory sites within the CNS. Additionally, GM-CsF and M-CsF can induce the proliferation and activation of microglia (56,57). TNF-α also induces IL-6 expression by both primary rat and human astrocytes (24,25,28). Finally, TNF-α induces expression of its own gene in primary rat astrocytes, suggesting a positive feedback loop for TNF-α expression (IY Chung and EN Benveniste, *unpublished observation*).

TNF-α Expression by Glial Cells

Resident glial cells are capable of producing TNF-α upon exposure to multiple stimuli. Primary rat astrocytes express TNF-α mRNA and secrete TNF-α protein in response to treatment with LPS (23,48,51), exposure to the cytokines interferon gamma (IFN-γ) and IL-1β (23), and exposure to a neurotropic virus, Newcastle disease virus (51). Primary rat astrocytes, in addition to producing soluble TNF-α, can express a membrane-bound form of TNF-α upon activation (IY Chung and EN Benveniste, *unpublished observation*). Primary human astrocytes produce TNF-α in response to LPS (38), and human astroglioma cell lines are capable of expressing TNF-α upon stimulation with LPS (38), IL-1β (31), and PMA plus calcium ionophore (58). Mouse microglia secrete TNF-α in response to LPS (41,56,59) and IFN-γ (56). Hetier et al. (59) also demonstrated that murine microglia express a membrane-bound form of TNF-α. These data collectively indicate that both activated astrocytes and microglia can produce TNF-α within the CNS.

INVOLVEMENT OF TNF IN ADC

Elevated levels of TNF-α have been demonstrated in the CSF of AIDS patients, and TNF-α staining in brains from AIDS patients localizes with some endothelial cells and astrocytes, but primarily with macrophages/microglia (45). TNF-α has been shown to activate and enhance HIV-1 replication in macrophages (60), and thus may contribute to the pathogenesis of ADC. Astrocytes have a direct role in this process, because TNF-α produced by these cells induces the expression of HIV-1 in macrophages (61). Furthermore, TNF-α can act synergistically with either IL-6 or GM-CsF to induce HIV-1 expression in macrophages (62). Because astrocytes can serve as a CNS source of these three cytokines (TNF-α, IL-6, GM-CsF) , the astrocyte may be involved in maintaining HIV expression in the CNS. See summary in Table 2.

TABLE 2. *Involvement of TNF-α in ADC*

Evidence
    Elevated levels in CSF
    TNF-α protein in ADC brains
Sources in CNS
    Astrocytes
    Microglia
    Infiltrating macrophages
    Endothelial cells
Effects
    Astrocytes
      Induce proliferation → Astrogliosis
      Induce cytokines → IL-6, CsFs, TNF-α
    Microglia
      Enhance HIV-1 replication?
    Oligodendrocytes
      Cell death → Demyelination
      Myelin damage → Myelin pallor
    Macrophages
      Induce expression of HIV-1

INTERLEUKIN 6 IN THE CENTRAL NERVOUS SYSTEM

Biological Action of IL-6 on Glial Cells

IL-6 is a pleiotropic cytokine involved in the regulation of inflammatory and immunologic responses. IL-6 has a mitogenic effect on bovine astrocytes (52), which may contribute to astrogliosis. Astrocytes respond to IL-6 by secreting nerve growth factor, which induces neural differentiation (25). IL-6 has been demonstrated to inhibit TNF-α production by monocytes (63). Since astrocytes can secrete TNF-α, and TNF-α induces IL-6 production by astrocytes (see below), IL-6 may be involved in the negative regulation of TNF-α expression in the CNS.

IL-6 Expression by Glial Cells

IL-6 is produced within the CNS by both astrocytes and microglia. Primary human, murine, and rat astrocytes can secrete IL-6 in response to a number of stimuli [including virus, IL-1, TNF-α, IFN-γ plus IL-1, LPS, calcium ionophore, and norepinephrine (24,25,28,51,64)], and human astroglioma cell lines express IL-6 mRNA in response to IL-1 (32). Mouse microglia will secrete IL-6 upon infection with virus or stimulation with the cytokine M-CsF (25), rat microglia express IL-6 upon stimulation with LPS (64), and microglial cell clones transformed by the *v-myc* oncogene constitutively secrete IL-6 (42). Similar to IL-1 and TNF-α, there are two endogenous CNS sources for IL-6, namely, astrocytes and microglia. These two CNS cell types are responsive to different stimuli for IL-6 production as both rat and murine microglia do not produce IL-6 in response to either IL-1, TNF-α, or norepinephrine, whereas astrocytes do (25,64).

INVOLVEMENT OF IL-6 IN ADC

Elevated CNS IL-6 levels have been demonstrated in ADC patients (45). IL-6 has been shown to up-regulate production of HIV in infected cells of the monocytic lineage and to act synergistically with TNF-α (65). IL-6 produced by human astrocytes can stimulate HIV-1 expression in a chronically infected promonocyte clone (U1.1.5) (66); thus, intracerebral production of IL-6 by astrocytes may contribute to HIV replication within the CNS. Another possible role of CNS IL-6 may relate to B-cell differentiation. There is evidence of B-cell stimulation during ADC due to the presence of HIV-1 specific immunoglobulin in the CSF of these patients (5). Production of IL-6

TABLE 3. *Involvement of IL-6 in ADC*

Evidence
  Elevated levels in CSF
Sources in CNS
  Astrocytes
  Microglia
  Infiltrating macrophages
  Endothelial cells
Effects
  Astrocytes
    Induce proliferation → Astrogliosis
  Microglia
    Enhance HIV-1 replication?
  Macrophages
    Induce expression of HIV-1
  B cells
    Involved in Ig synthesis?

by astrocytes and/or microglia may contribute in part to heightened humoral immune responses in ADC patients. See Table 3 for summary.

COLONY-STIMULATING FACTORS IN THE CENTRAL NERVOUS SYSTEM

Biological Action of CsFs on Glial Cells

Colony-stimulating factors (CsFs) are cytokines that regulate the survival, proliferation, and differentiation of hematopoietic cells, including mononuclear phagocytes. Because activation of microglia, the macrophage of the brain, is an important early response to brain trauma, there has been interest in how the activation and differentiation of microglia is induced. Numerous studies have examined the ability of CsFs to stimulate biologic activity of microglia. Frei et al (56) demonstrated that GM-CsF induced murine microglia to proliferate. Further *in vitro* studies by Giulian and Ingeman (57) also showed that rat microglia could proliferate in response to GM-CsF, and that GM-CsF induced more rapid phagocytosis by microglia. They also performed *in vivo* experiments in which recombinant GM-CsF was infused into the cerebral cortex of rats. GM-CsF stimulated both (a) the appearance of microglia at the site of injection and (b) the phagocytic capability of these cells. These findings indicate that GM-CsF can enhance inflammatory responses within the CNS by activation of microglia.

CsF Expression by Glial Cells

Astrocytes appear to be the major source of CsFs within the brain. Astrocytes express mRNA for both GM-CsF and G-CsF, and secrete these two

CsFs (35). Unstimulated astrocytes do not constitutively express these CsFs, but are induced to by both TNF-α and LPS (35,67). Human astroglioma cells lines can also express GM-CsF *in vitro* upon stimulation with IL-1 and TNF-α (29,30,55). Normal human astrocytes were recently shown to produce GM-CsF in response to both IL-1 and TNF-α (28). Similar observations have been made for murine astrocytes (68,69). These findings taken in concert indicate that astrocytes are the principal source of CsFs (specifically GM-CsF) within the CNS, and that this factor can activate numerous biological properties of microglia which are related to inflammatory processes and ADC.

INVOLVEMENT OF GM-CsF IN ADC

The disease ADC is due to HIV-1 infection of the CNS—and, in particular, infection of macrophages/microglia within this site (10). GM-CsF has been shown to enhance production of HIV-1 in primary human monocytes/macrophages (70); thus, this cytokine may contribute to HIV replication in the CNS. Additionally, TNF-α can synergize with GM-CsF to induce HIV expression in macrophages (62). Table 4 summarizes the effects of GM-CsF in ADC.

TRANSFORMING GROWTH FACTOR BETA IN THE CENTRAL NERVOUS SYSTEM

Biological Action of TGF-β on Glial Cells

TGF-β is produced by a wide variety of both normal and malignant cells, and generally exhibits numerous immunosuppressive functions such as inhibition of T-cell proliferation, down-regulation of MHC expression, and inhibition of proinflammatory cytokine production. TGF-β can modulate the activity of both astrocytes and microglia. TGF-β1 and TGF-β2 can inhibit

TABLE 4. *Involvement of GM-CsF in ADC*

Sources in CNS
  Astrocytes
  Activated T cells
Effects
  Microglia
    Induce proliferation
    Recruit microglia to sites of inflammation
    Enhance HIV-1 replication?
  Macrophages
    Induce proliferation
    Enhance HIV-1 replication

IFN-γ-induced class II MHC expression on both human astroglioma cells and rat astrocytes (71,72), can inhibit proliferation of rat astrocytes (73–75), and can act as chemotactic agents for both rat astrocytes and microglia (75,76). Primary rat astrocytes have been shown to express multiple subtypes of TGF-β receptors (Type I, Type II, and Type III) (75). Since TGF-β is produced by glial cells (see below), locally produced TGF-β may contribute to the recruitment and activation of glial cells (both astrocytes and microglia) at local inflammatory sites within the CNS.

TGF-β Expression by Glial Cells

TGF-β-like activity has been detected from a number of human glial tumors and astroglioma cell lines (77–79), suggesting that astrocytes may be a source of TGF-β within the CNS. The human glioblastoma cell lines tested could produce both latent and active forms of TGF-β, and exhibited heterogeneity with respect to the isoform of TGF-β expressed (78,79). Primary astrocytes are also capable of expressing TGF-β. Unstimulated rat astrocytes produce undetectable levels of TGF-β; however, treatment with exogenous TGF-β1 causes the astrocyte to secrete TGF-β (80). *In situ* hybridization conclusively identified the astrocyte as the cell in primary culture expressing TGF-β. This same group later demonstrated that rat astrocytes constitutively express mRNA for TGF-β1, which is increased upon exposure to exogenous TGF-β1, indicating that TGF-β1 levels can be regulated in an autocrine manner (75). da Cunha and Vitkovic (27) have also shown that primary rat astrocytes constitutively express mRNA for TGF-β1, but do not constitutively secrete TGF-β1 protein. However, upon stimulation with IL-1, the astrocytes secrete a latent form of TGF-β1. Interestingly, TGF-β1 mRNA levels do not increase, suggesting a post-transcriptional level of regulation for TGF-β1 expression. Further work from the Vitkovic laboratory has demonstrated that both primary rat oligodendrocytes and microglia can secrete TGF-β1 upon stimulation with IL-1α (33). Taken together, the above studies indicate that all three glial cell types—astrocytes, oligodendrocytes, and microglia—are capable of secreting TGF-β. Because TGF-β exerts many immunosuppressive effects, TGF-β produced by glial cells may act to restrict and/or down-regulate inflammatory processes within the CNS.

INVOLVEMENT OF TGF-β IN ADC

TGF-β1 has been identified in the brains of patients with AIDS, but not in control brain tissue (80). The TGF-β staining was localized to macrophages, microglia, and astrocytes, especially in areas of diseased brain. Moreover, HIV-1-infected monocytes secreted a factor which induced cultured astrocytes to secrete TGF-β. This factor in all likelihood is TGF-β itself (81).

TABLE 5. *Involvement of TGF-β in ADC*

Evidence
  TGF-β protein in ADC brains
Sources in CNS
  Astrocytes
  Microglia
  Infiltrating macrophages
  Oligodendrocytes
Effects
  Astrocytes
    Inhibit cytokine production
  Microglia
    Inhibit HIV-1 replication?
    Chemotactic agent
  Macrophages
    Inhibit HIV-1 replication

TGF-β, in turn, suppresses HIV replication in primary macrophages (82). Thus, HIV-1-induced TGF-β production by macrophages may act in an autocrine manner to inhibit HIV replication, or in a paracrine fashion to induce astrocytes to produce TGF-β. By either pathway, TGF-β may play an important role as a *negative regulator* of HIV expression in infected macrophages and/or microglia. This is in contrast to the other cytokines discussed thus far (IL-1, TNF-α, IL-6, GM-CsF) which all act to *enhance* HIV-1 expression. The effects of TGF-β are summarized in Table 5.

SUMMARY AND CONCLUSION

This chapter has summarized studies showing that cells of the immune system and glial cells of the CNS use many of the same cytokines as communication signals. Activated astrocytes and microglia are the principal sources of these cytokines in the CNS, although oligodendrocytes are capable of expressing IL-1 and TGF-β. There is a complex circuitry of interactions mediated by cytokines, especially in the event of blood–brain barrier damage and lymphoid/mononuclear cell infiltration into the CNS. Infiltrating activated macrophages produce cytokines such as IL-1, TNF-α, and IL-6, which would trigger glial cells to produce their own cytokines. The activation of astrocytes and microglia to secrete proinflammatory cytokines such as IL-1, TNF-α, IL-6, and GM-CsF may contribute to the propagation of intracerebral immune and inflammatory responses initiated by immune cells, as well as enhancement of HIV-1 expression in the CNS. The cytokine cascades ongoing in the CNS could ultimately be suppressed due to the presence of immunosuppressive cytokines such as TGF-β. Whether immune and inflammatory responses within the CNS are propagated or suppressed depends on a number of parameters, including (a) the activational status of these cells,

(b) cytokine receptor levels on glial and immune cells, (c) the presence of cytokines with both immune-enhancing and immune-suppressing effects (IFN-γ, IL-1, TNF-α, IL-6, TGF-β, CsFs), (d) the concentration and location of these cytokines in the CNS, and (e) the temporal sequence in which a particular cell is exposed to numerous cytokines (see Fig. 1). The ultimate

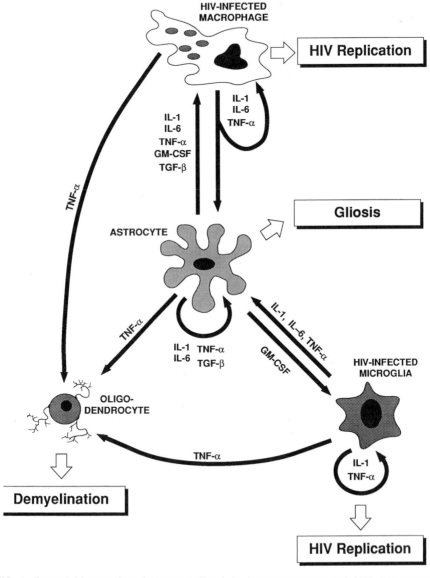

FIG. 1. Potential interactions between cells of the immune system and CNS that would contribute to ADC.

outcome of immunologic and inflammatory events in the CNS, as well as HIV expression, will be determined, in part, by an interplay of the above parameters.

ACKNOWLEDGMENTS

I thank Ms. Sue Wade for superb secretarial and editorial assistance in preparing this manuscript. This work was supported by National Multiple Sclerosis Society Grants 2205-A-3 and 2269-A-4 and by National Institutes of Health Grants AI-27290, NS-29719, and NS-31096.

REFERENCES

1. Levy JA. Isolation of AIDS-associated retroviruses from cerebrospinal fluid and brain of patients with neurological symptoms. *Lancet* 1985;9:586–588.
2. Petito CK, Cho E-S, Lemann E, Navia BA, Price RW. Neuropathology of acquired immune deficiency syndrome (AIDS): an autopsy review. *J Neuropathol Exp Neurol* 1986;45: 635–646.
3. Shaw GM, Harper ME, Hahn BH, et al. HTLV-III infection in brains of children and adults with AIDS encephalopathy. *Science* 1985;227:177–182.
4. Ho DD, Rota RR, Schooley RT, et al. Isolation of HTLV-III from the cerebrospinal fluid and neural tissues of patients with neurologic syndromes related to the acquired immune deficiency syndrome. *N Engl J Med* 1985;313:1493–1497.
5. Resnick L, diMarzo-Veronese F, Schupbach J, et al. Intra-blood-brain barrier synthesis of HTLV-III-specific IgG in patients with neurologic symptoms associated with AIDS or AIDS-related complex. *N Engl J Med* 1985;313:1498–1504.
6. Eilbott DJ, Peress N, Burger H, et al. Human immunodeficiency virus type 1 in spinal cords of acquired immunodeficiency syndrome patients with myelopathy: expression and replication in macrophages. *Proc Natl Acad Sci USA* 1989;86:3337–3341.
7. Gabuzda DH, Ho DD, de la Monte SM, Hirsch MS, Rota TR, Sobel RA. Immunohistochemical identification of HTLV-III antigen in brains of patients with AIDS. *Ann Neurol* 1986; 20:289–295.
8. Koenig S, Gendelman HE, Orenstein TM, et al. Detection of AIDS virus in macrophages brain tissue from AIDS patients with encephalopathy. *Science* 1986;233:1089–1093.
9. Wiley CA, Schreier RD, Nelson JA, Lampert PW, Oldstone MBA. Cellular localization of human immunodeficiency virus infection within the brains of acquired immune deficiency syndrome patients. *Proc Natl Acad Sci USA* 1986;83:7089–7093.
10. Watkins BA, Dorn HH, Kelly WB, et al. Specific tropism of HIV-1 for microglial cells in primary human brain cultures. *Science* 1990;249:549–553.
11. Merrill JE, Chen ISY. HIV-1, macrophages, glial cells, and cytokines in AIDS nervous system disease. *FASEB J* 1991;5:2391–2397.
12. Arai K, Lee F, Miyajima A, Miyatake S, Arai N, Yokota T. Cytokines: coordinators of immune and inflammatory responses. *Annu Rev Biochem* 1990;59:783–836.
13. de Giovine FS, Duff GW. Interleukin 1: the first interleukin. *Immunol Today* 1990;11:13–14.
14. Beutler B, Cerami A. The biology of cachectin/TNF—A primary mediator of the host response. *Annu Rev Immunol* 1989;7:625–655.
15. Brett J, Gerlach H, Nawroth P, Steinberg S, Godman G, Stern D. Tumor necrosis factor/ cachectin increases permeability of endothelial cell monolayers by a mechanism involving regulatory G proteins. *J Exp Med* 1989;169:1977–1991.
16. Pohlman TH, Stanness KA, Beatty PG, Ochs HD, Harlan JM. An endothelial cell surface factor(s) induced *in vitro* by lipopolysaccharide, interleukin 1, and tumor necrosis factor-alpha increases neutrophil adherance by a cd18-dependent mechanism. *J Immunol* 1986; 136:4548–4553.

17. Kriegler M, Perez C, DeFay K, Albert I, Lu SD. A novel form of TNF/cachectin is a cell surface cytotoxic transmembrane protein: ramifications for the complex physiology of TNF. *Cell* 1988;53:45–53.

18. van Snick JV. Interleukin-6: an overview. *Annu Rev Immunol* 1990;8:253–278.

19. Golde DW, Gasson JC. Hormones that stimulate the growth of blood cells. *Sci Am* 1988; July:62–70.

20. Massague J. The transforming growth factor-β family. *Annu Rev Cell Biol* 1990;6:597–632.

21. Giulian D, Lachman LB. Interleukin-1 stimulation of astroglial proliferation after brain injury. *Science* 1985;228:497–499.

22. Giulian D, Woodward J, Young DG, Krebs JF, Lachman LB. Interleukin-1 injected into mammalian brain stimulates astrogliosis and neovascularization. *J Neurosci* 1988;8: 2485–2490.

23. Chung IY, Benveniste EN. Tumor necrosis factor-α production by astrocytes: induction by lipopolysaccharide, IFN-γ and IL-1β. *J Immunol* 1990;144:2999–3007.

24. Benveniste EN, Sparacio SM, Norris JG, Grenett HE, Fuller GM. Induction and regulation of interleukin-6 gene expression in rat astrocytes. *J Neuroimmunol* 1990;30:201–212.

25. Frei K, Malipiero UV, Leist TP, Zinkernagel RM, Schwab ME, Fontana A. On the cellular source and function of interleukin-6 produced in the central nervous system in viral diseases. *Eur J Immunol* 1989;19:689–694.

26. Sparacio SM, Zhang Y, Vilcek J, Benveniste EN. Cytokine regulation of interleukin-6 gene expression in astrocytes involves activation of an NF-κ-B-like nuclear protein. *J Neuroimmunol* 1992;39:231–242.

27. da Cunha A, Vitkovic L. Transforming growth factor-beta (TGF-β1) expression and regulation in rat cortical astrocytes. *J Neuroimmunol* 1992;36:157–169.

28. Aloisi F, Care A, Borsellino G, et al. Production of hemolymphopoietic cytokines (IL-6, IL-8, colony-stimulating factors) by normal human astrocytes in response to IL-1β and tumor necrosis factor-α. *J Immunol* 1992;149:2358–2366.

29. Tweardy D, Mott P, Glazer E. Monokine modulation of human astroglial cell production of granulocyte colony-stimulating factor and granulocyte-macrophage colony-stimulating factor. I. Effects of IL-1α and IL-1β. *J Immunol* 1990;144:2233–2241.

30. Frei K, Piani D, Malipiero UV, Van Meir E, de Tribolet N, Fontana A. Granulocyte-macrophage colony-stimulating factor (GM-CSF) production by glioblastoma cells. *J Immunol* 1992;148:3140–3146.

31. Bethea JR, Chung IY, Sparacio SM, Gillespie GY, Benveniste EN. Interleukin-1β induction of tumor necrosis factor-alpha gene expression in human astroglioma cells. *J Neuroimmunol* 1992;36:179–191.

32. Yasukawa K, Hirano T, Watanabe Y, et al. Structure and expression of human B cell stimulatory factor-2 (BSF-2/IL-6). *EMBO J* 1987;6:2939–2945.

33. da Cunha AD, Jefferson JA, Jackson RW, Vitkovic L. Glial cell-specific mechanisms of TGF-β1 induction by IL-1 in cerebral cortex. *J Neuroimmunol* 1993;42:71–86.

34. Fontana A, Kristensen F, Dubs R, Gemsa D, Weber E. Production of prostaglandin E and an interleukin-1-like factor by cultured astrocytes and C6 glioma cells. *J Immunol* 1982; 129:2413–2419.

35. Malipiero UV, Frei K, Fontana A. Production of hemopoietic colony-stimulating factors by astrocytes. *J Immunol* 1990;144:3816–3821.

36. Fontana A, Hengartner H, de Tribolet N, Weber E. Glioblastoma cells release interleukin-1 and factors inhibiting interleukin-2-mediated effects. *J Immunol* 1984;132:1837–1844.

37. Lee JC, Simon PL, Young PR. Constitutive and PMA-induced interleukin-1 production by the human astrocytoma cell line T24. *Cell Immunol* 1989;118:298–311.

38. Velasco S, Tarlow M, Olsen K, Shay JW, McCracken JGH, Nisen PD. Temperature-dependent modulation of lipopolysaccharide-induced interleukin-1β and tumor necrosis factor α expression in cultured human astroglial cells by dexamethasone and indomethacin. *J Clin Invest* 1991;87:1674–1680.

39. Giulian D, Baker TJ, Shih L, Lachman LB. Interleukin-1 of the central nervous system is produced by ameboid microglia. *J Exp Med* 1986;164:594–604.

40. Hetier E, Ayala J, Denefle P, et al. Brain macrophages synthesize interleukin-1 and interleukin-1 mRNAs *in vitro*. *J Neurosci Res* 1988;21:391–397.

41. Chao CC, Hu S, Close K, et al. Cytokine release from microglia: differential inhibition by pentoxifylline and dexamethasone. *J Infect Dis* 1992;166:847–853.

42. Righi M, Mori L, De Libero G, et al. Monokine production by microglial cell clones. *Eur J Immunol* 1989;19:1443–1448.
43. Merrill JE, Matsushima K. Production of and response to interleukin-1 by cloned human oligodendroglioma cell lines. *J Biol Reg Homeost Agents* 1988;2:77–86.
44. Gallo P, Frei K, Rordorf C, Lazdins J, Tavolato B, Fontana A. Human immunodeficiency virus type 1 (HIV-1) infection of the central nervous system: an evaluation of cytokines in cerebrospinal fluid. *J Neuroimmunol* 1989;23:109–116.
45. Tyor WR, Glass JD, Griffin JW, et al. Cytokine expression in the brain during the acquired immunodeficiency syndrome. *Ann Neurol* 1992;31:349–360.
46. Osborn L, Kunkel S, Nabel GJ. Tumor necrosis factor α and interleukin 1 stimulate the human immunodeficiency virus enhancer by activation of the nuclear factor κB. *Proc Natl Acad Sci USA* 1989;86:2336–2340.
47. Selmaj KW, Raine CS. Tumor necrosis factor mediates myelin and oligodendrocyte damage *in vitro*. *Ann Neurol* 1988;23:339–346.
48. Robbins DS, Shirazi Y, Drysdale BE, Lieberman A, Shin HS, Shin ML. Production of cytotoxic factor for oligodendrocytes by stimulated astrocytes. *J Immunol* 1987;139:2593–2597.
49. Selmaj K, Raine CS, Farooq M, Norton WT, Brosnan CF. Cytokine cytotoxicity against oligodendrocytes: apoptosis induced by lymphotoxin. *J Immunol* 1991;147:1522–1529.
50. Benveniste EN, Sparacio SM, Bethea JR. Tumor necrosis factor-α enhances interferon-γ mediated class II antigen expression on astrocytes. *J Neuroimmunol* 1989;25:209–219.
51. Lieberman AP, Pitha PM, Shin HS, Shin ML. Production of tumor necrosis factor and other cytokines by astrocytes stimulated with lipopolysaccharide or a neurotropic virus. *Proc Natl Acad Sci USA* 1989;86:6348–6352.
52. Selmaj KW, Farooq M, Norton WT, Raine CS, Brosnan CF. Proliferation of astrocytes *in vitro* in response to cytokines. A primary role for tumor necrosis factor. *J Immunol* 1990;144:129–135.
53. Bethea JR, Gillespie GY, Chung IY, Benveniste EN. Tumor necrosis factor production and receptor expression by a human astroglioma cell line. *J Neuroimmunol* 1990;30:1–13.
54. Lachman LB, Brown DC, Dinarello CA. Growth promoting effect of recombinant interleukin-1 and tumor necrosis factor for a human astrocytoma cell line. *J Immunol* 1987;138:2913–2916.
55. Tweardy DJ, Glazer EW, Mott PL, Anderson K. Modulation by tumor necrosis factor-α of human astroglial cell production of granulocyte-macrophage colony-stimulating factor (GM-CSF) and granulocyte colony-stimulating factor (G-CSF). *J Neuroimmunol* 1991;32:269–278.
56. Frei K, Siepl C, Groscurth P, Bodmer S, Schwerdel C, Fontana A. Antigen presentation and tumor cytotoxicity by interferon-γ-treated microglial cells. *Eur J Immunol* 1987;17:1271–1278.
57. Giulian D, Ingeman JE. Colony-stimulating factors as promoters of ameboid microglia. *J Neurosci* 1988;8:4707–4717.
58. Bethea JR, Gillespie GY, Benveniste EN. Interleukin-1β induction of TNF-α gene expression: involvement of protein kinase C. *J Cell Physiol* 1992;152:264–273.
59. Hetier E, Ayala J, Bousseau A, Denefle P, Prochiantz A. Amoeboid microglial cells and not astrocytes synthesize TNF-α in swiss mouse brain cell cultures. *Eur J Neurosci* 1990;2:762–768.
60. Poli G, Kinter A, Justement JS, et al. Tumor necrosis factor α functions in an autocrine manner in the induction of human immunodeficiency virus expression. *Proc Natl Acad Sci USA* 1990;87:782–785.
61. Vitkovic L, Kalebic T, da Cunha A, Fauci AS. Astrocyte-conditioned medium stimulates HIV-1 expression in a chronically infected promonocyte clone. *J Neuroimmunol* 1990;30:153–160.
62. Rosenberg ZF, Fauci AS. Immunopathogenesis of HIV infection. *FASEB J* 1991;5:2382–2390.
63. Aderka D, Le J, Vilcek J. IL-6 inhibits lipopolysaccharide-induced tumor necrosis factor production in cultured human monocytes, U937 cells, and in mice. *J Immunol* 1989;143:3517–3523.
64. Norris JG, Benveniste EN. Interleukin-6 production by astrocytes: induction by the neurotransmitter norepinephrine. *J Immunol* 1993;45:137–146.

65. Poli G, Bressler P, Kinter A, et al. Interleukin 6 induces human immunodeficiency virus expression in infected monocytic cells alone and in synergy with tumor necrosis factor α by transcriptional and post-transcriptional mechanisms. *J Exp Med* 1990;172:151–158.

66. Vitkovic L, Wood GP, Major EO, Fauci AS. Human astrocytes stimulate HIV-1 expression in a chronically infected promonocyte clone via interleukin-6. *AIDS Res* 1991;7:723–727.

67. Ohno K, Suzumura A, Sawada M, Marunouchi T. Production of granulocyte/macrophage colony-stimulating factor by cultured astrocytes. *Biochem Biophys Res Commun* 1990;169:719–724.

68. Hao C, Guilbert LJ, Fedoroff S. Production of colony-stimulating factor-1 (CSF-1) by mouse astroglia *in vitro. J Neurosci Res* 1990;27:314–323.

69. Thery C, Hetier E, Evrard C, Mallat M. Expression of macrophage colony-stimulating factor gene in the mouse brain during development. *J Neurosci Res* 1990;26:129–133.

70. Koyanagi Y, O'Brien WA, Zhao JQ, Golde DW, Gasson JC, Chen ISY. Cytokines alter production of HIV-1 from primary mononuclear phagocytes. *Science* 1988;241:1673–1675.

71. Zuber P, Kuppner MC, de Tribolet N. Transforming growth factor-β2 down-regulates HLA-DR antigen expression on human malignant glioma cells. *Eur J Immunol* 1988;18:1623–1626.

72. Schluesener HJ. Transforming growth factors type β1 and β2 suppress rat astrocyte autoantigen presentation and antagonize hyperinduction of class II major histocompatibility complex antigen expression by interferon-γ and tumor necrosis factor-α. *J Neuroimmunol* 1990;27:41–47.

73. Toru-Delbauffe D, Baghdassarian-Chalaye D, Gavaret JM, Courtin F, Pomerance M, Pierce M. Effects of transforming growth factor β1 on astroglial cells in culture. *J Neurochem* 1990;54:1056–1061.

74. Lindholm D, Castren E, Kiefer R, Zafra F, Thoenen H. Transforming growth factor-β1 in the rat brain: increase after injury and inhibition of astrocyte proliferation. *J Cell Biol* 1992;117:395–400.

75. Morganti-Kossmann MC, Kossmann T, Brandes ME, Mergenhagen SE, Wahl SM. Autocrine and paracrine regulation of astrocyte function by transforming growth factor-β. *J Neuroimmunol* 1992;39:163–174.

76. Yao J, Harvath L, Gilbert DL, Colton CA. Chemotaxis by a CNS macrophage, the microglia. *J Neurosci Res* 1990;27:36–42.

77. Clark WC, Bressler J. Transforming growth factor-β-like activity in tumors of the central nervous system. *J Neurosurg* 1988;68:920–924.

78. Bodmer S, Strommer K, Frei K, et al. Immunosuppression and transforming growth factor-β in glioblastoma. *J Immunol* 1989;143:3222–3229.

79. Constam DB, Philipp J, Malipiero UV, ten Dijke P, Schachner M, Fontana A. Differential expression of transforming growth factor-β1, -β2, and -β-3 by glioblastoma cells, astrocytes, and microglia. *J Immunol* 1992;148:1401–1410.

80. Wahl SM, Allen JB, Francis NM. Macrophage- and astrocyte-derived transforming growth factor β as a mediator of central nervous system dysfunction in acquired immune deficiency syndrome. *J Exp Med* 1991;173:981–991.

81. Kekow J, Wachsman W, McCutchan JA, Cronin M, Carson DA, Lotz M. Transforming growth factor-β and non-cytopathic mechanisms of immunodeficiency in human immunodeficiency virus infection. *Proc Natl Acad Sci USA* 1990;87:8321–8325.

82. Poli G, Kinter AL, Justement JS, Bressler P, Kehrl JH, Fauci AS. Transforming growth factor β suppresses human immunodeficiency virus expression and replication in infected cells of the monocyte/macrophage lineage. *J Exp Med* 1991;173:589–597.

HIV, AIDS and the Brain, edited by
R. W. Price and S. W. Perry.
Raven Press, Ltd., New York © 1994.

4

HIV Neurons and Cytotoxic T Lymphocytes

Concepts About the AIDS Dementia Complex and Viral Persistence

Michael B. A. Oldstone

Viral Immunobiology Laboratory, Division of Virology, Department of Neuropharmacology, The Scripps Research Institute, La Jolla, California 92037

HIV DILEMMA: UNDERSTANDING PATHOGENESIS

AIDS dementia complex (ADC) is commonly associated with human immunodeficiency virus (HIV) infection in patients not treated with AZT (1–3). ADC and, perhaps, other disease manifestations of HIV infection are not due to a direct cytolytic attack by the virus, but are likely mediated by the host's immune response (i.e., immunopathologic in nature). This conclusion follows several observations. First, as we (4) and others (5; reviewed in ref. 6) noted, one rarely finds HIV genetic materials in neurons, although macrophages/microglia (commonly) and central nervous system (CNS) endothelial cells contain HIV nucleic acid sequences and proteins. Second, HIV infection readily induces both cell-mediated [cytotoxic T lymphocyte (CTL)] and humoral (antibody) immune responses (7–9). Third, the cerebrospinal fluids (CSFs) of ADC patients contain large numbers of anti-HIV CTLs. The anti-HIV specificities of CSF CTLs may differ from that found in peripheral blood, where the response (activity) can be less than that in the CSF (10). Such findings strongly suggest specific recruitment to, concentration in, and/or *in situ* generation in the CSF/CNS compartment. Fourth, in several other carefully studied viral infections, CTLs cause CNS disease (11–14). Fifth, autoimmune responses occur during HIV infection (15,16). Sixth, antibodies reactive against HIV proteins have also been noted to cross-react with a variety of host tissues or antigens (17,18)—examples of molecular mimicry (19). Seventh, HIV infects very few cells in contrast to the widespread disease produced. Finally, the cognitive disorders of HIV-positive patients diminish after treatment with 3'-azido-2',3'-dideoxythymidine (AZT) (1–3) as their psychometric testing scores improve (2) and the brain structure normalizes, as documented by positron emission tomographic (PET) and computed tomographic (CT) scans (1). This outcome strongly suggests that ADC is a partially reversible metabolic component of the disease rather than a structural defect, because neurons of the CNS, cells responsible for cognitive function, do not regenerate once injured or destroyed.

The four non-neuronal cell types in the CNS whose study appears promising for shedding light on ADC and other CNS disorders associated with HIV infection are astrocytes, microglia/macrophages, endothelial cells, and CTLs. While there is little evidence that astrocytes are infected with HIV, reactive astrocytosis is a hallmark of HIV infection (6,20). Astrocytes secrete a variety of factors (as displayed in Fig. 1), and these and/or other factors (21) not listed may well affect neuronal metabolism.

Microglia/macrophages and (to a lesser degree) CNS endothelial cells are infectable *in vivo* and *in vitro* with HIV (reviewed in refs. 6 and 22). These cells also release cytokines that may directly affect neurons or indirectly influence neuronal activity by their action on astrocytes. Anti-HIV-specific CTLs are generated in high numbers and frequencies in patients infected with HIV (7,9,10). Activated CTLs easily penetrate into the CNS, crossing the blood–brain barrier (23,24). Furthermore, virus-specific CTLs have been

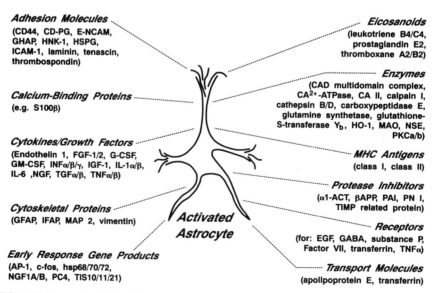

Adhesion Molecules
(CD44, CD-PG, E-NCAM, GHAP, HNK-1, HSPG, ICAM-1, laminin, tenascin, thrombospondin)

Calcium-Binding Proteins
(e.g. S100β)

Cytokines/Growth Factors
(Endothelin 1, FGF-1/2, G-CSF, GM-CSF, INFα/β/γ, IGF-1, IL-1α/β, IL-6 ,NGF, TGFα/β, TNFα/β)

Cytoskeletal Proteins
(GFAP, IFAP, MAP 2, vimentin)

Early Response Gene Products
(AP-1, c-fos, hsp68/70/72, NGF1A/B, PC4, TIS10/11/21)

Activated Astrocyte

Eicosanoids
(leukotriene B4/C4, prostaglandin E2, thromboxane A2/B2)

Enzymes
(CAD multidomain complex, CA^{2+}-ATPase, CA II, calpain I, cathepsin B/D, carboxypeptidase E, glutamine synthetase, glutathione-S-transferase Y_b, HO-1, MAO, NSE, PKCa/b)

MHC Antigens
(class I, class II)

Protease Inhibitors
(α1-ACT, βAPP, PAI, PN I, TIMP related protein)

Receptors
(for: EGF, GABA, substance P, Factor VII, transferrin, TNFα)

Transport Molecules
(apolipoprotein E, transferrin)

FIG. 1. Scheme showing various molecules associated with reactive astrocytes. Recently, tissue factor has been shown to be primarily made in the brain by astrocytes (21). (Courtesy of Dr. Lennart Mucke, The Scripps Research Institute, La Jolla, CA 92037.)

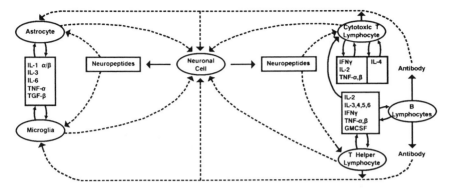

FIG. 2. Scheme showing several possible ways that astrocytes, microglia/macrophages, endothelial cells, and CTLs may play a role to compromise neuronal function.

shown to contribute to neurologic disease in several viral infections (11–14). Recently, CSF of HIV-1-infected subjects with ADC were noted to contain HIV-specific CTLs (10). In five of six persons studied, HIV-specific CTLs restricted by HLA class I glycoprotein molecules were recovered from the CSF and showed specificities for Gag, Pol, Env, and Nef proteins. Of interest was that four of the five persons possessed virus-specific CTLs in significantly higher numbers in the CSF than in the peripheral blood—indicating the specific recruitment to, or local induction of, CTLs within the CNS. Besides their direct lytic potential, CTLs also release a number of cytokines. While CTLs are found regularly in the blood during the acute stage and throughout the "clinically healthy state" of HIV infection, their fall late in infection is said to mirror the onset and degree of AIDS (7,9). Figure 2 schematizes several possible ways astrocytes, microglia/macrophages, endothelial cells, and CTL may play a role to compromise neuronal function.

CTL–VIRUS INTERACTIONS: IMMUNOLOGIC SURVEILLANCE AND IMMUNOSUPPRESSION

CTLs likely play the cardinal role in control of acute infections; in the absence of CTLs, persistent and/or latent infections are developed and maintained (reviewed in ref. 25). Viruses are cell-associated parasites, and their surface glycoproteins are usually not expressed (or are expressed to minimal degrees) on persistently infected cells. Under these conditions, antibodies are not efficient in lysing infected cells. Lysis requires both antibody and complement. Studies using purified proteins of the complement system and antibodies have shown that several million antibody molecules are needed to destroy virally infected cells, an ineffective and inefficient system (26,27). In contrast, T cells can detect significantly lower levels of viral antigens

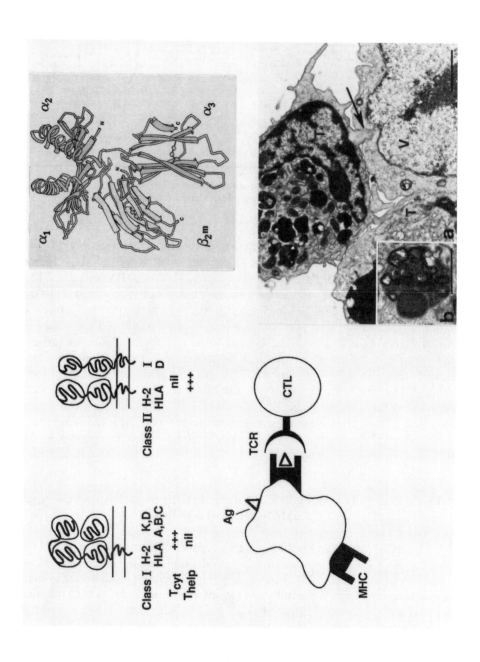

(peptides) expressed on infected cells usually requiring less than 100 molecules for their activation and activity. CTLs recognize viral sequences presented by cells that antiviral antibodies most often are unable to detect. Most important, CTLs are effective against nonglycosylated, nonstructural regulatory proteins that are transcribed early, well before structural viral proteins are made prior to virus assembly and release. Thus, CTLs possess the ability to recognize infected cells as foreign and destroy them during the phase of viral replication prior to assembly, and thereby eliminate the potential factories before they produce an infectious product.

CTLs recognize proteolytic fragments of viral proteins that are presented at the cell surface by MHC glycoprotein molecules (28–31) (Fig. 3).

Major histocompatibility complex (MHC) molecules are divided into class I and class II: Class I molecules are recognized by a CTL subset that bears the CD8 surface marker, and class II molecules are recognized by CTLs or T-helper cells that bear the CD4 surface marker. MHC class I utilizes primarily a cytosolic pathway and is found on nearly all cells in the body, with an exception being neurons. CTLs recognize viral peptide bound to the MHC glycoprotein, and the peptide sequence that binds is linear. The number of peptides per viral protein able to complex with the MHC glycoprotein in a manner that allows CTL recognition is limited and ranges from one to generally no more than three or four peptides per viral protein. Furthermore, the size of the peptide has been mapped experimentally and visualized by three-dimensional crystallography and usually consists of eight to nine amino acids. The three-dimensional structure of the MHC class I molecule reveals two alpha helices that border a floor of beta sheaths in which the peptide resides (31). The MHC heavy chain and its associated light chain (β_2-microglobulin) are encoded by different genes. Their synthesis and assembly occurs at the rough endoplasmic reticulum. It is currently believed that the assembled MHC molecule does not migrate to the cell surface until a specific peptide binds within the MHC alpha-1 and alpha-2 domains. During this scenario, the β2-microglobulin is conceived of as assisting to lock the peptide within the MHC groove, causing a change in confirmation that allows the complex

←——————————————————————————————

FIG. 3. Schemes and a photograph to explain principles of the CTL–virus-infected-cell interaction. **Upper left panel:** scheme showing MHC class I and II molecules and lists different functions in terms of cytotoxic (Tcyt) or helper (Thelp) T-cell activity. **Upper right panel:** Sketch of the three-dimensional x-ray crystallographic structure of HLA-A2. Viral peptide formed in the infected cells binds in the groove between the α_1 and α_2 arms. **Lower left panel:** Diagram depicting the MHC–peptide complex recognized by the receptor (TCR) of CTL. **Lower right panel:** Electron micrograph showing the interaction of a cloned LCMV-specific CTL pushing a process *(arrow)* deep into the cytoplasm of a virus-infected cell (V). Note the close cell–cell contact that is essential for CTL-mediated lysis. After contact, a variety of proteolytic enzymes and porforin are released by the CTL from granules **(inset b)** that cause approximately 9- to 15-nm lesions (holes) in the membranes of the target cell.

molecule to leave the endoplasmic reticulum. Once the MHC glycoprotein–peptide complex is on the cell surface, it is recognized by a CTL according to the latter's receptor composed of alpha and beta chains. If not recognized, the MHC–peptide complex likely dissociates, MHC glycoproteins recycle, and the peptide is degraded. Interestingly, neurons, according to studies on cultured cells, have a defect in the transcription of the heavy chain of MHC but not the light chain (β2-microglobulin) and thus fail to present peptides for recognition by CTLs (32). This is best viewed as a selective advantage for neurons, allowing them to escape immunologic assault. The downside is that this observation likely explains why DNA and RNA viruses often persist in such cells (32,33).

There are four major ways by which viruses can abort CTL activity. Two focus on how viruses alter the cell surface concentrations of MHC–peptide complexes. The third focuses on the generation of viral variants, namely, escape mutants that CTLs no longer recognize (34–37) [such variants that escape CTL recognition have been reported by McMichael and colleagues (36) to arise during HIV infection]. The fourth implicates the virus directly inactivating CTL activity through infection (38,39). A virus, like certain subgenera of human adenovirus (40,41) or cytomegalovirus (42), can down-regulate the surface expression of MHC class I antigen in infected cells. This is accomplished by a variety of different strategies. For example, an early adenovirus protein, E-19 (or a homologue), forms a complex with the nascent class I molecule in the endoplasmic reticulum and prevents the MHC protein from reaching the cell surface. Other adenoviruses use a different strategy by interfering with the transcription of the MHC molecule. A different approach is used by human cytomegalovirus. Analysis of this virus' nucleic acid sequences reveals the presence of an open reading frame whose predicted translation product has homology with the heavy chain of the MHC class I glycoprotein. Interestingly, cytomegalovirus virions bind to β2-microglobulin, and cytomegalovirus-infected cells fail to synthesize mature cellular class I MHC molecules, but mRNA levels remain unaltered. Thus, the cytomegalovirus MHC homologue presumably competes for and sequesters β2-microglobulin, thus preventing its binding to the MHC heavy chain. The consequence is that the MHC protein is prevented from reaching the surface of infected cells and renders such cells free from recognition by CTL.

Instead of altering MHC antigen presentation or transportation, viruses can infect cells of the immune system and abrogate their function (reviewed in ref. 43). By this means, either the CTLs can be removed through viral-induced lysis or, alternatively, the virus is not lytic but aborts CTL activity, or the virus can prepare the infected immune cell for lysis by CTLs.

Interestingly, most, if not all, viruses associated with persistent infection are known to infect lymphocytes and/or monocytes (43). The resulting interaction between the virus and the lymphoid cell may disable specific immune responsiveness, as has been shown for several RNA viruses [measles virus, lymphocytic choriomeningitis virus (LCMV) and HIV and DNA viruses (cytomegalovirus and hepatitis B virus). Such observations speak to the generalized concept that a common mechanism may exist by which viruses initiate persistence—that is, infection of effector T cells that ordinarily participate in clearing the virus. The obvious result would be a selective advantage for the virus by restricting immunosuppression against itself, although in some instances (such as infection with HIV) the lymphocyte defect leads to generalized immunosuppression and severe disease from opportunistic infectious agents.

Thus, in conclusion, viruses have developed a variety of strategies to subvert the host's immune response. Viruses that successfully escape from immune surveillance go on to persist where they can participate in a variety of late-onset or chronic disorders and diseases. Understanding the rules by which viruses play will enable the development of therapeutic approaches that will eventually lead to successful treatments to control infection.

ACKNOWLEDGMENTS

Research reported here was supported by Grants MH19185, DAM19-90-C-0070, NS12428, and AI09484. The author thanks Valerie Felts for manuscript preparation.

REFERENCES

1. Brunetti A, Berg G, DiChiro G, et al. Reversal of brain metabolic abnormalities following treatment of AIDS dementia complex with 3'-azido-2',3'-dideoxythymidine (AZT). *J Nucl Med* 1989;30:581–590.
2. Brouwers P, Moss H, Walter P, et al. Effect of continuous Zidovirdina therapy on neuropsychologic functioning in children with symptomatic human immunodeficiency virus infection. *J Pediatr* 1990;117:980–985.
3. Perry S. Organic mental disorders caused by HIV: update on early diagnosis and treatment. *Am J Psychiatry* 1990;147:696–710.
4. Wiley CA, Schrier RD, Nelson JA, Lampert PW, Oldstone MBA. Cellular localization of human immunodeficiency virus infection within the brains of acquired immune deficiency syndrome patients. *Proc Natl Acad Sci* 1986;83:7089–7093.
5. Koenig S, Gendelman H, Orenstein J, et al. Detection of AIDS virus in macrophages in brain tissue from AIDS patients with encephalitis. *Science* 1986;233:1089.
6. Wiley C, Nelson JA. Human immunodeficiency virus: infection of the nervous system. *Curr Top Microbiol Immunol* 1990;160:157–172.
7. Plata F. HIV-specific cytotoxic T lymphocytes. *Res Immunol* 1989;140:89–124.
8. Ho D, Rota T, Hirsh M. Antibody to lymphadenopathy-associated virus in AIDS. *N Engl J Med* 1985;312:649.
9. Walker BD, Plata F. Cytotoxic T lymphocytes against HIV. *AIDS* 1990;3:177–184.
10. Jassoy C, Johnson RP, Navia BA, Worth J, Walker B. Detection of a vigorous HIV-1-specific CTL response in CSF from infected persons with AIDS dementia complex. *J Immunol* 1992;149:3113–3119.
11. Joly E, Mucke L, Oldstone MBA. Viral persistence in neurons explained by lack of major histocompatibility complex class I expression. *Science* 1991;253:1283–1285.
12. Bainziger J, Hengartner H, Zinkernagel R, Cole G. Induction or prevention of immunopath-

ologic disease by cloned cytotoxic T cell lines specific for lymphocytic choriomeningitis virus. *Eur J Immunol* 1986;16:387.

13. Klavinskis LS, Tishon A, Oldstone MBA. Efficiency and effectiveness of cloned virus-specific cytotoxic T lymphocytes *in vivo. J Immunol* 1989;143:2013–2016.

14. Chan W, Javanovic T, Lukic H. Infiltration of immune T cells in brain of mice with herpes simplex virus induced encephalitis. *J Neuroimmunol* 1989;23:195.

15. Ziegler JL, Stites DP. Hypothesis: AIDS in an autoimmune disease directed at the immune system and triggered by a lymphotropic retrovirus. *Clin Immunol Immunopathol* 1986;41: 305–313.

16. Morrow WJ, Isenberg DA, Sobol RE, Stricker RB, Kieber-Emmons T. AIDS virus infection and autoimmunity: a perspective of the clinical, immunological and molecular origins of the autoallergic pathologies associated with HIV disease. *Clin Immunol Immunopathol* 1991;58:163–180.

17. Yamada M, Zurbriggen A, Oldstone MBA, Fujinami RS. Common immunologic determinant between human immunodeficiency virus type 1 gp41 and astrocytes. *J Virol* 1991;65: 1370–1376.

18. Golding H, Shearer GH, Hillman K, et al. Common epitope in HIV-1 gp41 and HLAII elicits immunosuppressive autoantibodies capable of contributing to immune dysfunction in HIV-1-infected individuals. *J Clin Invest* 1989;83:1430–1435.

19. Oldstone MBA. Molecule mimicry and autoimmune disease. *Cell* 1987;50:819–820.

20. Navia B, Cho S, Price R. The AIDS dementia complex. II. *Neuropathol Ann Neurol* 1986; 19:525.

21. Eddleston M, de la Torre JC, Oldstone MBA, Loskutoff DJ, Edgington TS, Mackman N. Tissue factor mRNA is expressed in astrocytes of the central nervous system—potential roles in cerebral hemostatis and infection. *J Clin Invest* 1993;92:349–358.

22. Moses A, et al. HIV infection of human brain capillary endothelial cells occur via a CD4-independent mechanism. *Science,* submitted 1992.

23. Wekerle H, Linington C, Meyerman R. Cellular immune reactivity within the CNS. *Trends Neurosci* 1986;9:271.

24. Hickey WF, Hsu BL, Kimura H. T lymphocyte entry into the central nervous system. *J Neurosci Res* 1991;28:254–260.

25. Oldstone MBA. Molecular anatomy of viral persistence. *J Virol* 1991;65:6381–6386.

26. Sissons JPG, Oldstone MBA, Schreiber RD. Antibody-independent activation of the alternative complement pathway by measles virus-infected cells. *Proc Natl Acad Sci USA* 1980; 77:559–562.

27. Sissons JGP, Schreiber RD, Perrin LH, Cooper NR, Muller-Eberhard HJ, Oldstone MBA. Lysis of measles virus-infected cells by the purified cytolytic alternative complement pathway and antibody. *J Exp Med* 1979;150:445–454.

28. Zinkernagel RM, Doherty PC. Restriction of *in vitro* T cell-mediated cytotoxicity in lymphocytic choriomeningitis within a syngeneic or semiallogeneic system. *Nature* 1974;248: 701–702.

29. Townsend ARM, Rothbard J, Gotch FM, Bahadur G, Wraith D, McMichael AJ. The epitopes of influenza nucleoprotein recognized by cytotoxic T lymphocytes can be defined with short synthetic peptides. *Cell* 1986;44:959–968.

30. Rotzschke O, Falk K, Deres K, Schild H, Norda M, Melzger J, Jung G, Rammensee H-G. Isolation and analysis of naturally processed viral peptides as recognized by cytotoxic T cells. *Nature* 1990;348:252–254.

31. Bjorkman PJ, Saper MA, Samraoui B, Bennett WS, Strominger JL, Wiley DC. Structure of the human class I histocompatibility antigen, HLA-A2. *Nature* 1987;329:506–511.

32. Joly E, Mucke L, Oldstone MBA. Viral persistence in neurons explained by lack of major histocompatibility complex class I expression. *Science* 1991;253:1283–1285.

33. Joly E, Oldstone MBA. Neuronal cells are deficient in loading peptides onto MHC class I molecules. *Neuron* 1992;8:1185–1190.

34. Pircher HD, et al. Viral escape by selection of cytotoxic T lymphocyte-resistant virus variants *in vivo. Nature* 1990;354:453.

35. Aebischer T, et al. *In vitro* selection of lymphocytic choriomeningitis virus escape mutant by CTL. *Proc Natl Acad Sci USA* 1991;88:11045.

36. Phillips RE, et al. Human Immunodeficiency virus genetic variation that can escape cytotoxic T cell recognition. *Nature* 1991;354:453.

37. Lewicki H, Tishon A, Borrow P, Evans C, Oldstone MBA. Virus variants escape CTL immunosurveillance: mutation at CTL receptor recognition. Manuscript submitted, 1993.
38. Salvato M, Borrow P, Shimomaye E, Oldstone MBA. Molecular basis of viral persistence: a single amino acid change in the glycoprotein of lymphocytic choriomeningitis virus is associated with suppression of the antiviral cytotoxic T lymphocyte response and establishment of persistence. *J Virol* 1991;65:1863–1869.
39. Matloubian M, Somasundaram T, Kolkehar SR, Selvakumar R, Ahmed R. Genetic basis of viral persistence: single amino acid change in the viral glycoprotein affects ability of lymphocytic choriomeningitis virus to persist in adult mice. *J Exp Med* 1990;172:1043–1048.
40. Nilsson T, Jackson M, Peterson PA. Short cytoplasmic sequences serve as retention signals for transmembrane proteins in the endoplasmic reticulum. *Cell* 1989;58:707–718.
41. Tanaka K, Isselbacher KJ, Khoury G, Jay G. Reversal of oncogenesis by the expression of a major histocompatibility complex class I gene. *Science* 1985;228:26–30.
42. Browne H, Smith G, Beck S, Minson T. A complex between the MHC class I homologue encoded by human cytomegalovirus and β2-microglobulin. *Nature* 1990;347:770–772.
43. McChesney MB, Oldstone MBA. Viruses perturb lymphocyte functions: selected principles characterizing virus induced immunosuppression. *Annu Rev Immunol* 1987;5:279–304.

HIV, AIDS and the Brain, edited by
R. W. Price and S. W. Perry.
Raven Press, Ltd., New York © 1994.

5

Macrophages and Microglia in HIV-Related CNS Neuropathology

Dennis W. Dickson, Sunhee C. Lee, William Hatch,
Linda A. Mattiace, Celia F. Brosnan, and William D. Lyman

*Department of Pathology (Neuropathology) and The Rose F. Kennedy Center for
Research in Mental Retardation and Human Development, Albert Einstein
College of Medicine, Bronx, NY 10461*

Functional and structural neurological disorders of the central nervous system (CNS) are common in the acquired immunodeficiency syndrome (AIDS) (1–4). Included in the spectrum of CNS pathology in AIDS are: disorders associated with systemic disease (e.g., hypoxic and metabolic encephalopathies); opportunistic infections of the meninges and brain; CNS lymphoma; cerebrovascular disease; and pathology directly attributable to human immunodeficiency virus type 1 (HIV-1) infection. This review will focus only on the latter.

HIV-1 INFECTION OF THE CNS

The evidence for direct HIV-1 infection of the nervous system is overwhelming, including: localization of HIV-1 to intrinsic cells of the CNS by immunocytochemistry (5–7) and *in situ* hybridization (8); demonstration of viral genome in brain tissue (3,9); and culture of virus from CSF or brain tissue (10). Most evidence suggests that the major cell types vulnerable to productive HIV-1 infection in the CNS are macrophages and microglia (3,7). Discussion of the relationship of macrophages to microglia is beyond the scope of this review, but most evidence suggests that both cell types are derived from bone marrow precursors (11,12). Intrinsic microglia are derived from precursor cells that migrate into the CNS early in gestation and become highly ramified cells throughout both gray and white matter (13). In this differentiated state, ramified microglia have a slow turnover rate and limited proliferative potential (11). Less differentiated macrophages in the CNS are located in the perivascular compartment (12,14). Perivascular cells have a more rapid turnover rate and are apparently replenished from circulating monocytes throughout the lifetime of the individual (12,14). It is unclear to what extent intrinsic microglia contribute to the perivascular macrophage population and whether perivascular cells can enter the parenchyma and differentiate into ramified intrinsic microglia in the adult. These issues are relevant to a more complete understanding of the pathobiology of HIV-1 infection of the CNS.

Although immunocytochemical studies have demonstrated HIV-1 antigens in perivascular macrophages and intrinsic microglia, the mechanism of HIV-1 infection of macrophages and microglia is not completely understood. It is currently unresolved whether HIV-1 enters the CNS as cell-free virus (viremia) or is carried into the CNS within infected cells (cell-associated HIV-1). It is tempting to speculate that HIV-1 enters the CNS in the normal process of turnover of the perivascular macrophage and that subsequent dissemination of virus to intrinsic microglia is via cell-to-cell spread, but most of the steps in this process remain unproven.

MECHANISM OF HIV-1 INFECTION OF MICROGLIA

Monocytotropic strains of HIV-1 have a propensity to infect macrophages and microglia and to produce CNS disease (15). The mechanism of microglial infection is unclear because microglia have low levels of CD4 antigen expression, which is the receptor for HIV-1 (16,17). CD4 has been easier to detect in rodent microglia, where cellular activation is associated with up-regulation of CD4 (18). If an analogous situation exists for human microglia, activation of these cells during systemic illness or local CNS disease processes may be associated with increased susceptibility to HIV-1 infection. A potential marker for microglial activation is class II major histocompatibility antigen (HLA-DR) expression. HLA-DR expression is increased in human microglia during systemic infectious and inflammatory conditions (19), possibly due to soluble factors such as interferon gamma (IFN-γ) (20).

Other possible mechanisms of HIV-1 infection of microglia could involve non-CD4-mediated binding of virus to target cell membranes (21–24) or antibody-mediated uptake (25,26), because microglia can express immunoglobulin Fc receptors (27). The possibility of antibody-mediated enhanced uptake of virus is of more than theoretical importance given the efforts to develop vaccines, which are expected to elicit antibody responses to HIV-1 antigens. If antibody-mediated uptake is a major means of infection of microglia, a possibly untoward outcome of vaccination may be increased susceptibility to CNS dysfunction. On the other hand, it has recently been demonstrated that microglia can be productively infected *in vitro* (28–30), and that at least in some cases this infection can be blocked with soluble CD4 or antibodies to CD4 (30). In addition, recent reports shed doubt on the clinical significance of Fc receptors as infectivity receptors (26). Other mechanisms of viral binding and entry may also exist, as suggested by recent reports that HIV-1 can infect cells expressing galactosyl ceramide or a derivative and that such binding is not blocked by CD4, but is dependent upon the major viral coat glycoprotein, gp120 (31).

Although a great deal is known about the pathogenesis of CNS dysfunction in AIDS, complete understanding of this disease remains elusive. It has been noted that clinical manifestations are often disproportionate to neuropathology and that neuropathology is often disproportionate to evidence of productive viral infection. This has led to the hypothesis that much of the CNS dysfunction in AIDS is due to indirect mechanisms. Evidence to be presented in this review suggests that productive microglial infection may be sufficient to account for most of the HIV-related CNS neuropathology and that infected microglia are detected not only associated with overt pathology, but also with subtle or inapparent pathological changes.

METHODS TO DETECT PRODUCTIVE HIV-1 INFECTION IN THE CNS

The method used in this laboratory to detect productive HIV-1 infection in the CNS of AIDS patient has been immunocytochemistry with antibodies to viral structural proteins (7). For safety reasons we have elected to perform these studies on fixed and paraffin-embedded tissue samples. Given these technical constraints, we have found only one commercially available antibody to be effective in demonstrating HIV-1 antigens, namely, a monoclonal antibody to gp41 (clone 41.4; Genetic Systems, Seattle, WA). Although *in situ* hybridization is a useful adjunct in this regard, better localization is obtained with immunocytochemistry. Furthermore, a positive signal with *in situ* hybridization does not exclude latent infection. We have not addressed the issue of latent CNS infection, although it is acknowledged that such an infection may theoretically be associated with significant cellular dysfunction.

CNS PATHOLOGY ASSOCIATED WITH PRODUCTIVE INFECTION OF MICROGLIA

HIV-1 Encephalitis

One of the most common pathological changes in the brains of patients dying with AIDS is subacute microglial nodule encephalitis, referred to as *HIV-1 encephalitis*. The cardinal histological features of HIV-1 encephalitis are microglial nodules with multinucleated cells (32,33) and perivascular macrophages. Inflammatory cell infiltrates and perivascular lymphocytic cuffing, which are typical features of many viral encephalitides, are not a prominent feature (34). Microglial reactions in a variety of pathological conditions, including HIV-1 encephalitis, can be effectively demonstrated with RCA lectin histochemistry. Using this method, microglial nodules are readily demonstrated (Fig. 1). Double-labeling studies have consistently shown that the cells in such microglial nodules reactive for HIV-1 antigens are microglia (Fig. 1).

Microglial nodules are a relatively nonspecific feature of a number of viral and spirochetal CNS infections. Their distribution in AIDS is archetypal, with predilection for the cerebral white matter, the deep gray matter (basal ganglia and thalamus), and brainstem (35). A pathognomonic feature of HIV-1 encephalitis is the multinucleated cell; however, immunocytochemistry has proven to be a more sensitive means of demonstrating HIV-1 as the cause of the encephalitis than has detection of multinucleated cells. Many cases with microglial nodule encephalitis have few or no multinucleated cells, yet have positive immunocytochemistry for HIV-1 antigens.

HIV Leukoencephalopathy

Cerebral white matter pathology in AIDS exhibits several distinct, but frequently concurrent, patterns of change (36,37). Diffuse or perivascular attenuation and variable degrees of vacuolation of myelin are common. Astrocytic gliosis is usually prominent, while perivascular chronic inflammation is minimal. Multinucleated cells and microglial proliferation are detected, but may be minimal. Immunocytochemistry reveals extensive astrocytic gliosis and infection of ramified microglia and perivascular cells. In most cases, microglia in the white matter display more HIV-1 immunoreactivity than do those in the cerebral cortex. It is, in fact, unusual to detect many infected microglia in the cerebral cortex even in advanced cases of HIV-1 encephalitis. If perivascular macrophages are the site of entry of HIV-1 into the CNS, it is unclear why the white matter and deep gray matter should be preferentially affected, while the cerebral cortex is relatively spared. The capillary density is higher in cortical gray matter than in white matter, but perivascular macrophages are more readily apparent, even in normal brains, in the larger blood vessels in the white matter and the basal ganglia.

Necrotizing Lesions of the Brain and Spinal Cord

Necrotizing lesions are relatively frequent in AIDS (38,39), but their pathogenesis is often obscure. In some cases, infarcts are related to emboli or systemic vascular disease; in other cases, intrinsic cerebrovascular disease is suspected. HIV-1 antigen is often markedly increased in macrophages found in necrotic lesions, regardless of their underlying pathogenesis. Furthermore, there is often a gradient of infection that accompanies such lesions,

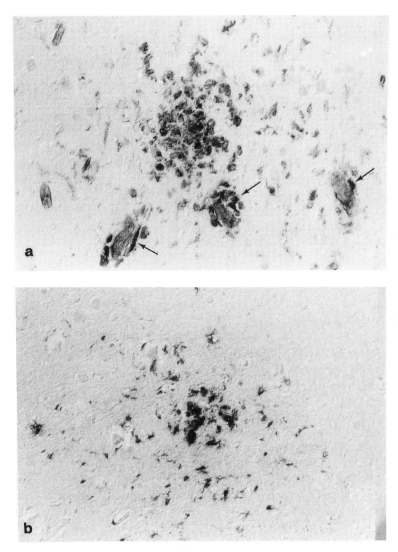

FIG. 1. A section of the brain of a patient with AIDS stained with RCA lectin histochemistry demonstrates one of the lesions that is typical of HIV encephalitis, a microglial nodule **(a)**. Note that RCA-positive perivascular cells are also stained *(arrows)*. An adjacent section stained with a monoclonal antibody to gp41 demonstrates that many of the cells in the microglial nodule are infected with HIV-1 **(b)**.

with viral antigen densest near the lesion and decreasing the further one goes from the lesion.

Part of the normal tissue response to brain injury is mobilization of microglia, recruitment of phagocytes from the blood, or both. The relative proportion of cells from each source has been a subject of much research that has culminated in the "graded response" hypothesis (40), which is a widely held tenet. With small injuries or lesions not associated with gross damage to the blood–brain barrier (e.g., cellular reaction to neurons undergoing experimental axotomy), intrinsic microglia are the major source of responding phagocytes (40,41). With larger lesions or lesions associated with disruption of the blood–brain barrier, most of the phagocytes are derived from circulating monocytes. The presence of gp41-positive macrophages in necrotic lesions in AIDS may be due to activation of latent virus in intrinsic microglia or recruitment of monocytes carrying HIV-1 (the Trojan Horse hypothesis). It is worth noting that some of the phagocytes in necrotic lesions are process-bearing cells (7), which may tend to favor their origin from intrinsic microglia.

In the axotomy model, microglia respond to injuries by proliferating (41). Microglia grown *in vitro* also have proliferative potential, especially in response to colony-stimulating factors (42). If proliferation is needed for efficient HIV-1 replication, microglia responding to necrotic lesions may have an augmented propensity for productive infection. The brain of a patient who suffered a large internal capsule infarct 5 months before he died was recently studied in our laboratory with RCA lectin histochemistry for microglia and macrophages and gp41 immunocytochemistry. HIV-1 immunoreactivity was prominent not only in many of the macrophages responding to the infarct, but also in macrophages lower in the neuroaxis that were engaged in active Wallerian degeneration. Infected microglia were detected in degenerating brainstem tracts, but not in immediately adjacent gray and white matter. Animal studies suggest that macrophages responding to remote neuronal injuries, such as those in Wallerian degeneration, may be preferentially derived from intrinsic microglia. Thus, this experiment of nature suggests that at least some HIV-1-infected macrophages in the CNS are derived from intrinsic microglia.

An unusual manifestation of HIV-1 infection in the spinal cord is a necrotizing myelitis. This process is sometimes associated with a vasculitis of obscure etiology, but possibly related to HIV-1 and herpetic viral infections. In these lesions, HIV-1 antigen is readily detected in macrophages and even within intramural cells of affected blood vessels (43). These findings contrast with those of vacuolar myelopathy (see below), where the degree of tissue damage is less severe and viral antigen is difficult to detect. It is interesting to note that secondary viral infections have been shown previously to be associated with unusually severe forms of CNS infection in AIDS. It is speculated that productive HIV-1 infection is enhanced in this situation by *trans*-

activating factors such as nuclear factor κB, a DNA binding protein whose expression is increased in response to inflammatory cytokines (44).

HIV-1 INFECTION IN THE ABSENCE OF DETECTABLE CNS PATHOLOGY

Perhaps the most significant observation that has been obtained from immunocytochemical studies of AIDS brains with monoclonal antibodies to

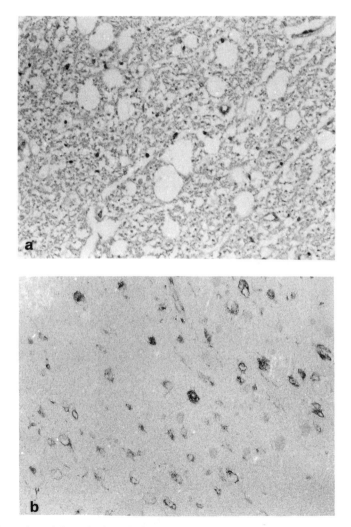

FIG. 2. A section of the spinal cord of a patient with vacuolar myelopathy displays typical myelin vacuolation **(a)**. An adjacent section stained with RCA lectin histochemistry demonstrates many densely stained oval granular foamy macrophages **(b)**.

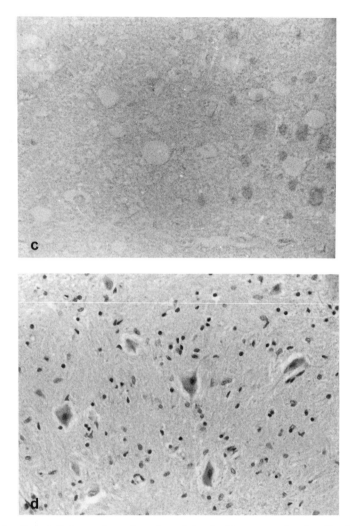

FIG. 2. *Continued.* But an adjacent section stained with a monoclonal antibody to gp41 fails to reveal significant HIV-1 immunoreactivity **(c).** In contrast, a section of the dentate nucleus of the cerebellum reveals at most only mild gliosis **(d).**

HIV-1 structural proteins is that brains with minimal or subtle neuropathology sometimes have extensive viral burden (7,27,43). We have frequently detected marked gp41 immunoreactivity in brains that had only mild gliosis. The distribution of the viral antigens in these cases was not random; instead, it paralleled (to some extent) the distribution of infection in HIV-1 encephalitis. Of particular note has been the consistent localization of HIV-1 antigens in microglia in specific regions of the deep gray matter. The pattern of distri-

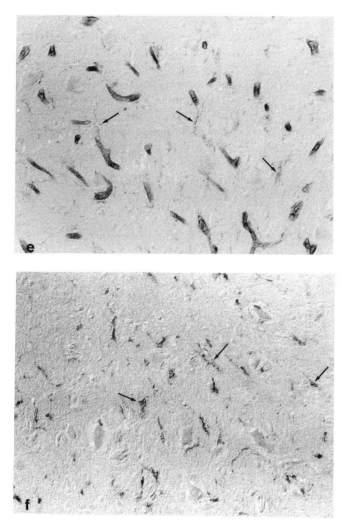

FIG. 2. *Continued.* The RCA stain shows weakly stained (but delicate) ramified microglia *(arrows)* and extensive microvasculature typical of gray matter **(e).** Despite the relatively normal appearance of the dentate nucleus, gp41, immunostaining demonstrates that many of the intrinsic microglia *(arrows)* in the dentate nucleus are infected **(f).**

bution of HIV-1 antigen in these cases is similar to the distribution of pathology in multisystem atrophies (35). Vulnerable regions were: the dentate nucleus in the cerebellum (Fig. 2); the red nucleus and substantia nigra in the midbrain; the subthalamic nucleus and thalamic fasciculus in the diencephalon; and the globus pallidus and corpus striatum in the forebrain. With routine histopathologic methods of analysis, in addition to immunocytochemistry for macrophage and astrocytic reactions, these regions are usually unremarkable. The explanation for the distribution of HIV-1 infection remains a mystery, but it suggests that microglia in certain brain regions may be more vulnerable to HIV-1 than microglia in other areas. This may relate to differences in viral receptor density or proliferative potential of the microglia or to other factors specific to these brain regions, such as their rich innervation by peptidergic systems or high iron content. Alternatively, HIV-1 infection may be enhanced in microglia responding (activated and/or proliferating microglia) to injury of neurons in these regions that are selectively vulnerable to some as-yet-to-be-defined neurotoxin (see below).

CNS PATHOLOGY WITH MINIMAL OR NO EVIDENCE OF ACTIVE INFECTION

Neocortical Pathology in AIDS

Several recent studies have demonstrated neuronal or synaptic loss (45,46) and dendritic abnormalities (47) in the cerebral cortex of patients with AIDS. Infected microglia usually do not co-localize with this pathology. The explanation for this neurotoxicity is unknown, but several hypotheses have been proposed, including effects of diffusable small molecules such as viral coat protein, nitric oxide, and quinolinic acid (see below). There is, however, no convincing evidence for productive infection of neurons.

Vacuolar Myelopathy

Vacuolar myelopathy is a disorder of the posterior and lateral funiculi of the thoracic spinal cord that is characterized pathologically by vacuolation of myelin and relative preservation of axons (48), with gliosis and collections of lipid phagocytes in the regions of vacuolation. In most cases of vacuolar myelopathy there are no inflammatory cells, microglial nodules, or multinucleated cells. Vacuolar myelopathy shares pathological features with toxic–metabolic myelopathy due to vitamin B_{12} deficiency (subacute combined degeneration). Although there are reports of HIV-1 infection of the spinal cord in such cases (49), more often little or no evidence of active viral infection is found (3,50) (Fig. 2). The myelopathy that is common in pediatric AIDS is usually not associated with myelin vacuolation, but rather with corticospinal tract degeneration (51). It has also been very difficult to detect any HIV-1 antigens in the spinal cord of pediatric AIDS patients (3).

The noninflammatory spinal cord syndromes in AIDS are probably not a direct manifestation of HIV-1 infection of the spinal cord microglia. Because the myelin pathology in vacuolar myelopathy is similar to myelin damage produced *in vitro* with tumor necrosis factor alpha (TNF-α) (52), a cytokine-mediated process remains the best hypothesis for this disorder.

Pediatric HIV-1 Encephalopathy

Infants and children with HIV-1 infection often have neurological manifestations characterized by spasticity and developmental delay or loss of milestones. Accompanying the progressive neurological deterioration, many children develop mineralization of the basal ganglia (53) and an acquired microcephaly. Although some children have productive HIV-1 infection with readily detectable HIV-1 antigens in their brains, many children have very low levels or undetectable immunoreactivity (3,54).

Astrocytic gliosis usually accompanies brain atrophy and basal ganglia mineralization. In some cases, the major cellular reaction is, in fact, astrocytic, with minimal evidence of productive HIV-1 infection of microglia. The pathogenesis of these changes is unclear, but diffusable small molecules or even associated metabolic, nutritional, or endocrinologic disorders may play a role. In the setting of systemic HIV-1 infection, increased levels of inflammatory cytokines, including TNF-α, have been demonstrated (55,56). Some of these cytokines have significant effects on astrocytes, at least *in vitro* (57). For example, the macrophage-derived cytokines interleukin 1β (IL-1β) and TNF-α induce astrocytic proliferation and morphological changes similar to those seen in gliotic brains (57). In concert, activated astrocytes produce growth factors [e.g., granulocyte-monocyte colony-stimulating factor (GM-CSF)] that promote microglial growth and development (57).

MECHANISMS OF HIV-RELATED CNS PATHOLOGY

Although some of the initial studies suggested that neuroglia (astrocytes and oligodendroglia) might be infected by HIV-1, most of the subsequent studies indicated that microglia are the primary target of active retroviral infection. It has been suggested that some cell types (e.g., astrocytes) may have a restricted form of infection associated with low-level or no production of structural proteins (e.g., gp41), but production of regulatory proteins (e.g., *tat, nef,* or *rev*) (58). The recent observations that similar immunoreactivity can be detected in normal astrocytes (59) suggest that these findings must be interpreted with caution.

The evidence for infection of ramified and ameboid microglia, in addition to evidence for infected multinucleated giant cells, is more compelling. Since infection in microglia can be detected with antibodies to structural proteins of HIV-1, including gp41, it suggests that microglial infection is productive and not lytic. Ultrastructural studies of multinucleated cells from brain lesions show intact cells with viral budding into internal membrane-bound compartments (60) (Fig. 3). Productive HIV-1 infection in CD4$^+$ lymphocytes is associated with cellular proliferation. It has been unclear how infection in microglia could be productive, since microglia have limited prolifera-

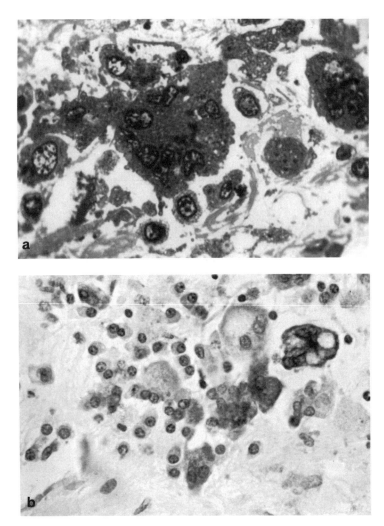

FIG. 3. A cluster of multinucleated cells in this brain are demonstrated in this toluidine blue-stained plastic section of frontal white matter **(a).** The multinucleated cells and microglia in this lesion displayed variable immunoreactivity with anti-gp41 **(b).**

tive potential. Studies that have demonstrated HIV-1 production in response to cytokine-mediated activation of monocytes offers an alternative explanation for the ability of HIV-1 to proliferate in nondividing cells. On the other hand, *in vitro* studies of human fetal and adult microglia suggest that microglia may have additional proliferative potential which had been overlooked in more static observational studies and that microglia proliferate in

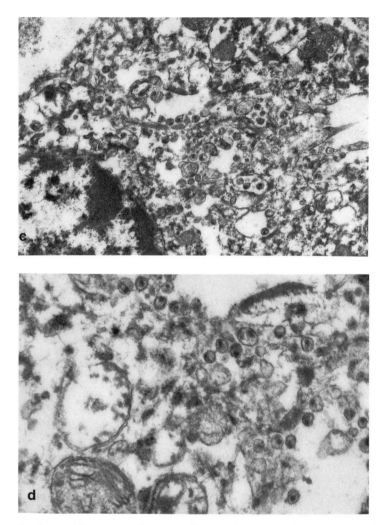

FIG. 3. *Continued.* Ultrastructural examination of this same region revealed multinucleated cells with numerous intracellular viral particles consistent with HIV-1 **(c)**, most of which appeared to be within membrane-bound spaces in the cytoplasm **(d)**.

response to colony-stimulating factors, especially GM-CSF (42). Analogous to peripheral blood monocytes grown in the presence of colony stimulating factors (15), human fetal microglia have been shown to be susceptible to infection by monocytotropic strains of HIV-1, which produce a nonlytic infection characterized by viral budding predominantly into internal membrane-bound cytoplasmic compartments (Fig. 4).

Infection of macrophages and presumably microglia is associated with cel-

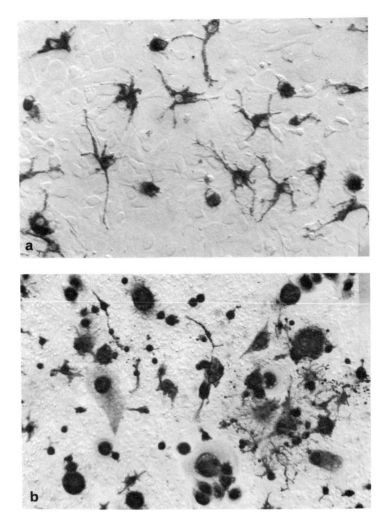

FIG. 4. Microglia grown *in vitro* and stained in this photomicrograph with a monoclonal antibody to CD68 (a macrophage antigen) display ramified morphology when cultured with a confluent layer of astrocytes (unstained cells in background) **(a).** When a similar culture was exposed overnight to HIV-1$_{JR-FL}$, washed thoroughly, and then cultured for 16 additional days, microglia became multinucleated and many lost their ramified morphology **(b).**

lular activation and production of a number of potentially toxic factors (61,62). Macrophages are considered to be the major cellular source for quinolinic acid in the brain because they contain the rate-limiting enzyme indoleamine-2,3-dioxygenase (63). Quinolinic acid production in macrophages is increased by IFN-γ, which is elevated in AIDS and may be partly responsible

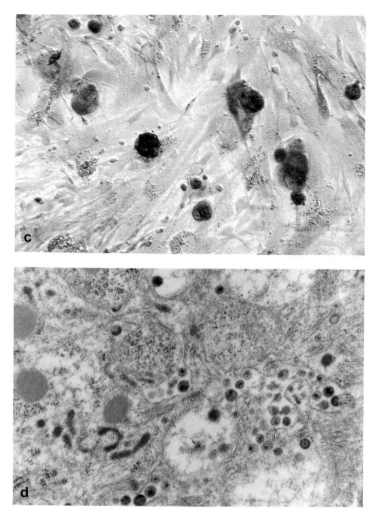

FIG. 4. *Continued.* A similar *in vitro*-infected culture stained with monoclonal antibody to gp41 demonstrates presence of viral antigens in the multinucleated cells, but not the astrocytes **(c)**. At the ultrastructural level, retroviral particles were detected within membrane-bound spaces of microglia **(d)**, but not astrocytes.

for the increased HLA-DR expression in microglia in AIDS. Elevated levels of quinolinic acid in serum and cerebrospinal fluid have been shown to be highly correlated with AIDS dementia (64).

Other products of infected microglia that may be toxic to the CNS include viral coat protein (gp120) (65–67) and TNF-α (68). TNF-α produces myelin vacuolation *in vitro* that is very similar to that in vacuolar myelopathy. Toxic cytokines derived from infected microglia or the systemic circulation may

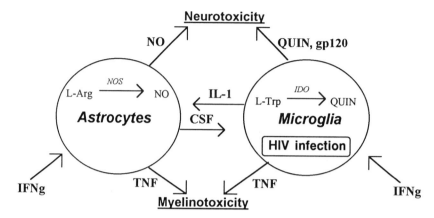

FIG. 5. A schematic diagram of some of the documented interactions between human astrocytes and microglia that may be relevant to HIV-related CNS pathology illustrates that infected and activated microglia (and macrophages) may be the major source for several neurotoxic substances, including quinolinic acid and viral coat protein, gp120. Quinolinic acid production by macrophages has been shown to be up-regulated in response to IFN-γ, which is elevated in the systemic circulation and within the CNS compartment during systemic and CNS viral infections. Astrocytes have been shown to be highly sensitive to IL-1β, especially in the context of IFN-γ. When exposed to IL-1β, astrocytes produce a number of soluble factors that may mediate CNS pathology, including nitric oxide and TNF-α. The latter molecule, which is also produced by activated microglia, has been shown to produce *in vitro* vacuolation of myelin. Although rodent microglia and macrophages may produce nitric oxide, evidence from our laboratory (69) suggests that astrocytes are the primary source of NO in the human CNS; recent studies suggest that NO may be toxic to neurons. NO, nitric oxide; QUIN, quinolinic acid; L-Arg, L-arginine; NOS, nitric oxide synthase; IL-1, interleukin 1; CSF, colony-stimulating factor; L-Trp, L-tryptophan; IDO, indoleamine-2,3-dioxygenase; TNF, tumor necrosis factor; IFNg, interferon gamma.

also be the mechanism that best explains diffuse gliosis seen in the brains of adults and children with AIDS, especially when little viral antigen can be detected.

Although nitric oxide has recently been recognized as a potential neurotoxin, recent evidence suggests that microglia are not the major source for nitric oxide in humans (69). This differs from rodents, where microglia may be capable of producing nitric oxide. On the other hand, the evidence suggests that astrocytes produce nitric oxide, especially in response to activation by IL-1β, which can be derived from microglia (69) (Fig. 5).

Further studies are needed to study the functional changes associated with HIV-1 infection of microglia and whether there are developmental or microenvironmental factors that determine susceptibility to infection with respect to observed differences in microglial infection related to patient age and neuroanatomy. A better understanding of microgliogenesis and the cell biology of microglia will undoubtedly increase our understanding of HIV-related CNS pathology.

ACKNOWLEDGMENTS

The constructive criticism and helpful advice of Dr. Cedric S. Raine is greatly appreciated, as is the assistance with electron microscopy by Yvonne Kress, immunocytochemistry by Grace Gong and Meng-Liang Zhao, and tissue culture studies by Wei Liu. Without the help of Dr. William Rashbaum in Obstetrics and Gynecology, the studies of fetal microglia would have been impossible. Drs. Katsuhiro Kure, Karen Weidenheim, and Kenneth Hutchins have all assisted in neuropathologic studies of AIDS. Their contribution is gratefully acknowledged. Research for this chapter has been supported by NIMH Grant MH47667.

REFERENCES

1. Budka H. Neuropathology of human immunodeficiency virus infection. *Brain Pathol* 1991; 1:163–175.
2. Dickson DW, Belman AL, Park YD, et al. Central nervous system pathology in pediatric AIDS: an autopsy study. *APMIS* 1989;97(suppl 8):40–57.
3. Kure K, Llena J, Lyman WD, Soeiro R, Weidenheim KM, Hirano A, Dickson DW. Human immunodeficiency virus-1 infection of the nervous system: an autopsy study of 268 adult, pediatric and fetal brains. *Hum Pathol* 1991;22:700–710.
4. Levy RM, Bredesen DE, Rosenbaum ML. Neurological manifestations of the acquired immunodeficiency syndrome (AIDS): experience at UCSF and review of the literature. *J Neurosurg* 1985;62:475–495.
5. Wiley CA, Schrier RD, Nelson JA, Lampert PW, Oldstone MBA. Cellular localization of human immunodeficiency virus infection within the brains of acquired immune deficiency syndrome patients. *Proc Natl Acad Sci USA* 1986;83:7089–7093.
6. Vaseux R, Brousse N, Jarry A, et al. AIDS subacute encephalitis: identification of HIV-infected cells. *Am J Pathol* 1987;126:403–410.
7. Kure K, Lyman WD, Weidenheim KM, Dickson DW. Cellular localization of an HIV-1 antigen in subacute AIDS encephalitis using an improved double-labeling immunohistochemical method. *Am J Pathol* 1990;136:1085–1092.
8. Stoler MH, Eskin TA, Benn S, Angerer RC, Angerer LM. Human T-cell lymphotropic virus type III infection of the central nervous system: a preliminary in situ analysis. *JAMA* 1986;256:2360–2364.
9. Shaw GM, Harper ME, Hahn BH, et al. HTLV-III infection in brains of children and adults with AIDS encephalopathy. *Science* 1985;227:177–182.
10. Ho DD, Rota TR, Schooley RT, et al. Isolation of HTLV-III from cerebrospinal fluid and neural tissues of patients with neurologic syndromes related to the acquired immunodeficiency syndrome. *N Engl J Med* 1985;313:1493–1497.
11. Matsumoto Y, Fujiwara M. Absence of donor-type major histocompatibility complex class I-bearing microglia in the rat central nervous system of radiation bone marrow chimeras. *J Neuroimmunol* 1987;17:71–82.
12. Hickey WF, Kimura H. Perivascular microglial cells of the CNS are bone marrow-derived and present antigen *in vivo*. *Science* 1988;239:290–292.
13. Mattiace LA, Brosnan CF, Dickson DW. Distribution and characterization of microglia in the normal human fetal brain. *Soc Neurosci Abstr* 1991;17:734.
14. Graeber MB, Streit WJ, Kreutzberg WJ. Identity of ED2-positive perivascular cells in rat brain. *J Neurosci Res* 1989;22:103–106.
15. Gendelman HE, Orenstein JM, Baca LM, Weiser B, Burger H, Kalter DC, Meltzer MS. The macrophage in the persistence and pathogenesis of HIV infection. *AIDS* 1989;3:475–495.
16. Maddon PJ, Dalgleish AG, McDougal JS, Clapham PR, Weiss RA, Axel R. The T4 gene

encodes the AIDS virus receptor and is expressed in the immune system and the brain. *Cell* 1986;47:333–348.

17. Funke I, Hahn A, Rieber EP, Weiss E, Rieth-Muller G. The cellular receptor (CD4) for the human immunodeficiency virus is expressed on neurons and glial cells in human brain. *J Exp Med* 1987;165:1230–1235.

18. Perry VH, Gordon S. Modulation of CD4 antigen on macrophages and microglia in rat brain. *J Exp Med* 1987;164:594–604.

19. Mattiace LA, Davies P, Dickson DW. Detection of HLA-DR on microglia in post-mortem human brain is a function of clinical and technical factors. *Am J Pathol* 1990;136:1101–1114.

20. Vass K, Lassmann H. Intrathecal application of interferon gamma: progressive appearance of MHC antigens within the rat nervous system. *Am J Pathol* 1990;137:789–800.

21. Claphan PR, Weber JN, Whitby D, et al. Soluble CD4 blocks infectivity of diverse strains of HIV and SIV for T cells and monocytes but not for brain and muscle cells. *Nature* 1989; 337:368–373.

22. Harouse JM, Kunsch C, Hartle HT, Laughlin MA, Hoxie JA, Wigdahl B, Gonzalez-Scarano F. CD4-independent infection of human neural cells by human immunodeficiency virus type 1. *J Virol* 1989;63:2527–2533.

23. Takeda A, Tuazon CU, Ennis FA. Antibody-enhanced infection by HIV-1 via Fc receptor-mediated entry. *Science* 1988;242:580–583.

24. Kunsch C, Hartle HT, Wigdahl B. Infection of human fetal dorsal root ganglion cells with human immunodeficiency virus type 1 involves an entry mechanism independent of the CD4 T4 epitope. *J Virol* 1989;63:5054–5061.

25. McKeating JA, Griffiths PD, Weiss RA. HIV susceptibility conferred to human fibroblasts by cytomegalovirus-induced Fc receptor. *Nature* 1990;343:659–661.

26. Connor RI, Dinces NB, Howell AL, Romet-Lemonne JL, Pasquali JL, Fanger MW. Fc receptors for IgG (Fc gamma Rs) on human monocytes and macrophages are not infectivity receptors for human immunodeficiency virus type 1 (HIV-1): studies using bispecific antibodies to target HIV-1 to various myeloid cell surface molecules, including Fc gamma R. *Proc Natl Acad Sci USA* 1991;88:9593–9597.

27. Dickson DW, Mattiace LA, Kure K, Hutchins K, Lyman WD, Brosnan CF. Biology of disease: microglia in human disease, with an emphasis on acquired immune deficiency syndrome. *Lab Invest* 1991;64:135–156.

28. Peudenier S, Hery C, Montagnier L, Tardieu M. Human microglia cells: characterization in cerebral tissue and in primary culture, and study of their susceptibility to HIV-1 infection. *Ann Neurol* 1991;29:152–161.

29. Watkins BA, Dorn HH, Kelly WB, Armstrong RG, Potts BJ, Michaels F, Kufta CV, Dubois-Dalcq M. Specific tropism of HIV-1 for microglial cells in primary brain cultures. *Science* 1990;249:549–551.

30. Jordan CA, Watkins BA, Kufta C, Dubois-Dalcq M. Infection of brain microglial cells by human immunodeficiency virus type 1 is CD4 dependent. *J Virol* 1991;65:736–742.

31. Bhat S, Spitalnik SL, Gonzalez-Scarano F, Silberberg DH. Galactosyl ceramide or a derivative is an essential component of the neural receptor for human immunodeficiency virus type 1 envelope glycoprotein gp120. *Proc Natl Acad Sci USA* 1991;88:7131–7134.

32. Budka H. Multinucleated giant cells in brain: a hallmark of the acquired immunodeficiency syndrome (AIDS). *Acta Neuropathol (Berl)* 1986;69:253–256.

33. Dickson DW. Multinucleated giant cells in acquired immunodeficiency syndrome: origin from endogenous microglia? *Arch Pathol Lab Med* 1986;110:967–968.

34. Weidenheim KM, Epshteyn I, Lyman WD. Immunocytochemical identification of T-cells in HIV-1 encephalitis: implications for pathogenesis of CNS disease. *Mod Pathol* 1993;6 *(in press)*.

35. Kure K, Weidenheim KM, Lyman WD, Dickson DW. Morphology and distribution of HIV-1-positive microglia in subacute AIDS encephalitis: pattern of involvement resembling a multisystem degeneration. *Acta Neuropathol (Berl)* 1990;80:393–400.

36. Smith TW, DeGirolami U, Henin D, Bolgert F, Hauw J-J. Human immunodeficiency virus (HIV) leukoencephalopathy and the microcirculation. *J Neuropathol Exp Neurol* 1990;49: 357–366.

37. Schmidbauer M, Huemer M, Cristina S, Trabatton GR, Budka DH. Morphological spectrum distribution and clinical correlation of white matter lesions in AIDS brains. *Neuropathol Appl Neurobiol* 1992;18:489–501.

38. Mizusawa H, Hirano A, Llena JF. Cerebrovascular lesions in acquired immune deficiency syndrome (AIDS). *Acta Neuropathol (Berl)* 1988;76:451–457.
39. Park YD, Belman AL, Kim TS, et al. Stroke in pediatric acquired immunodeficiency syndrome (AIDS). *Ann Neurol* 1990;28:553–560.
40. Streit WJ, Graeber MB, Kreutzberg GW. Functional plasticity of microglia: a review. *Glia* 1988;1:301–307.
41. Graeber MB, Streit WJ, Kreutzberg WJ. Formation of microglia-derived brain macrophages is blocked by adriamycin. *Acta Neuropathol (Berl)* 1989;78:348–358.
42. Lee SC, Liu W, Roth P, Dickson DW, Berman JW, Brosnan CF. Macrophage colony-stimulating factor in human fetal astrocytes and microglia: differential regulation by cytokines and lipopolysaccharide, and modulation of class II MHC on microglia. *J Immunol* 1993;150:594–604.
43. Dickson DW, Less SC, Mattiace LA, Yen S-HC, Brosnan CF. Microglia and cytokines in neurological disease, with special reference to AIDS and Alzheimer's disease. *Glia* 1993; 7:75–83.
44. Griffin GE, Leung K, Folks TM, Kunkel S, Nabel GJ. Activation of HIV gene expression during monocyte differentiation by induction of NF-κB. *Nature* 1989;339:70–73.
45. Ketzler S, Weis S, Haug H, Budka H. Loss of neurons in the frontal cortex in AIDS brains. *Acta Neuropathol (Berl)* 1990;80:92–94.
46. Masliah E, Ge N, Morey M, DeTeresa R, Terry RD, Wiley CA. Cortical dendritic pathology in human immunodeficiency virus encephalitis. *Lab Invest* 1992;66:285–291.
47. Wiley CA, Masliah E, Morey M, Lemere C, DeTeresa R, Grafe M, Hansen LA, Terry RD. Neocortical damage during HIV infection. *Ann Neurol* 1991;29:651–657.
48. Petito CK, Navia BA, Cho E-S, Jordan BD, George DC, Price RW. Vacuolar myelopathy pathologically resembling subacute combined degeneration in patients with the acquired immunodeficiency syndrome. *N Engl J Med* 1985;312:874–879.
49. Eilbott DJ, Peress N, Burger H, Laneve D, Orenstein J, Gendelman HE, Seidman R, Weiser B. Human immunodeficiency virus type 1 in spinal cords of acquired immunodeficiency syndrome patients with myelopathy: expression and replication in macrophages. *Proc Natl Acad Sci USA* 1986;86:3337–3341.
50. Rosenblum M, Scheck AC, Cronin K, Brew BJ, Khan A, Paul M, Price RW. Dissociation of AIDS-related vacuolar myelopathy and productive HIV-1 infection of the spinal cord. *Neurology* 1989;39:892–896.
51. Dickson DW, Belman AL, Kim TS, Horoupian DS, Rubinstein A. Spinal cord pathology in pediatric acquired immunodeficiency syndrome. *Neurology* 1989;39:227–235.
52. Selmaj KW, Raine CS. Tumor necrosis factor mediates myelin and oligodendrocyte damage *in vitro*. *Ann Neurol* 1988;23:339–346.
53. Belman AL, Lantos G, Horoupian DS, Novick BE, Ultmann MH, Dickson DW, Rubinstein A. AIDS: calcification of the basal ganglia in infants and children. *Neurology* 1986;36: 1192–1199.
54. Vaseux R, Lacroix-Ciaudo C, Blanche S, Cumont M-C, Henin D, Gray F, Boccon-Gibod L, Tardieu M. Low levels of human immunodeficiency virus replication in the brain tissue of children with severe acquired immunodeficiency syndrome encephalopathy. *Am J Pathol* 1992;140:137–144.
55. Mintz M, Rapaport R, Oleske JM, Connor EM, Kenigsberger MR, Denny T, Epstein LG. Elevated serum levels of tumor necrosis factor are associated with progressive encephalopathy in children with acquired immunodeficiency syndrome. *Am J Dis Child* 1989;143: 771–774.
56. Grimaldi LME, Martin GV, Franciotta DM, Brustia R, Castagna A, Pristera R, Lazzarin A. Elevated alpha-tumor necrosis factor levels in spinal fluid from HIV-1 infected patients with central nervous system involvement. *Ann Neurol* 1991;29:21–25.
57. Lee SC, Liu W, Dickson DW, Brosnan CF, Berman JW. Cytokine production by human fetal astrocytes and microglia. *J Immunol* 1993;150:2659–2667.
58. Haseltine WA. Molecular biology of the human immunodeficiency virus type 1. *FASEB J* 1991;5:2349–2360.
59. Parmentier HK, van Wichen DF, Gmelig Meyling FHJ, Goudsmit J, Schuurman H-J. Epitopes of human immunodeficiency virus regulatory proteins *tat*, *nef*, and *rev* are expressed in normal human tissue. *Am J Pathol* 1992;141:1209–1216.

60. Sharer LR, Epstein LG, Cho E-S, Joshi VV, Meyenhofer ME, Rankin LE, Petito CK. Pathologic features of AIDS encephalopathy in children: evidence of LAV/HTLV-111 infection of brain. *Hum Pathol* 1986;17:271–284.
61. Merrill JE, Koyanagi Y, Chen ISY. Interleukin-1 and tumor necrosis factor alpha can be induced from mononuclear phagocytes by human immunodeficiency virus type 1 binding to the CD4 receptor. *J Virol* 1989;63:4404–4408.
62. Molina J-M, Scadden DT, Byrn R, Dinarello CA, Groopman JE. Production of tumor necrosis factor alpha and interleukin 1 beta by monocytic cells infected with human immunodeficiency virus. *J Clin Invest* 1989;84:733–743.
63. Heyes MP, Saito K, Markey S. Human macrophages convert L-tryptophan into the neurotoxin quinolinic acid. *Biochem J* 1992;283:633–635.
64. Heyes MP, Brew BJ, Saito K, et al. Inter-relationships between quinolinic acid, neuroactive kynurenines, neopterin and β_2-microglobulin in cerebrospinal fluid and serum of HIV-1-infected patients. *J Neuroimmunol* 1992;40:71–80.
65. Brenneman DE, Westbrook GL, Fitzgerald SP, Ennist DL, Elkins KL, Ruff MR, Pert CB. Neuronal cell killing by the envelope protein of HIV and its prevention by vasoactive intestinal peptide. *Nature* 1988;335:639–642.
66. Dreyer EB, Kaiser PK, Offermann JT, Lipton SA. HIV-1 coat protein neurotoxicity prevented by calcium channel antagonists. *Science* 1990;248:364–367.
67. Lipton SA. Requirement for macrophages in neuronal injury induced by HIV envelope protein gp120. *NeuroReport* 1992;3:913–915.
68. Lee SC, Liu W, Brosnan CF, Dickson DW. Characterization of primary human fetal dissociated central nervous system cultures with an emphasis on microglia. *Lab Invest* 1992;67:465–476.
69. Lee SC, Dickson DW, Liu W, Brosnan CF. Activation of nitric oxide synthase in human astrocytes by IL-1β and IFNγ. *J Neuroimmunol* 1993;46:19–24.

HIV, AIDS and the Brain, edited by
R. W. Price and S. W. Perry.
Raven Press, Ltd., New York © 1994.

6

Cellular Neuropathology in HIV Encephalitis

Eliezer Masliah, Cristian L. Achim, Nianfeng Ge,
Richard DeTeresa, and Clayton A. Wiley

*Departments of Neurosciences and Pathology, University of California at
San Diego, School of Medicine, LaJolla, CA 92093*

During the progress of acquired immunodeficiency syndrome (AIDS), approximately 75 percent of the patients develop alterations of the nervous system (1–7). While a high proportion of central nervous system (CNS) pathology is associated with opportunistic infections, approximately 20–30 percent of cases at autopsy reveal neuropathological evidence of human immunodeficiency virus encephalitis (HIVE), characterized by the presence of multinucleated giant cells (MNGCs) and microglial nodules which contain HIV antigens (e.g., gap protein p24 or envelope protein gp41) and HIV-specific nucleic acids (5,8). In addition, HIVE is accompanied by white matter pallor and gliosis (1,9). Extensive immunocytochemical and *in situ* hybridization studies in human and animal models of lentiviral encephalitis have shown that the virus is predominantly found within monocytic/microglial cells (3,4,9–14). However, there is little evidence of infection of neurons or glia. It is still not clear if the neurological alterations found in patients with HIVE without opportunistic infections are related to the direct effect of virus on CNS cells or to an indirect mechanism mediated by glial or monocytic/microglial cells. In this regard it is of prime importance to define to what extent different neuronal populations are affected in HIVE. The topographical distribution of the damage will help elucidate whether neurodegeneration proceeds in a retro or anterograde fashion. The main objective of the present study is to review the current knowledge of the damage to neurons and their processes in HIVE and to propose possible mechanisms of cortical damage based on the specificity and characteristics of the neuronal lesions.

NEURONAL POPULATIONS AFFECTED IN HIVE

Previous studies have shown extensive neuropathological changes in subcortical gray and white matter (2,3,5,9,11,12,15) in HIVE. More subtle alterations in the neocortex with frontal and temporal lobe atrophy, accompanied by: (a) spongiform degeneration in laminae 1–3 and (b) neuronal loss with astrocytosis, have been recently reported (16–19). Ketzler et al. (18) have shown an 18 percent loss of neurons and a 31 percent reduction of the perikaryon volume in the fronto-orbital cortex in AIDS brains. Recently we have used morphometric techniques and found a 30–50 percent decrease in the number of large neurons (200–500 μm^2) in the frontal, parietal, and temporal cortex of HIVE cases accompanied by 20 percent reduction in neocortical width (16). The areas of neuronal loss were often accompanied by astrocytosis, which in morphometric studies was characterized by an increase in the number of cells smaller than 40 μm^2 (16). Previous studies by Budka et al. have described this condition as diffuse poliodystrophy (5).

Children infected with HIV frequently develop HIVE, but less commonly develop opportunistic CNS infections (4,7). HIVE in children is characterized by large necrotizing cortical and subcortical lesions. In these cases, HIV involvement in the nervous system is accompanied by extensive neuronal loss and damage to the neocortex (20,21). The HIV-related lentivirus, simian immunodeficiency virus (SIV), produces variable damage in the adult

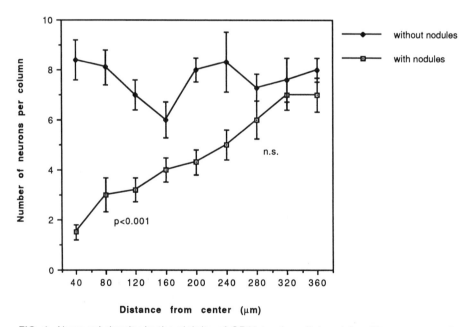

FIG. 1. Neuronal density in the vicinity of GP41+ microglial nodules. The presence of microglial nodules in the cortical gray matter accentuated the already existing neuronal loss in cases with HIVE. The closer to the nodules, the greater the pyramidal cell loss. However, this effect disappear 300 μm away from the nodule, suggesting the possible diffusion of neurotoxins from the nodule.

monkey brain, whereas young monkeys show extensive cortical damage similar to that reported in HIVE in both children and adults (22).

Detailed immunocytochemical studies with an antibody against HIV gp41 have shown that in the neocortex and spinal cord, the HIV-positive microglial cells are attached to the neuronal membrane and surround the neuronal perikarya, suggesting that infected microglia may be responsible for neuronal damage (5). Hypothetically, if diffusable putative neurotoxic factors are released from HIV-bearing microglial cells, one should find a gradient of neuronal damage—that is, progressively heavier neuronal damage in the proximity of the HIV-positive microglial nodules. Preliminary quantitative studies in the frontal cortex on HIVE cases with abundant microglial nodules, but without evidence of opportunistic infections, have shown greater neuronal loss in the proximity to the nodules as compared to neuronal groups further away from the nodules (Fig. 1).

Morphometric studies of the neuronal density in various regions of the hippocampus stained with cresyl violet have shown a slight decrease in pyramidal neurons in the CA1 region, with fewer alterations in CA2–CA4 (Fig. 2). In order to identify neuronal populations affected in HIVE and determine

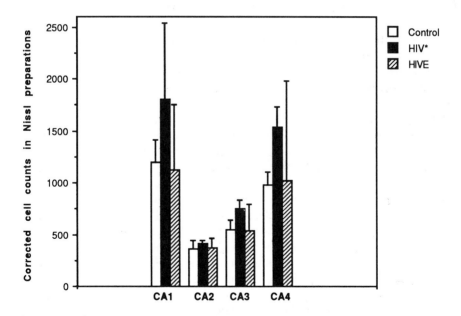

* HIV seropositive cases without encephalitis

FIG. 2. Pyramidal cell counts in the hippocampus in HIVE. No statistically significant changes were observed when control cases were compared to HIV-seropositive cases with or without encephalitis. Sections were stained with cresyl violet and counted as previously described with the Quantimet 970 (16).

how neuronal damage relates to the severity of HIV infection within the nervous system, we quantified parvalbumin (PV+) and neurofilament (NF+) immunoreactive neurons in frontal cortex and hippocampus. We found that in the neocortex, the density of NF+ and PV+ neurons was not correlated with the severity of HIVE, and therefore changes in these neuronal subsets did not account for previously reported neuronal loss (23). However, neuritic processes of PV+ neurons were fragmented, atrophic, and in some cases distended. In contrast to the frontal cortex, there was a trend toward decreased density of PV+ neurons in the hippocampus that only reached significance in the CA3 layer where there was a 50–90 percent decrease in PV+ neurons. This decrease was tightly correlated with the severity of HIVE (23). Double-immunolabeling immunocytochemical analysis confirmed neuritic damage to interneurons. These results suggest that HIVE differentially involves specific subpopulations of neurons. Since direct HIV infection of neuronal cells was not detected, damage to PV+ cells and fibers may be indirectly mediated by cytokines or HIV antigen released by infected microglia (24).

NEURITIC ALTERATIONS IN HIVE

Confocal laser imaging and electron microscopic analysis showed vacuolated areas of the neuropil in relation to dendritic processes (2,16,25) (Fig. 3). In order to further characterize and quantify alterations in the dendritic tree of neocortical pyramidal neurons, we performed a modified Golgi impregnation technique on formalin fixed blocks from the frontal cortex of HIVE cases, HIV-seropositive control cases without encephalitis, and five HIV-seronegative controls. Apical dendrites of pyramidal neurons from HIVE cases were dilated, vacuolated, and tortuous with decreased length and branching. Basal and oblique dendrites also showed these alterations, but to a lesser extent. Computer-aided quantification of dendritic spines in pyramidal neurons in two frontal cortex cases showed a 40–60 percent decrease throughout the entire length of dendrites in HIVE (25). Laser confocal imaging of Golgi-impregnated sections displayed aberrant spines in regions of abnormal second-order dendritic branches. These observations support the role of primary dendritic damage in HIVE, in contrast to other neurodegenerative disorders (like Alzheimer's disease) where the primary pathology is presynaptic (26). The percent of neocortical area occupied by dendrites [immunostained for microtubule associated protein (MAP-2)] and presynaptic terminals (immunostained with anti-synaptophysin) were quantified with the aid of a computer. In the frontal cortex, 28 percent of the neuropil area from seronegative control brains stained with MAP-2. No significant differences were observed when measurements from age-matched controls were compared to AIDS patients with minimal to no HIVE ($p = 0.52$). However,

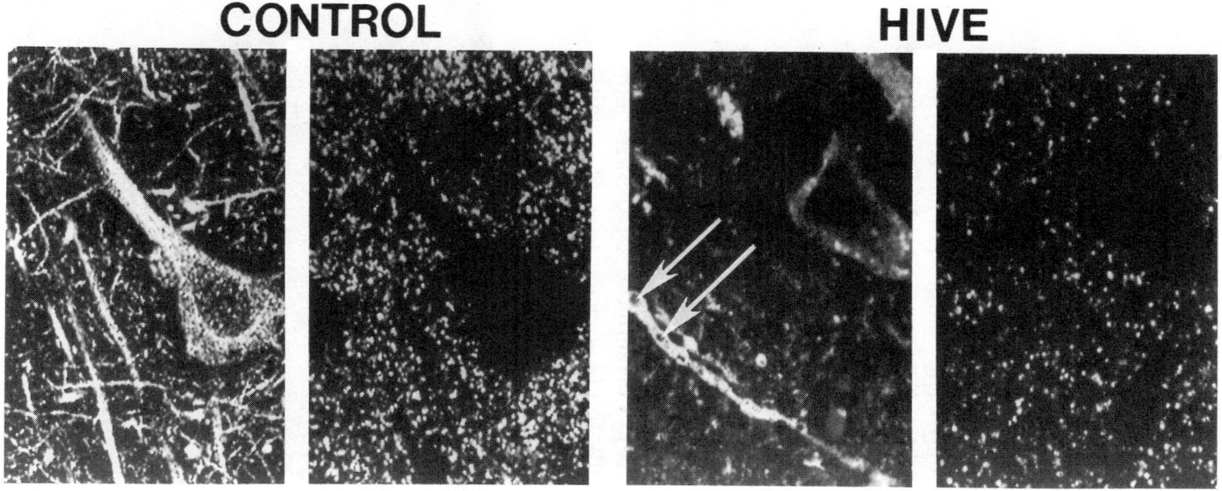

FIG. 3. Dendritic alterations in HIVE. Laser confocal imaging of dendrites (**left**) and presynaptic terminals (**right**). In the control cases, anti-MAP2 immunolabeled pyramidal neurons as well as abundant apical dendrites and their ramifications. Anti-synaptophysin immunolabeled the neuropil with a punctate pattern. In severe HIVE cases, the immunolabeled dendrites were dilated and vacuolated with an overall loss in their complexity.

comparison of these measurements to AIDS patients with moderate to severe HIVE showed a statistically significant 36 percent loss of the area occupied by MAP-2-immunolabeled dendrites ($p < 0.01$, unpaired, two-tailed t-test) (2).

In control cases, anti-synaptophysin-immunolabeled presynaptic boutons occupied 22 percent of the frontal cortex neuropil area. In AIDS cases with minimal to no HIVE the presynaptic boutons occupied 20 percent of the area. However, comparison of synaptophysin measurements from brains with moderate to severe HIVE showed a 23 percent loss of neocortical pre-synaptic area (17% total neocortical area) compared to the brains of non-infected age-matched controls ($p < 0.01$, unpaired, two-tailed t-test) (2). Consistent with these findings, laser confocal imaging of sections double-immunolabeled with anti-synaptophysin and anti-MAP-2 showed that cases with abundant gp41 immunoreactivity displayed tortuous dendrites with ex-tensive areas of vacuolation and overall decrease in density of ramifications. The decrease in neocortical dendritic area was also closely correlated with a decrease in the neocortical presynaptic complexity. Studies in experimental models of spongiform retroviral encephalopathy (a model system that mimics some aspects of nervous system damage by retrovirus in humans) have shown vacuolization and damage to dendritic processes similar to the one observed in HIVE (27,28). Furthermore, neurofilament-positive damaged neurites were occasionally found adjacent to gp41-positive macrophage/mi-croglial cells (Fig. 4).

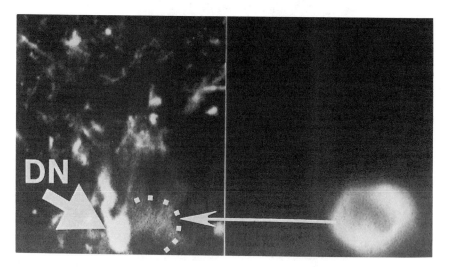

FIG. 4. Dystrophic neuritic (DN) alterations in the proximity of GP41 + macrophages. Laser confocal imaging of neurites immunolabeled with an antibody against neurofilament **(left)** were closely associated to GP41 + macrophages. The image is shown in the same optical plane but split into the two channels **(right)**. The arrow indicates the actual location of the macrophage when the images were merged.

Immunoelectron microscopic studies of the neuritic alterations in the HIVE hippocampus, immunolabeled with an antibody against parvalbumin, showed that these abnormal structures contained mitochondria, distended vesicles, and some laminated bodies (Fig. 5).

SPECTRUM OF HIV-ASSOCIATED CORTICAL ALTERATIONS

In the previous two sections, we reviewed the characteristics of the neuronal damage in HIVE. These morphometric studies suggested that there were various degrees of neuronal involvement in cortical regions in HIVE. In this regard, it is necessary to ask to what extent the severity of neuronal damage is related to the abundance of the virus in the brain, as well as to the presence of HIV-related lesions (gliosis, microglia nodules, etc.). Using the semiquantitative scoring system for detection of gp41-stained cells, we evaluated the presence of HIV in successive sections from regions immunostained for glial fibrillary acidic protein (GFAP), an astrocytic marker (2). A composite score for the presence of HIV within the brain was derived by adding the three regional scores as follows: absent or minimal expression of gp41, 0–1; moderate, 2–3; severe, 4–6. While all cases with MNGCs had moderate to high scores for gp41, more than three-quarters of the cases with moderate to high gp41 did not have MNGC. The least staining was observed in cortical gray matter (CGM), where less than 30 percent of the cases showed evidence of gp41. Most of the staining in cortical white matter (CWM) was limited to occasional positive cells, with only 15 percent of the cases showing abundant gp41 in this region. Of the three sites compared, deep gray matter (DGM) (in particular the inner globus pallidus) contained the greatest viral staining, with more than 45 percent of the cases showing abundant gp41 and only 20 percent of the cases showed no evidence of gp41 (2).

Linear regression analysis was performed comparing regional and global gliosis, HIV distribution, and neocortical presynaptic and dendritic areas. Presence of gp41 in the neocortical gray matter strongly correlated with presence of gp41 in the cortical white matter but not with the presence of gp41 in the deep gray matter (2). Decreased dendritic and presynaptic areas were closely associated with the presence of gp41 immunoreactivity in the entire cerebrum (gp41 total) and in the neocortical gray and white matter individually. In contrast, the association of neocortical pre- and postsynaptic changes with presence of gp41 in the subcortical gray matter was less strong, and the statistical significance depended upon inclusion of cases with minimal gp41. When less infected cases were not included in the regression analysis, the correlation was not significant, suggesting that cerebral cortex damage did not vary with severity of basal ganglia damage (2). In contrast to the above correlations, gliosis as measured by GFAP immunoreactivity did not show significant correlations with the degree of synaptic/dendritic pathology.

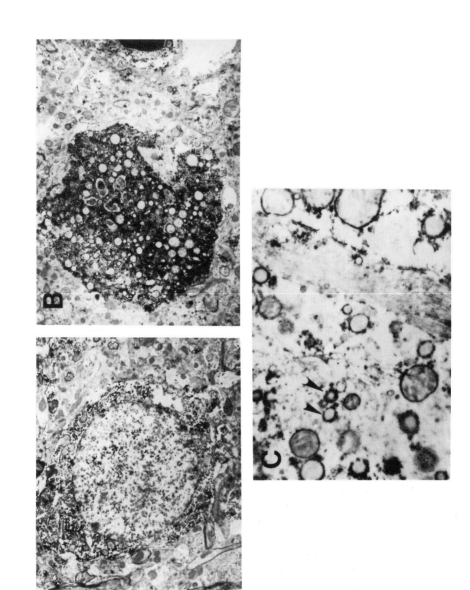

Studies are underway to evaluate the correlation between the neuronal and neuritic lesions in HIVE and the amount of HIV-1 present in the brain, quantified by the polymerase chain reaction technique and by *in situ* hybridization. Furthermore, future studies will be necessary to define the correlation between the severity of the cognitive impairment in patients with HIVE and degree of cortical and subcortical damage and viral burden in the brain.

POSSIBLE MECHANISMS OF NEURONAL DAMAGE IN HIVE

The cognitive and motor alterations associated with HIVE have been previously described as "subcortical" (15,29,30). Without question, severe damage to subcortical structures is commonly observed in HIVE, and this might account for some of the motor alteration. However, memory loss and other cognitive alterations observed in patients with HIVE might be associated with the prominent loss of dendritic arbor (2,25), loss of large pyramidal neurons (16–19), and damage to interneurons of the neocortex and hippocampus (23).

Many different factors associated with HIV (including structural and transcriptional proteins) or HIV-infected macrophages (protease-resistant low-molecular-weight factors, cytokines, metabolic products, etc.) (24,31–35) have been described as neurotoxic in a variety of assays. Given the dendritic pathology noted above and the distribution of NMDA receptors on dendritic membranes, it is intriguing to note that some of the neurotoxic effects have been blocked by N-methyl-D-aspartate (NMDA) antagonists (34,35). The specificity of these effects awaits development of an experimental model in which quantitative effects can be analyzed. Recent studies have suggested that the damage to neurons and their processes in HIVE might be mediated by cytokines produced by infected microglia or astrocytes (24). Among the possible candidates are the monokines interleukin 1 (IL-1), interleukin 6 (IL-6), tumor necrosis factor alpha (TNF-α), and transforming growth factor beta (TGF-β) (36). Cytokines are among the most potent factors mediating intercellular communication and could modulate interactions between the immune and nervous systems (37). Cytokines released by macrophages/microglia, the predominant immune cell within the brain, have been proposed to modulate neuronal survival and death (24). Since macrophages are the only

---

FIG. 5. Immunoelectron microscopic analysis of parvalbumin positive neurites in HIVE. Immunoelectron microscopic localization of PV immunoreactivity in HIVE hippocampus. **A:** PV+ neuron displayed a strong immunoreactivity in its endomembrane system. **B:** A PV+ dystrophic neurite showed intense immunoreactivity in the granular material surrounding mitochondria and laminated bodies. **C:** PV immunostaining was observed around small vesicles *(arrowheads)* in the dystrophic neurite. (A, B: ×5000. C: ×13,000.)

immune cells found in HIVE, their secretion of cytokines could modulate neurologic damage if nervous system cells possessed appropriate receptors (38). We examined the distribution of cytokine receptors in fetal human brain tissue cultured *in vitro* as microspheres in vibratome sections of frontal cortical from AIDS autopsies. The autopsy material and the cultured brain microspheres were studied by confocal laser microscopy and immunocytochemistry/fluorescence using phycoerythrin-labeled cytokines and antibodies against cellular and viral markers. By immunofluorescent/laser confocal microscopy, IL-1β binding sites were identified on the surface of macrophages and neuronal processes. This binding could be blocked by preincubation

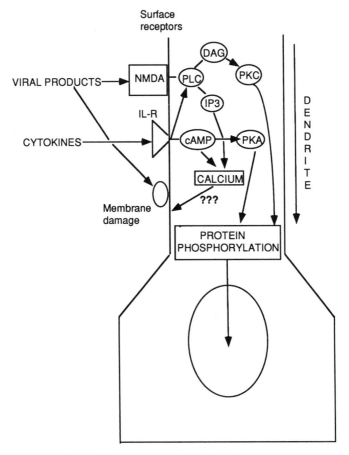

FIG. 6. Mechanisms of dendritic damage in HIVE. Putative viral products and cytokines with a potential neurotoxic effect might mediate this condition through specific receptors in the dendrite surface that activates enzymes that induce the release of calcium and phosphorylation of substrates. DAG, diacylglycerol; IP3, inositol-1,4,5-triphosphate; PKA, cAMP-dependent protein kinase; PKC, protein kinase C; PLC, phospholipase C.

with excess unlabeled IL-1β. Neuritic process binding sites were retained in a patch-like fashion on the cell surface. Processes immunolabeled for GFAP did not show IL-1β binding. In vibratome sections of AIDS brain tissues, binding sites appeared to be distributed on neuritic processes that were MAP2-positive. Preliminary quantitative analysis indicate increased IL-1β binding in HIVE correlating with macrophage infiltration, microglia activation, high levels of HIV proteins, and neuritic damage (38). Once a cytokine binds to its receptor, a cascade of intracellular events is triggered; among them, activation of PKC and calcium release and phosphorylation of specific proteins (39,40) (Fig. 6). In this regard, dendritic damage mediated by HIV could be triggered by overphosphorylation of substrates or calcium imbalance (Fig. 6). *In vitro* studies have shown that calcium blockers decrease HIV neurotoxicity, suggesting a possible role of calcium in HIVE neurodegeneration (34). However, it is still not clear by which intracellular pathway HIV toxin or toxins released from microglia or astrocytes mediate neurodegeneration in HIVE.

ACKNOWLEDGMENTS

The authors wish to thank Mrs. Margaret Mallory for her expert technical assistance. This work was supported by the following: a grant from the University of California AIDS Task Force; NIH grants NS-25178, MH45294, MH43298, and NS-00928 to CAW; Training Grants NS-07078 and UARP-F91SD050 to CLA; AG08201, AG08205, AG05131 to RDT; and AG10689-01, a grant from the Alzheimer Disease Association, to EM.

REFERENCES

1. Sharer LR. Pathology of HIV-1 infection of the central nervous system. A review. *J Neuropathol Exp Neurol* 1992;51:3–11.
2. Masliah E, Achim CL, Ge N, DeTeresa R, Terry RD, Wiley CA. Spectrum of human immunodeficiency virus-associated neocortical damage. *Ann Neurol* 1992;32:321–329.
3. Kure K, Llena JF, Lyman WD, et al. Human immunodeficiency virus-1 infection of the nervous system. An autopsy study of 268 adult, pediatric, and fetal brains. *Hum Pathol* 1991;22:700–710.
4. Brustle O, Spiegel H, Leib SL, et al. Distribution of human immunodeficiency virus (HIV) in the CNS of children with severe HIV encephalomyelopathy. *Acta Neuropathol* 1992; 84:24–31.
5. Budka H. Neuropathology of human immunodeficiency virus infection. *Brain Pathol* 1991; 1:163–175.
6. Achim CL, Schrier RD, Wiley CA. Immunopathogenesis of HIV encephalitis. *Brain Pathol* 1992;1:177–184.
7. Dickson DW, Belman AL, Park YD, et al. Central nervous system pathology in pediatric AIDS: an autopsy study. *APMIS* 1989;8:40–57.
8. Budka H, Wiley CA, Kleihues P, et al. HIV-associated disease of the nervous system: review of nomenclature and proposal for neuropathology-based terminology. *Brain Pathol* 1991;1:143–152.
9. Budka H, Costanzi G, Cristina S, et al. Brain pathology induced by infection with the

human immunodeficiency virus (HIV). A histological, immunocytochemical, and electron microscopical study of 100 autopsy cases. *Acta Neuropathol (Berl)* 1987;75:185–198.

10. Cvetkowich TA, Lazar E, Blumberg BM, et al. Human immunodeficiency virus type 1 infection of neural xenografts. *Proc Natl Acad Sci USA* 1992;89:5162–5166.

11. Kure K, Lyman WD, Weidenheim KM, Dickson DW. Cellular localization of an HIV-1 antigen in subacute AIDS encephalitis using an improved double-labeling immunohistochemical method. *Am J Pathol* 1990;136:1085–1092.

12. Wiley CA, Schrier RD, Nelson JA, Lampert PW, Oldstone MB. Cellular localization of human immunodeficiency virus infection within the brain of acquired immune deficiency syndrome patients. *Proc Natl Acad Sci USA* 1986;83:7089–7093.

13. McArthur JC, Becker PS, Parisi JE, et al. Neuropathological changes in early HIV-1 dementia. *Ann Neurol* 1989;26:681–684.

14. Kure K, Weidenheim KM, Lyman WD, Dickson DW. Morphology and distribution of HIV-1 gp41-positive microglia in subacute AIDS encephalitis. *Acta Neuropathol (Berl)* 1990;80:393–400.

15. Navia BA, Cho F, Petito CK, Price RW. The AIDS dementia complex. II. Neuropathology. *Ann Neurol* 1986;19:525–535.

16. Wiley CA, Masliah E, Morey M, et al. Neocortical damage during HIV infection. *Ann Neurol* 1991;29:651–657.

17. Artigas J, Niedobitek F, Grosse G, Heise W, Gosztonyi G. Spongiform encephalopathy in AIDS dementia complex: report of five cases. *AIDS* 1989;2:374–381.

18. Ketzler S, Weis S, Haug H, Budka H. Loss of neurons in the frontal cortex in AIDS brain. *Acta Neuropathol* 1990;80:92–94.

19. Everall IP, Luthert PJ, Lantos PL. Neuronal loss in the frontal cortex in HIV infection. *Lancet* 1991;337:1119–1121.

20. Clague CPT, Ostrowski MA, Deck JHN, Harnish DG, Colley EA, Stead RH. Severe diffuse necrotizing cortical encephalopathy in acquired immune deficiency syndrome (AIDS): an immunocytochemical and ultrastructural study. *J Neuropathol Exp Neurol* 1988;47:346.

21. Giangaspero F, Scanabissi E, Baldacci MC, Betts CM. Massive neuronal destruction in human immunodeficiency virus (HIV) encephalitis: a clinico-pathological study of a pediatric case. *Acta Neuropathol (Berl)* 1989;78:662–665.

22. Lackner AA, Smith MO, Munn RJ, et al. Localization of simian immunodeficiency virus in the central nervous system of rhesus monkeys. *Am J Pathol* 1991;139:609–621.

23. Masliah E, Ge N, Achim C, Hansen LA, Wiley CA. Selective neuronal vulnerability in HIV encephalitis. *J Neuropathol Exp Neurol* 1992;51:585–593.

24. Merrill JE, Chen ISY. HIV-1, macrophages, glial cells, and cytokines in AIDS nervous system disease. *FASEB J* 1991;5:2391–2397.

25. Masliah E, Ge N, Morey M, DeTeresa R, Terry RD, Wiley CA. Cortical dendritic pathology in human immunodeficiency virus encephalitis. *Lab Invest* 1992;66:285–291.

26. Masliah E, Terry RD, Alford M, DeTeresa R, Hansen LA. Cortical and subcortical patterns of synaptophysin-like immunoreactivity in Alzheimer disease. *Am J Pathol* 1991;138:235–246.

27. Baszler TV, Zachary JF. Murine retroviral-induced spongiform neuronal degeneration parallels resident microglial cell infection: ultrastructural findings. *Lab Invest* 1990;63:612–623.

28. Nagra RM, Burrola PG, Wiley CA. Development of spongiform encephalopathy in retroviral infected mice. *Lab Invest* 1992;66:292–302.

29. McArthur JC. Neurological manifestations of AIDS. *Medicine* 1987;66:407–437.

30. Price RW, Brew B, Sidtis J, Rosenblum M, Scheck AC, Cleary P. The brain in AIDS: central nervous system HIV-1 infection and AIDS dementia complex. *Science* 1988;239:586–592.

31. Glowa JR, Panlilio LV, Brenneman DE, Gozes I, Fridkin M, Hill JM. Learning impairment following intracerebral administration of the HIV envelope protein gp120 or a VIP antagonist. *Brain Res* 1992;570:49–53.

32. Lipton SA. Models of neuronal injury in AIDS: another role for the NMDA receptor? *Trends Neurol Sci* 1992;15:75–79.

33. Pulliam L, Herndier BG, Tang NM, McGrath MS. Human immunodeficiency virus-infected macrophages produce soluble factors that cause histological and neurochemical alterations in cultured human brains. *J Clin Invest* 1991;87:503–512.

34. Dreyer EB, Kaiser PK, Offermann JT, Lipton SA. HIV-1 coat protein neurotoxicity prevented by calcium channel antagonists. *Science* 1990;248:364–367.
35. Lipton SA. HIV-related neurotoxicity. *Brain Pathol* 1992;1:193–199.
36. Tyor WR, Glass JD, Griffin JW, et al. Cytokine expression in the brain during the acquired immunodeficiency syndrome. *Ann Neurol* 1992;31:349–360.
37. Miyajima A, Miyatake S, Schreurs J, et al. Coordinate regulation of immune and inflammatory responses by T cell-derived lymphokines. *FASEB J* 1988;2:2462–2473.
38. Achim CA, Wiley CA, Ge N, Masliah E. Cytokine receptor localization in human central nervous system *in vivo* and *in vitro:* correlation with HIV infection. *J Neuropathol Exp Neurol* 1992;51:374.
39. Yamato K, el-Hajjaoui Z, Simon K, Koeffler HP. Modulation of interleukin-1 beta RNA in moncytic cells infected with human immunodeficiency virus-1. *J Clin Invest* 1990;86: 1109–1114.
40. Rosoff PM, Savage N, Dinarello CA. Interleukin-1 stimulates diacylglycerol production in T lymphocytes by a novel mechanism. *Cell* 1988;54:73–81.

HIV, AIDS and the Brain, edited by
R. W. Price and S. W. Perry.
Raven Press, Ltd., New York © 1994.

7

Neuropathology and Pathogenesis of SIV Infection of the Central Nervous System

Leroy R. Sharer

Department of Laboratory Medicine and Pathology, New Jersey Medical School, Newark, NJ 07103

ANIMAL MODELS OF AIDS

After the discovery in 1983 of human immunodeficiency virus type 1 (HIV-1), the lentivirus that causes acquired immunodeficiency syndrome (AIDS) (1), it become imperative to develop an animal model of the disease, in order to study issues of pathogenesis and treatment. Several animal lentiviruses had been studied for some time, including equine infectious anemia virus, visna/maedi virus of sheep, and caprine arthritis–encephalitis virus (CAEV). It was recognized that the latter two caused neurological disease in their respective hosts, and it was soon appreciated that HIV-1 was also associated with an encephalopathy.

The obvious choice for an animal model was one that employed HIV-1 itself. Several problems were encountered in developing such a model, however. HIV-1 was found capable of infecting two nonhuman primate species, chimpanzees and gibbon apes, but in both cases the animals remained clinically well (2). Numerous other species were inoculated with the virus, but it was not possible to infect them. After a few years there appeared reports of infection of rabbits by HIV-1, but little information was provided about central nervous system (CNS) disease in this species (3). Recently there has been a report of the successful infection of pig-tailed macaques *(Macaca nemestrina)* with HIV-1, with signs of acute disease in the infected animals (4). The report, however, did not indicate if there was any neurological dysfunction or neuropathological change. Two rodent models, the HIV-1 transgenic mouse (5) and the severe combined immunodeficiency disease (SCID) mouse reconstituted with human immune cells and subsequently infected with HIV-1 (6), have also been developed, but there is limited information about CNS disease in these models.

Other animal lentiviruses, including visna/maedi and CAEV, have been advanced as animal models for CNS disease in AIDS. However, these diseases are not generally associated with immunodeficiency, and the neuropathology of these disorders is unlike that of HIV-1. More recently, feline immunodeficiency virus (FIV) has been proposed as a model for HIV-1 encephalitis, but there are insufficient data about the model at this time (7).

THE SIMIAN IMMUNODEFICIENCY VIRUSES

The simian immunodeficiency viruses (SIVs) are a group of African nonhuman primate lentiviruses that can cause an AIDS-like disease in an appropriate Asian simian host. The first of the SIVs to be discovered, now called SIVmac, was reported in rhesus macaques *(Macaca mulatta)* at the New England Regional Primate Research Center in 1985 (8). SIVs have been isolated from other Asian macaque species, including SIVmne, which was recovered from *M. nemestrina* (9). An isolate closely related to SIVmac, in terms of genomic organization and homogeneity, was obtained from sooty mangabey monkeys *(Cercocebus atys)* of African origin; in this species, the animals that are infected with SIV, termed SIVsmm, have no symptoms (10). The SIVmac and SIVsmm isolates are closely related not only to each other but also to HIV-2. Hirsch et al. (11) have proposed that HIV-2 diverged from these SIVs as recently as 30–40 years ago.

More distantly related to these SIVs are isolates from African green (vervet) monkeys *(Cercopithecus aethiops),* termed SIVagm (12). Even more remotely related to all these SIVs is an isolate from a chimpanzee *(Pan troglodytes)* from the wild, from Gabon, termed SIVcpz (13). It is of interest that this isolate appears to be more closely related to HIV-1 than it is to any other SIV, since none of the other SIVs has significant genomic homogeneity with HIV-1. It should be noted that there has been accidental transmission of SIVsmm to a human laboratory worker (14). This episode should not be surprising, since various SIVs can be readily propagated in human lymphocytes *in vitro*.

When either SIVmac or SIVsmm is injected into a macaque species of Asian origin, the animals frequently develop AIDS, characterized by progressive depletion of CD4 lymphocytes, opportunistic infections, wasting, and death. At autopsy, besides various viral, fungal, parasitic, and bacterial opportunistic infections, these animals exhibit lymphocyte depletion in lymph nodes and spleen as well as multinucleated (syncytial) giant cells (MGCs) in multiple organs, including the gastrointestinal tract, lungs, and brain. The lesions in brain constitute an immunodeficiency virus-like encephalitis, with remarkable similarities to lesions of HIV-1 encephalitis in humans.

PATHOLOGY OF SIV MENINGOENCEPHALITIS

The earliest reports of SIVmac infection of rhesus macaques indicated that there were lesions in the brain that contained MGCs (Fig. 1) (8). We

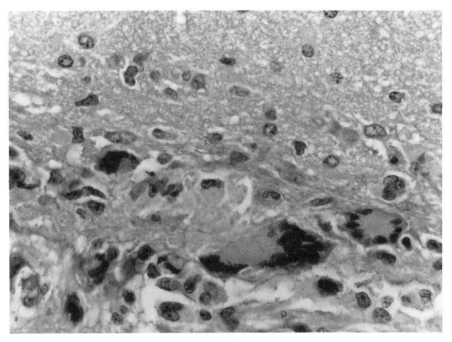

FIG. 1. Multinucleated (syncytial) giant cells (MGCs) in subependymal region, occipital lobe; rhesus monkey infected with SIV. Note the similarity to MGCs seen in the brains of humans with HIV-1 encephalitis. (Hematoxylin and eosin, ×600.)

and others noted the resemblance to the MGCs associated with HIV-1 (15), and it was therefore proposed that SIV encephalitis was a model for HIV-1 encephalitis in humans. CNS lesions were particularly severe in juvenile rhesus monkeys, and this suggested a similarity to HIV-1 encephalitis in children (15). The two disease, SIV encephalitis and HIV-1 encephalitis, do indeed have many similarities, although there are important differences as well.

Gross examination of the brain of a rhesus macaque infected with SIV is often unrevealing, although there may be mild enlargement of the lateral ventricles. The most characteristic microscopical lesion in the CNS associated with SIV infection is the inflammatory cell infiltrate, consisting chiefly of infected macrophages (Fig. 2) as well as MGCs (15). This lesion is generally perivascular; and although it can be found anywhere in the CNS, it is most frequently encountered in the central white matter of the cerebral hemispheres, the basal ganglia, and the pons. These macrophage infiltrates have been likened to granulomas (16), although granulomas are not generally a feature of viral infections of the CNS. Karyorrhexis is often seen in the lesions, which may contain small numbers of lymphocytes as well. The

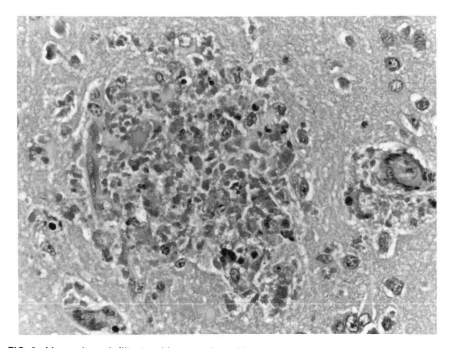

FIG. 2. Macrophage infiltrate with necrosis and karyorrhexis, frontal cortex; rhesus monkey infected with SIV. Note MGCs to the right of the infiltrate. (Hematoxylin and eosin, ×375.)

macrophages and MGCs contain both SIV viral antigen, on immunocytochemistry, and SIV-specific nucleic acid sequences, by *in situ* hybridization (Fig. 3); and lentiviral particles can be demonstrated within them, on ultrastructural examination. Microglia are also infected by SIV (17), but virus cannot be demonstrated in neuroectodermal cells (neurons, astrocytes, and oligodendrocytes), by standard techniques.

The macrophage infiltrates are often surrounded by reactive, gemistocytic astrocytes, and in rare instances they may be accompanied by vacuolation of the neuropil (18). Perivascular accumulations of lymphocytes can be seen in the parenchyma, usually occurring early in the course of disease. We have observed lymphocytes about vessels as early as 2 weeks after experimental infection, before the occurrence of infected perivascular macrophages (Fig. 4) (19). White matter or myelin pallor is an unusual phenomenon, and when it does occur it is usually restricted to the immediate vicinity of the macrophage infiltrates and is not diffuse. White matter astrocytosis, as viewed for example with immunocytochemistry for glial fibrillary acidic protein (GFAP), cannot be confidently distinguished in the SIV-infected macaque brain, because of the normal background astrocytic prominence in the white matter of uninfected rhesus macaques (Fig. 5) (19). In the uninfected macaque, the astro-

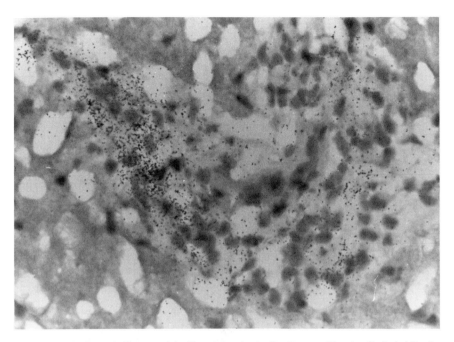

FIG. 3. Macrophage infiltrate, with silver granules indicating positive *in situ* hybridization for SIV-specific nucleic acid sequences; cerebellar white matter of rhesus monkey infected with SIV. [Frozen section, with ^{35}S-labeled probe for SIV (19); hematoxylin and eosin counterstain, ×600.]

cytes of the cerebral white matter have copious cytoplasm and tapering processes that are GFAP-positive, an appearance that in the brains of human children and adults would be considered to be pathological. Decreased neuronal density in the cerebral cortex, which has been reported in the brains of humans with HIV-1 encephalitis (20), has not as yet been documented in the simian model.

A prominent feature of SIV infection of the macaque brain is lymphocytic leptomeningitis, with MGCs that can be demonstrated to harbor the virus (Fig. 6) (15). MGCs containing SIV antigen and specific nucleic acid sequences can be found in the leptomeninges as early as 2 weeks after experimental infection (19). It would appear that the cerebrospinal fluid (CSF) compartment is infected independently of the CNS compartment. Inflammation of the stroma of the choroid plexus, also with MGCs, occurs as well.

If SIV encephalitis of the macaque CNS is to serve as an animal model for HIV-1 encephalitis, it must have some resemblance to the human disorder. Table 1 lists similarities between the simian and the human immunodeficiency virus encephalitides, while the most important differences are given in Table 2. The major difference between the two disorders is the relative

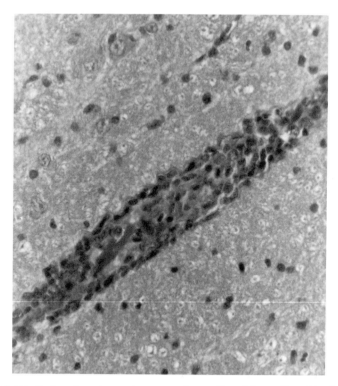

FIG. 4. Perivascular lymphocytes and mononuclear cells, white matter of basis pontis, 2 weeks following experimental infection of rhesus macaque with SIV (19). This and other infiltrates were negative for SIV antigen, on immunocytochemistry. No SIV-positive macrophages could be detected in parenchyma at this time point, although positive cells were found in leptomeninges. (Hematoxylin and eosin, ×375.)

lack, in the simian model, of prominent white matter pathology, the importance of which has been stressed in human subjects with HIV-1 by many investigators, based on both clinical imaging and pathological studies (21). It could be argued that because this feature is missing, SIV is not a suitable model for HIV-1 encephalitis; however, this must be weighed against the numerous similarities between the two encephalitides. The cellular pathology of SIV encephalitis is startlingly reminiscent of HIV-1 encephalitis, particularly the productively infected MGCs. The topographies of the two encephalitides—and, more important, the cell tropisms of the two viruses—are virtually identical.

Most of the early reports of SIV-related AIDS in macaque species gave little information about the neurological status of the affected animals, other than to mention terminal obtundation. Thus it was initially uncertain whether SIV infection had a clinical correlate for either HIV-1-associated dementia or cognitive/motor impairment. More recently a study has documented the

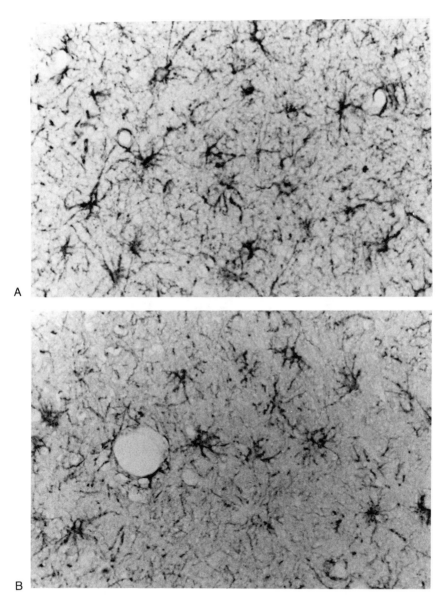

FIG. 5. A: Astrocytes in cerebral deep white matter of a juvenile rhesus macaque infected with SIV. Note prominent cell bodies and tapering processes. **B:** Astrocytes in cerebral deep white matter of control, uninfected juvenile rhesus macaque. The appearance of the astrocytes is virtually indistinguishable from that of part A. [A, B: immunocytochemistry for glial fibrillary acidic protein (GFAP), nickel-enhanced diaminobenzidine chromogen, no counterstain, ×375.]

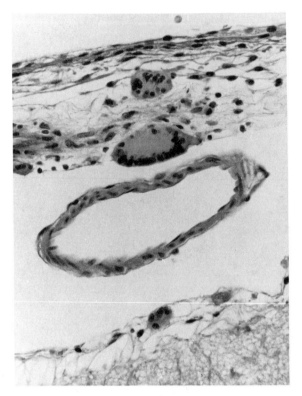

FIG. 6. MGCs and mononuclear cells in leptomeninges of rhesus monkey infected with SIV. One of the MGCs has tapering processes extending from the nuclei, so-called "nuclear bridges." (Hematoxylin and eosin, ×325.)

TABLE 1. *Similarities between HIV-1 and SIV encephalitides*

1. Infected cells are chiefly of monocyte origin, including macrophages, microglial cells, and multinucleated giant cells.
2. Topographic distribution of lesions: most frequent in cerebral white matter, basal ganglia, and pons.
3. No evidence of direct infection of cells of neuroectodermal origin.
4. Mild, diffuse astrocytosis demonstrable in cerebral cortex.

TABLE 2. *Differences between HIV-1 encephalitis and SIV encephalitis*

HIV-1	SIV
1. White matter pallor and gliosis	1. Minimal white matter change
2. Minimal or mild leptomeningitis	2. Prominent leptomeningitis, with MGCs

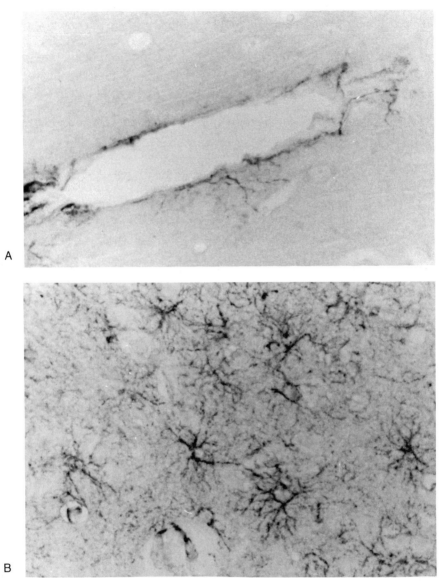

FIG. 7. A: Middle layers of cerebral cortex of control, uninfected rhesus macaque (same animal as in Fig. 5B). Only a few astrocytes can be discerned, adjacent to a blood vessel. **B:** Prominent astrocytes in middle layers of cerebral cortex of rhesus monkey with SIV encephalitis (same animal as in Fig. 5A). Cortical astrocytosis was diffuse in this animal and was not confined to regions of inflammation. (A, B: immunocytochemistry for GFAP, nickel-enhanced diaminobenzidine chromogen, no counterstain, ×430.)

development of cognitive and motor deficits in a group of eight rhesus monkeys that had been trained on a test battery prior to infection with the SIVsmm isolate Delta/B670 (22). Seven of the eight animals developed motor impairment, while three (including the single animal that did not have motor involvement) had cognitive deficits, both at a time when the animals were relatively free of systemic illness related to SIV. Control animals included two monkeys that were not inoculated with SIV, as well as two inoculated animals that failed to develop productive infection and were considered uninfected. None of the four uninfected controls had any cognitive or motor impairment over the 1-year period of observation. CSF quinolinic acid levels were positively correlated with the onset of motor skill impairment but not with cognitive impairment (23). At necropsy in the infected animals there were varying degrees of CNS involvement by SIV encephalitis, with no obvious correlation between either the severity or the location of the lesions and the degree of impairment during life. All eight of the infected animals had astrocytosis in the cerebral cortex, while only one of the uninfected (and uninoculated) animals had a comparable degree of gliosis (Figs. 7 and 8) (23–25). In a more recent experiment, one productively infected rhesus monkey that had no deficits on testing also had no gliosis in the cerebral cortex (25). These findings suggest that there is either a direct or an indirect effect

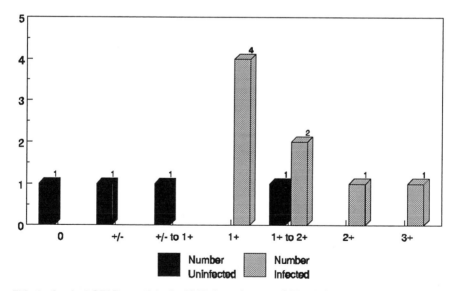

FIG. 8. Cortical GFAP reactivity in SIV-infected versus SIV-uninfected rhesus macaques. The x axis indicates the degree of GFAP staining, from 0 to 3 +, while the y axis indicates the number of animals with each degree of change. Only one uninfected, control animal had notable GFAP reactivity in cerebral cortex, compared with eight of eight infected monkeys.

of SIV on the cerebral cortex, as had been proposed for humans with HIV-1 infection and that this effect is related to the cognitive/motor deficits.

In addition to SIV encephalitis, SIV-infected macaques may develop opportunistic infections of the CNS, the most common of which is simian cytomegalovirus (simian CMV) encephalitis, which is a necrotizing inflammatory disease with prominent meningitis and a polymorphonuclear leukocytic response (26). Opportunistic infections with simian virus-40 (SV-40) have also occurred, both with (27) and without (L Sharer, *unpublished observations*) lesions resembling progressive multifocal leukoencephalopathy (PML) in humans. Lymphomas, sometimes associated with simian Epstein–Barr virus infection, have also been observed in both the CNS and the peripheral nervous system. Surprisingly, encephalitis due to Herpesvirus simiae has not been reported, despite the high prevalence of this virus in macaque species.

PATHOGENESIS OF SIV MENINGOENCEPHALITIS

Infection of the CNS by an SIV isolate appears to depend on the development of macrophage tropism of the particular isolate, since lymphocytetropic strains do not appear to enter the CNS compartment (28,29). Similar experimental data exist for HIV-1 infection of the human CNS (30,31). Several studies have indicated that SIV enters both the CSF and the CNS compartments early in the course of experimental infection, within the first few weeks (19,32). An analogy has been made (19) with the occasional patient who develops aseptic meningitis, acute encephalopathy, or both shortly after infection with HIV-1, often preceding seroconversion (33). Infection of the CNS compartment would appear to occur from the bloodstream, rather than from the CSF, in view of the later finding of perivascular mononuclear cells and infected macrophages (19). Ringler and colleagues (34) have presented evidence that the endothelial cell adhesion molecule VCAM-1 is up-regulated in blood vessels in the brain of macaques with SIV encephalitis. More recently, his group has demonstrated *in vitro* adhesion of macrophage cells to these vessels in frozen sections of brain tissue from monkeys with SIV encephalitis, with blocking of macrophage adhesion by anti-VCAM-1 antibodies (D. Ringler, *personal communication*). It is likely that SIV enters the CNS during normal monocyte trafficking, with passage of virus into the CNS via infected monocytes. Although infected cells must pass through or between them, the endothelial cells themselves would not appear to be directly infected by SIV at any point, based on our own observations (19) as well as those of Lackner et al. (17).

In summary, the SIV macaque model has proved useful for the study of issues of pathogenesis that relate to HIV encephalopathy in humans. Although there are differences between SIV encephalitis in macaques and HIV encephalitis in humans, the similarities continue to outweigh them. We can anticipate further advances from this animal model of human disease.

ACKNOWLEDGMENTS

Collaboration of the following is gratefully acknowledged: at the Tulane (Delta) Regional Primate Research Center: Dr. Gary B. Baskin and Dr. Michael Murphey-Corb; at the Laboratory of Cell Biology, National Institutes of Mental Health: Dr. Lee Eiden, Dr. Elizabeth Murray, Dr. Diane Rausch, and Dr. Judit Lendvay; at the University of Mainz, Germany: Dr. Eberhard Weihe and Dr. Donatus Nohr; at the University of Rochester School of Medicine: Dr. Leon G. Epstein; and at New Jersey Medical School: Dr. Jennifer Michaels, Mr. Scott Diegmann, and Ms. Dana Settembre. Research for this chapter was funded in part by PHS Grant NS 25121 from the NIH.

REFERENCES

1. Barré-Sinoussi F, Chermann JC, Rey F, et al. Isolation of a T-lymphotropic retrovirus from a patient at risk for acquired immune deficiency syndrome (AIDS). *Science* 1983;220: 868–871.
2. Watanabe M, Ringler DJ, Fultz PN, et al. A chimpanzee-passaged human immunodeficiency virus isolate is cytopathic for chimpanzee cells but does not induce disease. *J Virol* 1991;65:3344–3348.
3. Kulaga H, Folks T, Rutledge R, Truckenmiller ME, Gugel E, Kindt TJ. Infection of rabbits with human immunodeficiency virus 1. *J Exp Med* 1989;169:321–326.
4. Agy MB, Frumkin LR, Corey L, et al. Infection of *Macaca nemestrina* by human immunodeficiency virus type-1. *Science* 1992;257:103–106.
5. Leonard JM, Abramczuk JW, Pezen DS, et al. Development of disease and virus recovery in transgenic mice containing HIV proviral DNA. *Science* 1988;242:1665–1670.
6. Namikawa R, Kaneshima H, Lieberman M, Weissman IL, McCune JM. Infection of the SCID-hu mouse by HIV-1. *Science* 1988;242:1684–1686.
7. Hurtrel M, Ganière J-P, Guelfi J-F, et al. Comparison of early and late feline immunodeficiency virus encephalopathies. *AIDS* 1992;6:399–406.
8. Letvin NL, Daniel MD, Sehgal PK, et al. Induction of AIDS-like disease in macaque monkeys with T-cell tropic retrovirus STLV-III. *Science* 1985;230:71–73.
9. Benveniste RE, Morton WR, Clark EA, et al. Inoculation of baboons and macaques with simian immunodeficiency virus/Mne, a primate lentivirus closely related to human immunodeficiency virus type 2. *J Virol* 1988;62:2091–2101.
10. Murphey-Corb M, Martin LN, Rangan SR, et al. Isolation of an HTLV-III-related retrovirus from macaques with simian AIDS and its possible origin in asymptomatic mangabeys. *Nature* 1986;321:435–437.
11. Hirsch VM, Olmsted RA, Murphey-Corb M, Purcell RH, Johnson PR. An African primate lentivirus (SIVsm) closely related to HIV-2. *Nature* 1989;339:389–392.
12. Allan JS, Short M, Taylor ME, et al. Species-specific diversity among simian immunodeficiency viruses from African green monkeys. *J Virol* 1991;65:2816–2828.
13. Huet T, Cheynier R, Meyerhans A, Roelants G, Wain-Hobson S. Genetic organization of a chimpanzee lentivirus related to HIV-1. *Nature* 1990;345:356–359.
14. Khabbaz RF, Rowe T, Murphey-Corb M, et al. Simian immunodeficiency virus needlestick accident in a laboratory worker. *Lancet* 1992;340:271–273.
15. Sharer LR, Baskin GB, Cho E-S, Murphey-Corb M, Blumberg BM, Epstein LG. Comparison of simian immunodeficiency virus and human immunodeficiency virus in the immature host. *Ann Neurol* 1988;23S:108–112.

16. Letvin NL, King NW. Immunologic and pathologic manifestations of the infection of rhesus monkeys with simian immunodeficiency virus of macaques. *J AIDS* 1990;3:1023–1040.
17. Lackner AA, Smith MO, Munn RJ, et al. Localization of simian immunodeficiency virus in the central nervous system of rhesus monkeys. *Am J Pathol* 1991;139:609–621.
18. Sharer LR, Baskin GB, Michaels J, Diegmann S. Vacuoles in SIV myelitis [Abstract]. *J Neuropathol Exp Neurol* 1990;49:352.
19. Sharer LR, Michaels J, Murphey-Corb M, et al. Serial pathogenesis study of SIV brain infection. *J Med Primatol* 1991;20:211–217.
20. Wiley CA, Masliah E, Morey M, et al. Neocortical damage during HIV infection. *Ann Neurol* 1991;29:651–657.
21. Sharer LR. Pathology of HIV-1 infection of the central nervous system [Review]. *J Neuropathol Exp Neurol* 1992;51:3–11.
22. Murray EA, Rausch DM, Lendvay J, Sharer LR, Eiden LE. Cognitive and motor impairments associated with SIV infection in rhesus monkeys. *Science* 1992;255:1246–1249.
23. Rausch DM, Heyes MP, Murray EA, et al. Cytopathologic and neurochemical correlates of progression to motor/cognitive impairment in SIV-infected rhesus monkeys. Submitted for publication.
24. Sharer LR, Weihe E, Nohr D, et al. Cortical gliosis in SIV-infected macaques with documented cognitive-motor impairment [Abstract]. *J Neuropathol Exp Neurol* 1992;51:354.
25. Weihe E, Nohr D, Sharer L, Murray E, Rausch D, Eiden L. Cortical astrocytosis in juvenile rhesus monkeys infected with simian immunodeficiency virus. *Neuroreport* 1993;4: 263–266.
26. Baskin GB. Disseminated cytomegalovirus infection in immunodeficient rhesus monkeys. *Am J Pathol* 1987;19:345–352.
27. Horvath CJ, Simon MA, Bergsagel DJ, et al. Simian virus 40-induced disease in rhesus monkeys with simian acquired immunodeficiency syndrome. *Am J Pathol* 1992;140: 1431–1440.
28. Desrosiers RC, Hansen-Moosa A, Mori K, et al. Macrophage-tropic variants of SIV are associated with specific AIDS-related lesions but are not essential for the development of AIDS. *Am J Pathol* 1991;139:29–35.
29. Sharma DP, Zink MC. Anderson M, et al. Derivation of neurotropic simian immunodeficiency virus from exclusively lymphocytetropic parental virus: pathogenesis of infection in macaques. *J Virol* 1992;66:3550–3556.
30. Koyanagi Y, Miles S, Mitsuyasu RT, Merrill JE, Vinters HV, Chen ISY. Dual infection of the central nervous system by AIDS viruses with distinct cellular tropisms. *Science* 1987;236:819–822.
31. Epstein LG, Kuiken C, Blumberg BM, et al. HIV-1 V3 domain variation in brain and spleen of children with AIDS: tissue-specific evolution within host-determined quasispecies. *Virology* 1991;180:583–590.
32. Chakrabarti L, Hurtrel M, Maire M-A, et al. Early viral replication in the brain of SIV-infected rhesus monkeys. *Am J Pathol* 1991;139:1273–1280.
33. Michaels J, Sharer LR, Epstein LG. Human immunodeficiency virus type 1 (HIV-1) infection of the nervous system: a review. *Immunodeficiency Rev* 1988;1:71–104.
34. Sasseville VG, Newman WA, Lackner AA, et al. Elevated vascular cell adhesion molecule-1 in AIDS encephalitis induced by simian immunodeficiency virus. *Am J Pathol* 1992;141: 1021–1030.

HIV, AIDS and the Brain, edited by
R. W. Price and S. W. Perry.
Raven Press, Ltd., New York © 1994.

8

The SIV Model of AIDS Encephalopathy

Role of Neurotropic Viruses in Diseases

*Janice E. Clements, †Mark G. Anderson,
*M. Christine Zink, ‡Sanjay V. Joag, and ‡Opendra Narayan

*Department of Neurology, Johns Hopkins University School of Medicine,
Baltimore, MD 21205; †Department of Chemistry, University of Colorado,
Boulder, CO 80309; and ‡Department of Microbiology, University of Kansas
Medical Center, Kansas City, KS 66160

The simian immunodeficiency viruses (SIV_{mac}) cause pathological changes and clinical diseases in rhesus macaques that are strinkingly similar to the effects of human immunodeficiency virus (HIV) in humans (1–3). The SIV model provides a valuable system to investigate the mechanisms of pathogenesis of the multiple clinical syndromes characteristic of HIV infections in humans. SIV and HIV are members of the lentivirus family of retroviruses (4); they cause persistent infection and infect $CD4^+$ lymphocytes and cells of the macrophage lineage *in vivo* (5–9). The cell tropism of these viruses are reflected in the varied types of clinical diseases that are seen in infected hosts (2,5–7,10–12). The tropism of both HIV and SIV for $CD4^+$ lymphocytes is associated with functional loss of this subset of T cells. This results in the profound immunosuppression that results in the various opportunistic infections and oncogenic syndromes known collectively as the *acquired immunodeficiency syndrome* (AIDS) (8). A tropism of these viruses for monocytes and macrophages has been correlated with inflammatory and/or degenerative changes in specific organs such as the lung and brain. In these organs, giant-cell pneumonia or neuropathological changes accompany virus replication in macrophages in the affected tissues (13–17). These observations suggest that HIV and SIV isolates with a strict tropism for lymphocytes cause mainly AIDS, while viruses with a tropism for macrophages cause organ-specific diseases such as pneumonia and encephalopathy (5,14,15). HIV isolates with a dual tropism for T cells and macrophages have been isolated from the brain of patients who had the AIDS dementia complex (ADC).

This broadened cell tropism has been correlated with central nervous system (CNS) disease (14,16,18–20). Furthermore, recent studies have suggested that macrophage-tropic viruses isolated from the CNS represent a limited subset of macrophage-tropic viruses in an HIV-infected individual and have a selective tropism for resident brain macrophages called microglial cells (15,21). SIV infection of macaques provides an ideal model system to test this hypothesis.

MOLECULAR SIMILARITIES BETWEEN HIV AND SIV

The SIVs currently include four major subgroups of non-human-primate lentiviruses. Viruses in these four groups show distinct tropisms and pathogenic properties. The subgroups are based on the species from which the virus was isolated and include (a) macaque/mangabey (SIV_{mac}/SIV_{sm}), (b) African green monkey (SIV_{agm}), (c) Mandrill (SIV_{mnd}), and (d) Chimpanzee (SIV_{cpz}). At the molecular level, these four groups appear to be equidistant from each other when subjected to phylogenetic tree analyses (22). Viruses from two of the subgroups are closely related to the viruses that cause AIDS in humans: $SIV_{mac/sm}$ to HIV-2 and SIV_{cpz} to HIV-1. SIV_{mac} infection of rhesus macaques causes a disease that closely resembles the progressive pathologic changes observed in humans infected with HIV-1.

The genomic organization of SIV_{mac} and HIV-1 is compared in Fig. 1. There is little difference in their genomic structure; both viruses contain the structural *(gag* and *env)* genes as well as the enzymatic gene *(pol)*. Some differences are seen in the location of the auxiliary genes *vpu* (in HIV-1) and *vpx* (in SIV_{mac}). However, the *tat* and *rev* regulatory genes shown to be essential for HIV-1 replication are present and conserved in all strains of SIV_{mac}.

The envelope genes of HIV-1 and SIV_{mac} encode two glycoproteins: gp41, the transmembrane protein, serves as an anchor for gp120, the surface glycoprotein, which forms the knob-like structures on the outside of virions. These glycoproteins contain multiple regions or epitopes that affect viral entry and thereby contribute to viral tropism and potential cytopathicity. Epitopes in gp120 interact with the CD4 receptor on both CD4$^+$ lymphocytes and monocytes/macrophages, representing a major determinant of viral entry. In addition, gp120 contains epitopes that elicit neutralizing antibodies against the viruses. Changes in these epitopes on the surface glycoprotein have been associated with the altered cell tropism of HIV-1. The transmembrane glycoprotein contains a stretch of hydrophobic amino acids in both HIV-1 and SIV_{mac} that is involved in the fusion event between the virus and cell membrane. Changes in the transmembrane protein of HIV-1 are associated with altered cytopathicity of the virus in cell culture.

The long terminal repeat (LTR) of the viruses contain the signals that

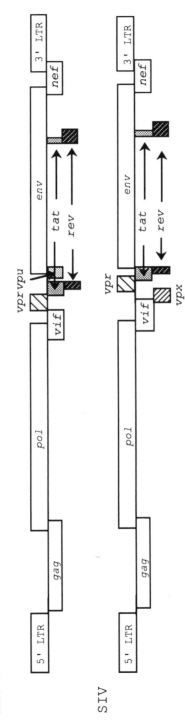

FIG. 1. Comparison of the organization of HIV-1 and SIV DNA.

regulate transcription of viral RNA (in the 5' LTR) and polyadenylation (in the 3' LTR). Cellular transcription factors bind to specific nucleotide sequences in the U3 region of the 5' LTR to control the level of transcription. Nucleotide sequence changes in this region can have effects at the transcriptional level that result in increased or decreased levels of viral replication in particular cells. Changes in the U3 region of the LTRs of HIV-1 isolates from the CNS of a patient with ADC have been shown to be associated with increased levels of expression in the brain of transgenic mice (23). In other retroviral systems the LTR has been associated with altered pathogenic potential and disease outcome in infected animals (24–26). Thus, changes in the envelope gene as well as the LTR may cause changes in cell tropism and virus replication that can lead to neurotropic and neurovirulent viruses.

NEUROADAPTATION OF SIV$_{mac}$239

A pathogenic molecular clone of SIV (SIV$_{mac}$239) was used to examine the role of macrophage-tropic virus in CNS disease. SIV$_{mac}$239 replicates only in lymphocytes *in vivo* and has been shown to cause an AIDS-like disease in macaques associated with depletion of T cells (1,2,6,27,28). Thus SIV$_{mac}$239, a molecularly cloned virus that was strictly T-cell-tropic and did not cause CNS disease, was used to determine if virus mutation and subsequent selection during infection in macaques would result in a macrophage-tropic virus that could cause CNS disease (Fig. 2) (28,29). Initial attempts to inoculate the virus intracerebrally (I.C.) were not successful in causing infection of the brain. However, virus-infected cells were found in the bone marrow, spleen, and peripheral blood probably due to the spillover of I.C.-inoculated virus into the bloodstream (30,31). Bone marrow cells from this animal showed evidence of virus replication in macrophage precursor cells and were therefore used to inoculate a subsequent animal, referred to as "10C" (Fig. 2). Rhesus macaque 10C died in less than 3 months with severe interstitial pneumonia with multinucleated giant cells. Using both *in situ* hybridization to detect SIV RNA and immunocytochemistry to show the presence of SIV protein, macrophages in the lung were shown to be infected with SIV$_{mac}$. Virus isolated from bone marrow and lung of 10C replicated in primary rhesus macrophage cultures. However, no virus was detected in the brain. Viral RNA could not be detected by *in situ* hybridization, nor could viral DNA be detected by the polymerase chain reaction (PCR) in the brain of this animal. Thus, *in vivo* passage of SIV$_{mac}$239 in rhesus macaques resulted in a broadened tropism of the virus from strictly T cells to include macrophages. The presence of macrophage-tropic SIV in this animal resulted in clinical disease in the lung. Neither virus nor virus-infected monocyte/macrophages crossed the blood–brain barrier to infect microglial cells in the brain.

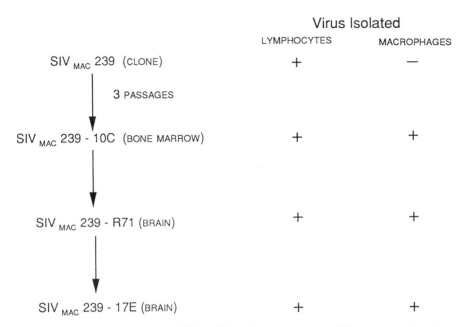

FIG. 2. The *in vivo* passages of SIV$_{mac}$239 in rhesus macaques. Virus isolated from the animals were titrated in lymphocyte cell lines or primary rhesus macaques macrophages.

Further passage *in vivo* of the macrophage-tropic virus was done to determine if virus that replicated in the CNS could be selected. Bone marrow cells from rhesus macaque 10C (Fig. 2) were used to inoculate two macaques I.C. Both animals developed SIV-induced pneumonia and encephalitis. In the brain, there were multifocal aggregates of mononuclear and multinucleated cells, and perivascular cuffs were observed throughout the neuropil. *In situ* hybridization and lectin histochemistry (RCA-1, a lectin that detects microglia) showed that virus was present mainly in macrophages. Virus isolated from brain homogenates replicated in both lymphocytes and primary rhesus macrophage cultures. In contrast, virus isolated from the peripheral blood leukocytes and spleen homogenates replicated only in lymphocytes. Thus, in both infected macaques, strictly lymphocyte-tropic viruses and macrophage-tropic viruses were present, although they were found replicating in different tissues.

To determine if the SIV strain in the brain of these animals was able to enter the brain after inoculation in the periphery, brain homogenate (from macaque R71) was used to infect two rhesus macaques in bone marrow and one animal I.C. (macaque 17E). All three animals were infected as determined by virus in blood and cerebrospinal fluid (CSF). Both lymphocytes and macrophages from these animals were found to be infected with SIV. Macaque 17E that was infected I.C. died 5 months after infection with severe disseminated SIV encephalitis. Brain homogenates had a high level of virus associated with infection of macrophages.

The two animals that were inoculated in the bone marrow did not develop disease after 6 months and were euthanized. Examination of brain, lungs, and spleen showed no histological evidence of virus infection, and no virus was isolated from these tissues. These studies demonstrate that a strictly T-lymphocyte-tropic virus can give rise to a macrophage-tropic virus after replication *in vivo* and that macrophage-tropism of SIV is necessary for infection and disease in both lung and brain. Thus, the macrophage-tropic/neurotropic SIV is virulent and replicates to high levels in macrophages in the brain but in these short-term infections failed to invade the brain after infection in the bone marrow.

MOLECULAR CHARACTERIZATION OF THE NEUROTROPIC VIRUS IN THE BRAINS OF MACAQUES R71 AND 17E

The envelope genes of SIV and HIV have been shown to be a major determinant of cellular tropism. This gene would be expected to contain the amino acid changes that would alter the tropism of $SIV_{mac}239$ from strictly lymphocyte-tropic to macrophage-tropic. The envelope genes of SIV viruses present in the brain of the two macaques R71 and 17E were examined to identify amino acid changes that occurred during neuroadaptation. This was done to determine if the viruses present in the brain of the two animals represented a wide heterogeneous group of isolates or were a limited number of closely related viruses. The viral envelope genes in the brain were examined directly by performing the PCR on DNA isolated from the brain of macaques R71 and 17E. The amplified products from multiple PCR samples were examined by direct nucleotide sequence analysis to determine the sequence of the population of envelope genes found in the brain (32).

Examination of the nucleotide sequences for the SIV envelope genes in the brain of macaque R71 revealed a relatively small number of amino acid changes when compared to the molecular clone of $SIV_{mac}239$ used for these studies. Sixteen amino acid changes (in the 730-amino-acid region analyzed) were detected in the population of envelope genes found in R71 brain. The amino acid changes were not localized in any specific region of the envelope gene but were dispersed throughout the surface glycoprotein (12/16 amino acid changes) as well as in the transmembrane glycoprotein (4/16).

To determine whether the changes found in the viruses in the brain of macaque R71 were stable and maintained in the next *in vivo* passage in monkey brain, DNA from brain of macaque 17E was amplified by PCR to analyze the nucleotide sequence of the envelope gene. The amino acid changes found in the viral DNA in 17E brain were very similar to those found in the R71 SIV viruses. Of the 16 amino acid changes found in the

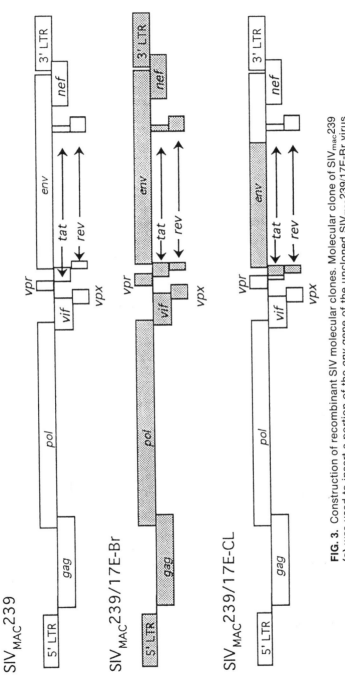

FIG. 3. Construction of recombinant SIV molecular clones. Molecular clone of SIV$_{mac}$239 **(a)** was used to insert a portion of the *env* gene of the uncloned SIV$_{mac}$239/17E-Br virus **(b)** to construct the infectious molecular clone SIV$_{mac}$239/17E-Cl **(c)**.

SIV$_{MAC}$239

SIV$_{MAC}$239/17E-Br

SIV$_{MAC}$239/17E-CL

TABLE 1. *Cell tropism of SIV_{mac} viruses[a]*

Virus	CEMx174	Macrophages
SIV_{mac} 239 (clone)	10^4	10^1
SIV_{mac} 239/R71$_{Br}$	10^4	10^3
SIV_{mac} 239/17E$_{Br}$	10^4	10^4
SIV_{mac} 239/17E (clone)	10^4	10^4

[a] $TCID_{50}$ of the viruses was determined in CEMx174 cells (a lymphocyte cell line) or in primary rhesus macaque macrophages.

17E SIV viruses, 14 were the same as found in the consensus sequence for the R71 SIV virus.

Thus, from the nucleotide sequence analysis, it is clear that a predominant SIV strain was present in the brain of macaque R71, and this strongly suggests that this virus has a selective advantage for replication in the brain. The identification of a closely related strain of SIV in the 17E brain further supports these ideas and shows that the virus strain present in R71 represents a stable virus genotype that was passaged to macaque 17E. Since the virus isolated from the brain is macrophage-tropic, it may indicate that the selective replication in the brain represents a tropism for resident brain macrophages, the microglial cells.

To determine if the envelope gene of the 17E strain would alter the cellular tropism of the parental strain of $SIV_{mac}239$, a recombinant molecular clone was constructed. The molecular clone contained the genome of $SIV_{mac}239$ with a portion of the envelope gene replaced with the envelope cloned from the brain of macaque 17E (Fig. 3). This molecular clone ($SIV_{mac}239/17E$) was examined for both production of virus and the cell tropism of the virus that was produced. The molecular clone was transfected into a human T-cell-line CEMx174 cells, and virus was detected. This virus was then examined for its ability to replicate in primary rhesus macrophages in comparison to the $SIV_{mac}239$ cloned virus as well as the viruses isolated from the brain from macaque 17E. The $SIV_{mac}239$ virus did not replicate in macrophages, but the viruses from the 17E brain and molecular clone ($SIV_{mac}239/17E$) replicated equally well in lymphocytes and in primary rhesus macrophages (Table 1). Thus, the amino acid changes identified in the envelope gene of the viruses isolated from the brain of macaques R71 and 17E confer a macrophage-tropism to the $SIV_{mac}239$ virus. It remains to be determined if the recombinant molecular clone will be neurovirulent like the viruses found in the brain or if additional changes in the LTR or other regions of the genome contribute to the neurovirulent phenotype of SIV.

CONCLUSIONS

Using the SIV model, the role of macrophage-tropic virus in CNS disease was investigated. Because these studies were initiated with an infectious molecular clone of SIV that was strictly T-lymphocyte-tropic, both the biological and molecular changes that occurred during *in vivo* passage and virus selection could be examined. Multiple passages *in vivo* of the lymphocyte-tropic virus $SIV_{mac}239$ resulted in a broadened tropism of the virus for macrophages. This broadened tropism of the virus resulted in an altered pattern of disease *in vivo*. Infection of rhesus macaques with $SIV_{mac}239$ resulted in AIDS-like disease but no detectable virus or pathology in brain or lung. In contrast, infection with the macrophage-tropic SIV isolate that emerged after two *in vivo* passages resulted in SIV-induced pneumonia and replication of a macrophage-tropic virus in lung. However, macrophage-tropism of the virus was not sufficient to confer the neurotropic phenotype or the SIV strain. Further *in vivo* passage was required for the selection of a neurovirulent strain of SIV. This suggested that the macrophage-tropic virus had to have an additional tropism for microglial cells, the cells of macrophage lineage found in the brain. It is interesting, however, that once a neurovirulent virus was selected *in vivo*, subsequent passage showed that it was stable and continued to caused CNS disease when inoculated into the brain. The ability of this neurovirulent virus to spread from non-neural sites to the brain—that is, its neuroinvasiveness in short-term studies (i.e., infection of rhesus macaques for 6 months)—was poor. These two viral properties neurotropism and neuroinvasiveness have been shown to be separable in a number of other viral systems (30). Thus, it is not surprising that these are separable phenotypes in SIV. Whether SIV, HIV, or any of the lentiviruses that usually cause CNS disease do so by natural spread of the virus to the brain [as is the case for polio and reoviruses (30)] or whether secondary factors are involved in attracting viral infected cells to the brain requires further studies in the SIV model.

The molecular characterization of the SIV envelope genes present in the brains of macaques R71 and 17E further confirm that a predominant neurotropic strain of SIV had been selected by passage *in vivo*. The closely related amino acid sequence of the envelope genes found in these animals also strongly suggests that the predominant viral genotype was stable on passage from R71 to 17E. The ability to confer macrophage-tropism using the amino acid changes found in 17E provides evidence for the role of these changes in the cell tropism and potential in the neurovirulence of the virus.

These studies on the SIV model of AIDS CNS disease are strikingly similar to the results emerging from studies of HIV strains in the brain of patients with ADC. HIV isolates from the brain have been associated with infection of macrophages and have a dual tropism for T lymphocytes and macrophages (5,13,14,16,18–20). In addition, the high level of genetic heterogenicity observed in the HIV isolates in an individual are in direct contrast to the relatively small number of HIV isolates found in the CNS (33,34). Thus, the SIV model serves as an excellent system in which to investigate the genetic basis for viral neurovirulence and to fully understand the stages and events that lead to SIV- and HIV-induced encephalopathies.

ACKNOWLEDGMENT

We thank Maryann Brooks for preparation of the manuscript. The work described was supported by grants from the NIH (AI27297, AI07394, and AI28748).

REFERENCES

1. Desrosiers RC. The simian immunodeficiency viruses. *Annu Rev Immunol* 1990;8:557–578.
2. Letvin NL, Daniel MD, Sehgal PK, Desrosiers RC, Hunt RD, Waldron LM, MacKey JJ, Schmidt DK, Chalifoux LV, King NW. Induction of AIDS-like disease in macaque monkeys with T cell tropic retrovirus STLV-III. *Science* 1985;230:71–73.
3. Ringler DJ, Hunt RD, Desrosiers RC, Daniel MD, Chalifoux LV, King NW. Simian immunodeficiency virus-induced meningoencephalitis: natural history and retrospective study. *Ann Neurol* 1988;23:S101–107.
4. Narayan O, Clements JE. Biology and pathogenesis of lentiviruses. *J Gen Virol* 1989;70: 1617–1639.
5. Cheng-Mayer C, Weiss C, Seto D, Levy JA. Isolates of human immunodeficiency virus type 1 from the brain may constitute a special group of the AIDS virus. *Proc Natl Acad Sci USA* 1989;86:8575–8579.
6. Desrosiers RC, Hansen-Moosa A, Mori K, Bouvier DP, King NW, Daniel M, Ringler DJ. Macrophage-tropic variants of SIV are associated with specific AIDS-related lesions but are not essential for the development of AIDS. *Am J Pathol* 1991;139:29–35.
7. Collman R, Hassan NF, Walker R, Godfrey B, Cutilli J, Hastings JC, Friedman H, Douglas SD, Nathanson N. Infection of monocyte-derived macrophages with human immunodeficiency virus type 1 (HIV-1): Monocyte-tropic and lymphocyte-tropic strains of HIV-1 show distinctive patterns of replication in a panel of cell types. *J Exp Med* 1989;170:1149–1163.
8. Fauci AS. The human immunodeficiency virus: infectivity and mechanisms of pathogenesis. *Science* 1988;239:617–622.
9. Lifson AR, Rutherford GW, Jaffe HW. The natural history of human immunodeficiency virus infection. *J Infect Dis* 1988;158:1360–1367.
10. Daniel MD, Letvin NL, King NW, Kannagi M, Sehgal PK, Hunt RD, Kanki PJ, Essex M, Desrosiers RC. Isolation of T-cell tropic HTLV-III-like retrovirus from macaques. *Science* 1985;228:1201–1204.
11. King NW, Chalifoux LV, Ringler DJ, Wyand MS, Sehgal PK, Daniel MD, Letvin NL, Desrosiers RC, Blake BJ, Hunt RD. Comparative biology of natural and experimental SIVmac infection in macaque monkeys: a review. *J Med Primatol* 1990;19:109–118.
12. Ringler DJ, Wyand MS, Walsh DG, Mackey JJ, Chalifoux LV, Popovic M, Minassian AA, Sehgal PK, Daniel MD, Desrosiers RC, King NW. Cellular localization of simian immunodeficiency virus in lymphoid tissues. I. Immunochemistry and electron microscopy. *Am J Pathol* 1989;134:373–383.
13. Koenig SC, Gendelman ME, Orenstein JM, Dalccanto MC, Pezeshkpour GH, Yungbluth M, Janotta F, Aksamit A, Martin MA, Fauci AS. Detection of AIDS virus in macrophages in brain tissue from AIDS patients with encephalopathy. *Science* 1986;233:1089–1093.
14. Koyanagi Y, Miles S, Mitsuyasu RT, Merrill JE, Vinters HV, Chen ISY. Dual infection of the central nervous system by AIDS viruses with distinct cellular tropisms. *Science* 1987; 236:819–822.
15. Michaels J, Price RW, Rosenblum MK. Microglia in the giant cell encephalitis of acquired immunodeficiency syndrome: proliferation, infection and fusion. *Acta Neuropathol* 1988; 76:373–379.

16. Price RW, Brew B, Sidtis J, Rosenblum M, Scheck AC, Cleary P. The brain in AIDS: central nervous system HIV-1 infection and AIDS dementia complex. *Science* 1988;239: 586–592.
17. Salahuddin SZ, Rose RM, Groopman JE, Markham PD, Gallo RC. Human T lymphotropic virus type III infection of human alveolar macrophages. *Blood* 1986;68:281–284.
18. Gartner S, Markovitz P, Markovitz DM, Betts RF, Popovic M. Virus isolation from and identification of HTLV-III/LAV-producing cells in brain tissue from a patient with AIDS. *JAMA* 1986;256:2365–2371.
19. Kato T, Hirano A, Llena JF, Dembitzer HM. Neuropathology of the acquired immune deficiency syndrome (AIDS) in 53 autopsy cases with particular emphasis on microglial nodules and multinucleated giant cells. *Acta Neuropathol* 1987;73:287–294.
20. Price RW, Brew BJ, Rosenblum M. The AIDS dementia complex and HIV-1 brain infection: a pathogenic model of virus-immune interaction. In: Waksman BH, ed. *Immunologic mechanism in neurologic and psychiatric disease*. New York: Raven Press, 1990;269–289.
21. Sharpless NE, O'Brien WA, Verdin E, Kufta CV, Chen ISY, Dubois-Dalcq M. Human immunodeficiency virus type 1 tropism for brain microglial cells is determined by a region of the env glycoprotein that also controls macrophage tropism. *J Virol* 1992;2588–2593.
22. Myers G, MacInnes K, Korber B. The emergence of simian/human immunodeficiency viruses. *AIDS Res Hum Retroviruses* 1992;8:373–386.
23. Corboy JR, Buzy JM, Zink MC, Clements JE. Expression directed from HIV long terminal repeats in central nervous system of transgenic mice. *Science* 1992;258:1804–1808.
24. Portis JL, Czub S, Garon CF, McAtee FJ. Neurodegenerative disease induced by the wild mouse ecotropic retrovirus is markedly accelerated by long terminal repeat as gag-pol sequences from nondefective friend murine leukemia virus. *J Virol* 1990;64:1648–1656.
25. Paquette Y, Kay DG, Rassart E, Robitaille Y, Jolicoeur P. Substitution of the U3 long terminal repeat region of the neurotropic Cas-Br-E retrovirus affects its disease-inducing potential. *J Virol* 1990;64:3742–3752.
26. Short MK, Okenquist SA, Lenz J. Correlation of leukemogenic potential of murine retroviruses with transcriptional tissue preference of the viral long terminal repeats. *J Virol* 1987; 61:1067–1072.
27. Kestler H, Kodama T, Ringler D, Marthas M, Pedersen N, Lackner A, Regier D, Sehgal P, Daniel M, King N, Desrosiers R. Induction of AIDS in rhesus monkeys by molecularly cloned simian immunodeficiency virus. *Science* 1990;248:1109–1112.
28. Sharma DP, Anderson M, Zink MC, Adams RJ, Donnenberg AD, Clements JE, Narayan O. Pathogenesis of acute infection in rhesus macaques with a lymphocyte-tropic strain of SIVmac. *J Infect Dis* 1992;166:738–746.
29. Sharma DP, Zink MC, Anderson A, Adams R, Clements JE, Joag SV, Narayan O. Derivation of neurotropic simian immunodeficiency virus from exclusively lymphocytetropic parental virus: pathogenesis of infection in macaques. *J Virol* 1992;66:3550–3556.
30. Johnson RT. *Viral infections of the nervous system*. New York: Raven Press, 1982;37–56.
31. Mims CA. Intracerebral injections and the growth of viruses in the mouse brain. *Br J Exp Pathol* 1960;41:52–59.
32. Anderson MA, Hauer D, Sharma DP, Joag SV, Narayan O, Zink MC, Clements JE. Analysis of envelope changes acquired by SIV$_{mac}$239 during neuroadaptation in rhesus macaques. *Virology* 1993;195:616–628.
33. Li Y, Hui H, Burgess CJ, Price RW, Sharp PM, BH, Shaw GM. Complete nucleotide sequence, genome organization and biological properties of human immunodeficiency virus type 1 *in vivo:* evidence for limited defectiveness and complementation. *J Virol* 1991;66: 6587–6600.
34. Li Y, Kappes JC, Conway JA, Price RW, Shaw GM, Mahn BH. Molecular characterization of human immunodeficiency virus type 1 cloned directly from uncultured human brain tissue: identification of replication-competent and defective viral genomes. *J Virol* 1991; 65:3973–3985.

HIV, AIDS and the Brain, edited by
R. W. Price and S. W. Perry.
Raven Press, Ltd., New York © 1994.

9

Peripheral Nerve Disorders in HIV Infection

Similarities and Contrasts with CNS Disorders

John W. Griffin, Steven L. Wesselingh, Diane E. Griffin, Jonathan D. Glass, and Justin C. McArthur

Department of Neurology, Johns Hopkins University, School of Medicine, Johns Hopkins Hospital, Baltimore, MD 21287

A diverse group of neuropathies contribute substantially to the neurologic morbidity associated with human immunodeficiency virus (HIV) infection. The most prevalent of these, the predominantly sensory neuropathy (PSN) of acquired immunodeficiency syndrome (AIDS), rivals AIDS dementia in incidence, and subclinical forms are nearly universal by the time of death from AIDS (1–3). The need to understand these neuropathies has taken on new urgency with the advent of antiretrovirals such as dideoxycytosine (ddC) and dideoxyinosine (ddI), which can themselves produce painful sensory neuropathies. It is likely that preexisting AIDS-associated nerve disease increases susceptibility to this drug-induced neurotoxicity. AIDS neuropathy can thereby limit the use of potentially life-sustaining antiretroviral agents. In addition to these direct clinical implications, understanding the pathogenesis of peripheral nerve diseases may provide insight into the CNS disorders associated with AIDS.

The nerve diseases associated with HIV infection, catalogued in Table 1, have instructive parallels to the nerve diseases associated with diabetes mellitus. Each of these underlying diseases affects over 1 million individuals in the United States alone. In both HIV infection and diabetes, a variable asymptomatic interval, usually of many years, is followed by (a) clinically manifested nerve disease in some individuals and (b) subclinical involvement in a great many asymptomatic individuals. There is a wide spectrum of specific disorders and clinical syndromes among the neuropathies in both diabetes and AIDS. They range from less common disorders that are self-limited

TABLE 1. *Neuropathic syndromes associated with HIV infection[a]*

Immune-mediated
  GBS
  CIDP
  "Axonal GBS"
  Vasculitic
  Ataxic dorsal radiculopathy
Infectious
  CMV polyradiculopathy
  CMV multiple mononeuropathy
  Herpes zoster
  MAI infiltration
Nutritional
  Multiple deficiencies
  B_{12} deficiency
Toxic
  ddl/ddC
Predominantly sensory
Neuropathy of AIDS

---

[a] HIV, human immunodeficiency virus; GBS, Guillain–Barré syndrome; CIDP, chronic inflammatory demyelinating polyneuropathy; CMV, cytomegalovirus; ddl, dideoxyinosine; ddC, dideoxycytosine; AIDS, acquired immunodeficiency syndrome; MAI,

(e.g., multiple mononeuropathies in diabetes and inflammatory demyelinating neuropathies in HIV infection) to the most prevalent groups (e.g., diabetic polyneuropathy and the AIDS sensory neuropathy), which are notoriously resistant to either definitive or symptomatic therapy. Both diabetic polyneuropathy and PSN of AIDS usually occur in advanced stages of the underlying disease and usually in association with other complications. In both, neuropathic pain is a major cause of morbidity and functional limitation. And finally, until recently, both have received less research attention from the neurology and neuroscience communities than their prevalence warrants, and much of the burden of care has devolved to the primary practitioners and internists dealing with the underlying diseases.

This chapter will review selected disorders of the peripheral nerves identified in HIV infection, with a special focus on the sensory neuropathy of AIDS.

INFLAMMATORY DEMYELINATING POLYNEUROPATHIES (IDPs)

The inflammatory demyelinating polyneuropathies, including both the acute (demyelinating Guillain–Barré syndrome) and chronic (inflammatory demyelinating polyneuropathy [CIDP]) forms, are among the most dramatic and treatable nerve diseases. They usually produce pronounced motor involvement, widespread loss of tendon reflexes, and varying degrees of large-fiber sensory loss and of polyradicular pain in the back and legs. A characteristic laboratory finding is elevated spinal fluid protein levels (4–7). Their precise pathogeneses are unknown, but almost certainly these disorders reflect an immune attack on peripheral nerves. The pathology usually includes lymphocytic infiltration (8) and macrophage-mediated demyelination (9). A variety of markers of immune activation are elevated in the serum and the cerebrospinal fluid (CSF) of affected patients (for review see ref. 10).

These disorders have similar clinical pictures in HIV-seronegative and -seropositive individuals. CIDP appears to have a higher incidence among HIV-infected individuals than it does among HIV-seronegative individuals. Whether HIV infection increases the likelihood of Guillain–Barré syndrome (GBS) is uncertain; with over 1 million HIV-infected individuals in North America, a small number of coincident cases will occur by chance. In any event, both disorders occur primarily in the earlier stages of infection, rather than at times when the CD4 counts are profoundly depressed. In the Johns Hopkins series of 17 HIV-seropositive patients with IDP (12 CIDP, 5 GBS), only 4 developed in individuals with AIDS. Most of the other 13 had lowered CD4:CD8 ratios, in the range of 0.4, but all of the pre-AIDS patients had CD4:CD8 ratios that were greater than 0.20 (11). GBS can occur at the time of seroconversion (12), and in many of our patients GBS or CIDP was the presenting symptom of HIV infection (13). As AIDS supervenes, CIDP tends to improve (11). A similar association with early stages of HIV infection has been noted in another immunopathogenetic disorder associated with HIV, idiopathic thrombocytopenic purpura (14), which can also remit as immune deficiency worsens (15,16).

The pathology of IDP in HIV infection is not qualitatively different from that of IDP in the absence of HIV infection. In most cases, at least some lymphocytic infiltrates are detected (8). The active demyelination is characterized by macrophage-mediated myelin "stripping" (11,17,18) (Fig. 1), with consequent segmental demyelination (Fig. 2). In demyelinating GBS, demyelination is a monophasic process followed by remyelination, whereas in CIDP we often see repeated cycles of demyelination and remyelination (11). In both GBS and CIDP, Wallerian-like degeneration and loss of myelinated fibers also develop.

In two of our CIDP cases, the sural nerves were examined at biopsy and the contralateral sural nerves, as well as the rest of the PNS, were studied in the autopsy tissue obtained 4 and 5 years after the biopsies. In both individuals, the CIDP improved as AIDS developed, and neither required therapy for CIDP during the last 2 years of life. At the time of biopsy, there was active demyelination, but at autopsy both had a much milder degree of ongoing demyelination; instead, there were numerous short remyelinated internodes and prominent whorls of supernumerary Schwann cells (onion bulbs), features associated with previous demyelination and remyelination (11).

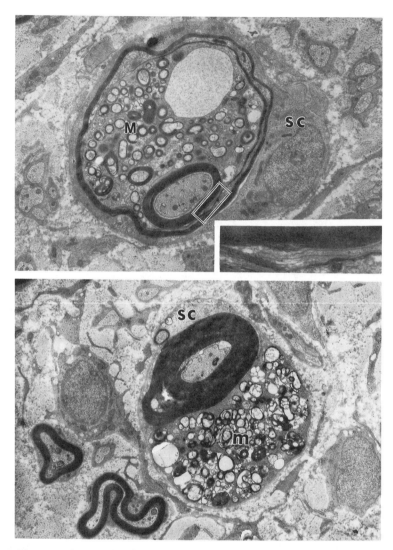

FIG. 1. Electron micrographs of transverse sections of sural nerve biopsies in HIV-infected individuals with CIDP. In the upper panel the myelinated fiber is in the early stages of macrophage-mediated demyelination. Note that a macrophage (M) containing myelin debris lies within the myelin sheath. Myelin lamellae are being separated by macrophage processes, as shown in the inset. The lower panel shows an earlier stage of demyelination. A macrophage (m) is within the Schwann cell basal lamina, but the myelin and axon remain relatively intact. The changes illustrated are similar to those seen in inflammatory demyelinating neuropathies in HIV-seronegative individuals.

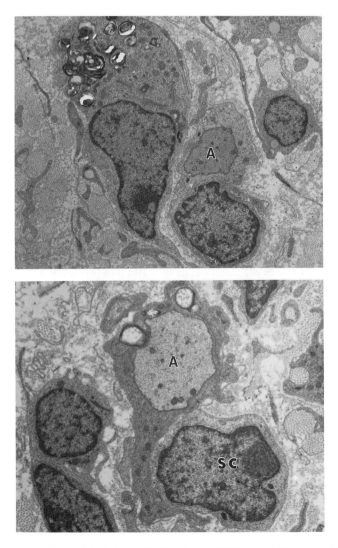

FIG. 2. Examples of completed demyelination in the CIDP in an HIV-infected individual. In the upper panel, the demyelinated axon (A) is ensheathed by Schwann cell cytoplasm. Note the nearby macrophage containing myelin debris. In the lower panel, this demyelinated axon (A) is ensheathed by a Schwann cell, and a second Schwann cell (containing a nucleus) reflects recent Schwann cell proliferation in response to demyelination. This Schwann cell (sc) lies below and to the right of the axon.

The immunopathology is quantitatively different in seropositive, compared to seronegative, cases of IDP. For example, the nerves in seronegative IDP have a predominantly CD4-positive T-cell infiltrate (19), whereas in HIV infection the CD8 cells usually exceed the CD4 cells (11). In both settings the CD4/CD8 ratio in the nerves parallels that in the blood, suggesting that many of the T cells enter the nerves nonspecifically (19). The pattern of cytokine expression in the nerves of most HIV-IDP cases has lower levels of interferon gamma (IFN-γ) than are found in comparable seronegative IDP cases (11). This discrepancy presumably reflects, in part, relatively lower numbers of T cells in the HIV-IDP nerves than in seronegative-IDP nerves. It may be exaggerated by a disproportionate reduction in the Th1 subclass of CD4-positive T cells, one of the cell types that produce IFN-γ. Early in the immune dysregulation of HIV infection, the Th1 subclass is preferentially lost (20), and a relatively greater proportion of CD4-positive cells are of the Th2 subclass which produces IL-4, IL-10, and other macrophage-deactivating lymphokines. Late in the course, both subsets of CD4 cells are lost, and T-cell-derived factors are reduced, as described in the section on PSN below.

Another distinction between seronegative and seropositive IDP is that many patients with HIV-associated IDP have a CSF pleocytosis (median, 25 cells/mm^2) (13), whereas most HIV-seronegative patients with IDP have few cells in the CSF (4–6). An unanswered question has been whether the pleocytosis simply reflects that frequently seen in the first few years of HIV infection, possibly associated with HIV entry into the CNS, or whether it is specific to the episode of IDP. In one reported patient, pleocytosis paralleled the course of GBS, suggesting that it has some relation to the neuropathy itself (21).

For the past 25 years, the term "Guillain–Barré syndrome" has often been used synonymously with acute inflammatory demyelinating polyneuropathy (8,22). It is increasingly clear, however, that some patients in North America and Europe (23), and many in northern China (24,25) and Latin America (26), have pronounced and fulminant axonal degeneration. These disorders presumably have an immunopathogenetic basis, and yet many are essentially noninflammatory (23,25). Such cases also occur in HIV-infected individuals. We followed a man with AIDS who developed acute, severe, paralytic, axonal neuropathy. He recovered partially, but died of AIDS 8 months later. The outstanding pathologic finding in the sural nerve biopsy at the time of neuropathic presentation was massive ongoing Wallerian-like degeneration (11). At autopsy, only a few myelinated fibers remained in the distal nerves. Taken together, the picture was consistent with monophasic Wallerian-like degeneration of myelinated fibers. We found virtually no active demyelination in the biopsy tissue, or evidence of remyelinated segments at autopsy, nor was there lymphocytic infiltration in either set of samples. Why might this particular disorder occur late in the course of AIDS (at a stage when, as indicated above, typical IDP is uncommon)? It is attractive to speculate that such noninflammatory cases could reflect antibody-mediated damage by T-cell-independent mechanisms. Similar atypical forms of GBS have been described among children in Mexico (26) and China (24,25). In the latter setting, serologic evidence suggests that the disease may follow *Campylobacter jejuni* infection (25), and thus might reflect shared epitopes between the organism and the axon or Schwann cell. T-cell-independent antibody-mediated disease could explain the development of this autoimmune disorder late in the course of AIDS.

In HIV-seropositive individuals, the clinical courses of both CIDP and GBS fit within the spectrum of their counterparts in seronegative individuals. The number of HIV-infected patients is too small to determine whether their natural histories are more or less severe. At least in the case of CIDP, the response to therapy resembles that of seronegative patients (13,27,28). Controlled trials have shown that plasmapheresis, intravenous immunoglobulin, and corticosteroids are efficacious in seronegative individuals. Plasmapheresis remains our first choice in seropositive individuals, but the therapy must be individualized. Although immunoglobulin therapy is easier to administer than plasmapheresis, particularly if venous access is limited, many HIV-infected individuals already have very high immunoglobulin levels, and so the potential for renal shutdown is a concern, particularly if abnormalities of renal function are present. Corticosteroids are an option but, because they can potentially decrease resistance to opportunistic infections, we use them as the third-line approach to therapy.

CYTOMEGALOVIRUS INFECTIONS OF NERVE

Cytomegalovirus (CMV) infection of nerve deserves special comment because it underlies some cases of demyelinating neuropathy, multiple mononeuropathy, and polyradiculitis, and, as discussed below, it has even been suggested as a cause of the painful predominantly sensory neuropathy. Before the advent of AIDS, direct CMV infection of nerve was almost unknown; today the spectrum of clinical manifestations continues to enlarge. The pleotrophic manifestations reflect in part the capacity of CMV to infect both endothelial cells (leading to angiopathic damage to nerve) and Schwann cells (contributing to Schwann cell death and demyelination).

Cytomegalovirus Polyradiculopathy

The most dramatic neuropathic syndrome produced by this opportunistic agent is CMV polyradiculopathy (29–35). The clinical picture is often sufficiently distinctive to suggest the diagnosis. Severely immunocompromised individuals typically develop abrupt pain in the back and lower extremities, with rapidly evolving flaccid paraparesis (30). The pathology is dominated by intensely inflammatory lesions of the lumbar roots, often including poly-morphonuclear leukocytes, inclusions in endothelial cells (3,29,35) and Schwann cells (31), necrotizing changes involving all cellular elements (29,35), and extensive Wallerian degeneration (29,35). The dorsal root ganglia and the spinal cord may become involved. Reflecting this pathology, the spinal fluid often contains high numbers of polymorphonuclear leukocytes (30), and cytology of spinal fluid can identify CMV inclusions (J Glass, *un-published observations*). For these reasons, spinal fluid examination is a keystone of diagnosis.

This disorder is at least partially treatable with gancyclovir or foscarnate, or both (30,36). Figure 3 illustrates the lumbar roots obtained at autopsy from a 45-year-old man who developed CMV polyradiculopathy 7 months before death, and was treated with gancyclovir. His polyradiculopathy stabi-lized and improved; however, 6 months later, off medication, he developed cranial neuropathies and CMV encephalitis. At autopsy, CMV inclusions were easily identified within Schwann cells of his cranial nerves. As shown in Fig. 3, however, his lumbosacral plexus was characterized by a striking remyelination of nerve fibers, as reflected by abnormally thin myelin sheaths, with no active CMV lesions. Such cases confirm the ability of CMV to pro-duce predominantly demyelinating lesions, at least on occasion, and the po-tential for substantial recovery with therapy. Therapy must be continued for very long periods.

Cytomegalovirus Multiple Mononeuropathy

Cytomegalovirus infection of nerve can also produce a picture of multifocal neuropathy or multiple mononeuropathy (35,37). Said et al. (35) described four cases with multifocal inflammatory lesions of peripheral nerve. In these lesions, the CMV inclusions were most often in endothelial cells, and many nerve fibers were undergoing Wallerian degeneration, presumably reflecting local infection of endothelial cells with necrotizing responses and inflamma-tory changes, culminating in multifocal nerve infarction. However, myelin changes, characterized by regions of excessive myelin folding and paranodal and segmental demyelination, were also identified (Fig. 3). An unusual find-ing was evidence of Schwann cell death, which left axons surrounded only by the original Schwann cell basal lamina. This change could reflect the ability of CMV to infect Schwann cells (3,29,31), but in sural nerve biopsies of such patients we have found foci in which most of the fibers have vacuo-lated degenerating Schwann cells and the unusual myelin changes illustrated in Fig. 3. Because it is unlikely that all of these fibers are infected, we have speculated that ischemia due to endothelial cell infection coupled with local production of cytokines toxic to Schwann cells may underlie these foci (37).

Cornblath et al. (37) have shown that some of these patients have electro-

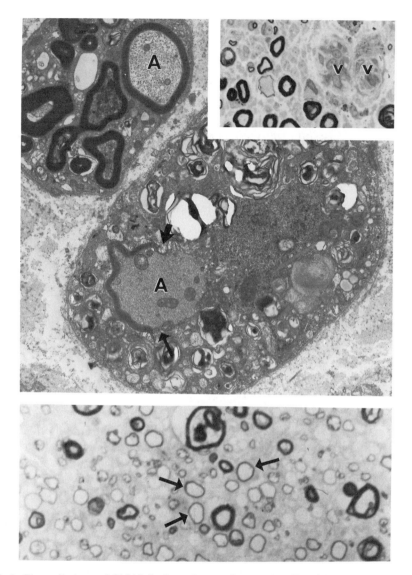

FIG. 3. The pathology of CMV infection of nerve **(upper panel)** and lumbar spinal roots **(lower panel).** The upper panel illustrates a sural nerve biopsy from an individual with multifocal demyelinating CMV neuropathy, with abundant CMV inclusions within the biopsied nerve segment. The pathology reflects a mixture of angiopathy [note the occluded endoneurial vessels (v)], myelinated fiber degeneration, and demyelination. An enlarged, thinly myelinated fiber is present in the inset. The electron micrograph in the upper panel illustrates the unusual features of demyelination in CMV neuropathy, with extensive myelin debris. The axons (A) are preserved, but Schwann cells and macrophages contain extensive myelin debris. The arrows identify regions in which myelin lamellae are being amputated. The lower panel illustrates the lumbar spinal root of an individual with typical CMV polyradiculopathy who was treated with gancyclovir and who partially recovered. At autopsy 6 months later, the lumbar roots were characterized by numerous thinly myelinated fibers, reflecting remyelination (examples illustrated by *arrows*).

physiologically definable multifocal demyelinating changes, so that CMV neuropathies might occasionally be confused with acute or chronic IDP (38). Unlike CIDP, CMV neuropathy typically occurs in patients with frank AIDS, often in association with systemic or retinal CMV, and the nerve involvement is patchy. Definitive diagnosis requires histologic demonstration of CMV lesions in the nerve. The recent advent of polymerase chain reaction (PCR) detection of CMV transcripts may simplify diagnosis of productive infection (39), but CMV is sufficiently common late in AIDS that demonstration of local inflammatory and destructive lesions is still best established histologically.

"Silent" CMV Infection of Nerve

Extensive pathological studies of unselected nerve specimens from AIDS autopsies have emphasized the frequency of CMV lesions (3,29,40). Cornford et al. (3) found that 29/115 (25 percent) of peripheral nerves had focal CMV lesions, with the inclusions usually being within endothelial cells and usually surrounded by a cuff of plasma cells. These lesions were more often in the epineurium or perineurium than in the endoneurial vessels, but they correlated with patchy fiber loss in the fascicles. Their incidence increased somewhat with duration of AIDS, and fiber loss in the sural nerves correlated with the presence of these lesions.

These studies have been taken to suggest that CMV might underlie the predominantly sensory neuropathy associated with AIDS. In a similar vein, Fuller et al. (41) suggested that CMV ganglionitis might underlie the neuropathic pain of PSN. Their hypothesis was based on the finding that there was a greater incidence of CMV in retina and other systemic sites in individuals with painful sensory neuropathy. Autopsy studies have not found prominent CMV lesions in the ganglia of affected individuals (2,3,42). It remains possible that CMV-induced damage to epineurial and perineurial endothelial cells might lead to angiopathic nerve damage and neuropathy. Focal ischemic lesions could cumulate over the length of the nerve, as occurs in vasculitis (43,44) and probably in diabetic neuropathy (45). Because of their rich collateral supply, the nerves are relatively insensitive to large-vessel disease, but quite susceptible to small-vessel disease. Such a mechanism could well apply to a subgroup of ''AIDS neuropathy'' cases; because of the therapeutic implications a prospective clinical and pathological study is warranted.

THE PREDOMINANTLY SENSORY NEUROPATHY OF AIDS (PSN)

Neuropathy, usually affecting sensory functions more than motor functions, is prevalent late in the course of AIDS (46–48). In some cases the onset is abrupt and the course subacute; in others the neuropathy develops slowly. By pathologic criteria, some nerve disease is almost universal by the time of death from AIDS (1,2), with a median reduction in myelinated fiber density of 27 percent. The high frequency of these pathologic changes and the wide range of severities undoubtedly account for the variations in reported incidence (30–80 percent) (46–48). Thus, clinical reports of the incidence of neuropathy in AIDS can be interpreted and compared only if the criteria for diagnosis and exclusion of neuropathy are specified. The Johns Hopkins series (46) revealed neuropathic symptoms and/or signs in approximately 30 percent of individuals with AIDS, a figure that predicts an estimated 30,000 new cases per year, roughly equal to new cases of AIDS dementia.

Clinically, sensory symptoms and findings predominate. A substantial fraction of individuals with PSN have intense neuropathic pain in the feet, especially on the soles, with variable, but often significant, functional limitations as a result. The typical clinical syndrome is of an ill patient with low CD4 counts who presents with complaints of spontaneous burning pain in the feet and hyperalgesia, including prominent mechanical hyperalgesia in many patients. Touch-evoked neuropathic pain causes some individuals with AIDS to walk in an antalgic fashion, often using one or two canes. Cooling the feet may provide relief. We have not encountered individuals with cold-exacerbated symptoms, a feature often associated with causalgic or sympathetically maintained pain. On examination, sensory thresholds are elevated and usually show impairment of both large-fiber modalities, such as vibratory sensibility, and small-fiber modalities, including warmth thresholds (48). Because of the pain, PSN is one of the most frequent causes for consultation by the HIV Neurology Service at Johns Hopkins. To date, neither definitive nor effective symptomatic treatments are available.

Motor dysfunction, reflected in atrophy of the intrinsic muscles of the feet and, less often, in mild dorsiflexor weakness at the ankles, can often be found if specifically sought. The degree of involvement of the autonomic nervous system remains unresolved. Although autonomic dysfunction in AIDS has been detected and measured in numerous laboratories (for review see ref. 49), these studies are difficult to interpret because of the paucity of disease control data in severely ill and cachectic patients. Almost certainly, the usual normal control data do not apply. Tendon reflexes are typically missing at the ankles, but are often exaggerated at the knees, reflecting coexisting myelopathy or intracranial disease. The electrophysiologic abnormalities reflect the predominant pathologic process, distally predominant axonal degeneration (46,47) (see below).

The interaction between PSN and neurotoxic agents has recently assumed particular importance because of the increased use of the antiretroviral agents ddC and ddI. Both of these agents produce in their own right a painful sensory neuropathy that is strikingly similar to PSN (50,51). Indeed, the extent to which ddI and ddC neurotoxicity reflects an "unmasking" of subclinical PSN is an issue that requires prospective evaluation, because there are several precedents for preexisting subclinical or mild nerve diseases conferring increased susceptibility to neurotoxic drugs. For example, individuals with heritable motor sensory neuropathies (Charcot–Marie–Tooth disease) can have devastating responses to administration of the usual doses of vincristine. Conceivably, the severity of the subclinical neuropathy associated with AIDS may dictate the extent of neurotoxic damage from ddI and ddC. A prospective study is warranted to examine the value of screening for specific neuropathic findings before instituting these agents.

Neuropathology of PSN

Autopsy studies have demonstrated a high incidence of pathologic abnormalities in the PNS of individuals with AIDS (1–3). At Johns Hopkins, we have dissected the peripheral nervous systems from a total of 190 individuals who died of AIDS. Quantitative studies compared 14 AIDS patients with clinically evident PSN, 7 of whom had severely painful neuropathies, to 12 autopsied AIDS cases with no clinically evident nerve disease. None of these autopsies had pathologic or immunocytochemical evidence of CMV within the nerves or ganglia. The results from these groups were compared to those from six normal controls, a group of HIV-positive patients with other types of neuropathy, and a group of seronegative individuals with predominantly sensory neuropathies of comparable severity. The major findings are summarized schematically in Fig. 4. We drew four conclusions:

1. *Neuropathy is almost universal by the time of death from AIDS*. Ongoing Wallerian-like degeneration of myelinated fibers was found in the distal sural nerves of all AIDS cases, whether or not neuropathy was recognized clinically. The median reduction in myelinated fiber density was 27 percent in both the "clinical neuropathy" and the subclinical groups (2).

2. *The peripheral fiber loss conformed to the pattern of distal axonal degeneration*. Nerve fiber degeneration in the cutaneous nerves could be due to degeneration of the whole primary sensory neuron, as seen in carcinomatous sensory neuronopathy and some other inflammatory, immune-mediated, and toxic neuropathies (for review see ref. 52), or could be due to selective Wallerian-like degeneration of the distal region of the fibers. Studies of the spatial distribution of nerve fiber loss demonstrated the latter pattern, as indicated in Fig. 4; in PSN there is an increasingly severe loss of nerve fibers from proximal to distal—from the dorsal root through the lumbosacral plexus, the sciatic nerve, the upper part of the sural nerve, and the low sural nerve at the ankle. The cell bodies of the sensory neurons in the dorsal root ganglia usually remained surprisingly normal, even in cases of severe distal fiber loss; there was only modest ongoing neuronal loss and reaction in the ganglia of most PSN patients (2,42).

The central processes of the lumbosacral dorsal root ganglion cells pass

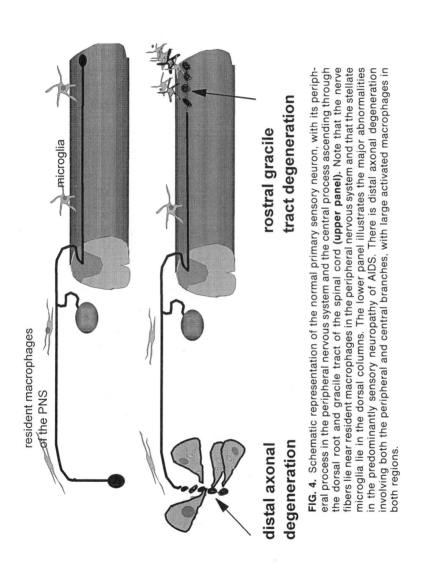

resident macrophages
of the PNS

microglia

distal axonal
degeneration

rostral gracile
tract degeneration

FIG. 4. Schematic representation of the normal primary sensory neuron, with its peripheral process in the peripheral nervous system and the central process ascending through the dorsal root and gracile tract of the spinal cord **(upper panel)**. Note that the nerve fibers lie near resident macrophages in the peripheral nervous system and that the stellate microglia lie in the dorsal columns. The lower panel illustrates the major abnormalities in the predominantly sensory neuropathy of AIDS. There is distal axonal degeneration involving both the peripheral and central branches, with large activated macrophages in both regions.

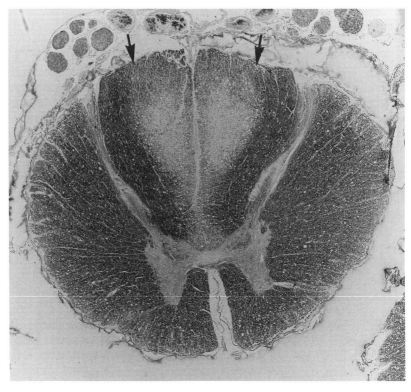

FIG. 5. Spinal cord of an individual with AIDS and sensory neuropathy. In the high thoracic spinal cord there is degeneration of the gracile tract in the medial portion of the dorsal column. The gracile tract is delineated by the arrows.

up the medial dorsal columns (gracile tracts) to terminate in the gracile nuclei. The central process of the lumbosacral dorsal root ganglion cells pass up the medial dorsal columns (gracile tracts) to terminate in the gracile nuclei. If the whole sensory neuron degenerates, the dorsal roots and the gracile tracts at all levels of the cord contain degenerating fibers. In "dying back" of sensory neurons, only the regions of the sensory axons farthest from the cell bodies (i.e., the rostral regions of the gracile tracts) degenerate. In severe cases of PSN, we have found Wallerian-like degeneration of the rostral gracile tract (2,53) (Figs. 4 and 5). The pathology of 12 of the 24 autopsied cases was complicated by associated vacuolar myelopathy, but in five cases of sensory neuropathy without vacuolar myelopathy we found some degree of Wallerian-like degeneration in the medial gracile tracts of the high thoracic cord. In two cases with severe sensory neuropathies, this rostral gracile tract degeneration was recognized on routine paraffin histology; in three other cases, examination of plastic sections was required. In these cases there was also immunocytochemical evidence of microglial/macrophage reaction in the rostral gracile tracts (see below). This pattern is compatible with "dying back" of large myelinated axons.

3. *Unmyelinated fiber loss is a feature of the sensory neuropathy of AIDS.* In both the clinical and subclinical neuropathies, loss of small myelinated and unmyelinated fibers was a common feature, and one that distinguished PSN from the "other neuropathy" groups studied (Fig. 6). The median reduction in unmyelinated fiber density was decreased by over 50 percent (2). In three patients, two specimens of sural nerve were obtained, one at biopsy and the second at autopsy from 7 months to 5 years later. These specimens clearly showed that the loss of unmyelinated fibers occurred during the late stages of AIDS (11). Because C fibers account for a high proportion of the unmyelinated fibers in cutaneous nerves, they are undoubtedly among the degenerating fibers in these nerves. Although we found no simple correlation between pain symptoms and numbers of remaining unmyelinated fibers, disease of the C fibers themselves might contribute to the neuropathic pain of PSN.

4. *There was a striking lack of axonal regeneration in the AIDS groups.* In most axonal neuropathies there is an admixture of degenerating and regenerating fibers. In PSN, axonal regeneration of either myelinated or unmyelinated fibers was virtually absent (2).

Immunopathology of PSN

We have recently published an immunocytochemical characterization of lymphocytes and macrophages in the peripheral nerves, dorsal root ganglia, and dorsal columns in PSN (54). T lymphocytes were uncommon; when present, they tended to be in discrete focal clusters (3,54), in agreement with the experience of Scaravilli et al. (42). We did not find widespread lymphocytic infiltration in the autopsy studies (1), presumably indicative of the T-lymphopenia characteristic of terminal AIDS. Other reports have emphasized the prominence of plasma (B) cells (3).

Much of the remainder of this review will focus on the macrophage responses in AIDS. A prominent change in the PSN nerves was the large extent of macrophage infiltration and the high degree of macrophage activation. The relevant background to these studies comes from a series of recent observations, made in our laboratory and others, on macrophage responses during experimental Wallerian degeneration.

1. *The immune system in normal nerves.* Although only occasional T cells are found in normal nerves, and the endothelial cells are major histocompatibility class (MHC) class II-negative, there is a recently recognized, but extensive, resident macrophage population (11,54–57). Approximately 9 percent of the total cells within the nerve fascicles are resident microglia (57). These

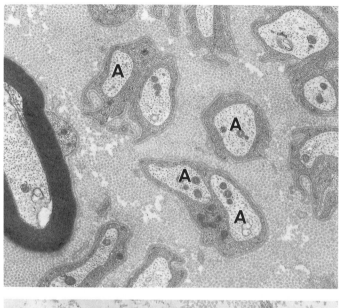

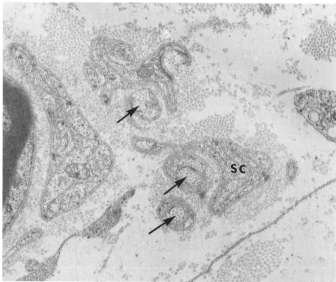

FIG. 6. Loss of unmyelinated nerve fibers in the predominantly sensory neuropathy of AIDS. The upper panel is an electron micrograph of a transverse section from a normal nerve, with a single myelinated fiber to the left. Unmyelinated axons (examples identified by A) are ensheathed by Schwann cells. In the lower panel the Schwann cells (sc) have a folded and lamellated appearance characteristic of denervated Schwann cells of unmyelinated fibers, and some forms empty pockets surrounding endoneurial collagen fibrils *(arrows)*.

cells are typically arrayed near endoneurial blood vessels but outside the basal lamina of the blood vessel. They are elongated and extend multiple ramified processes and have a striking resemblance to microglia of the central nervous system. They are constitutively MHC class II-positive, and also express CD4 and complement receptor 3 (CR3). This phenotype and their location near endoneurial vessels suggest that they are ideally suited to act as the "professional" antigen-presenting cells of the PNS (55).

2. *Responses of the immune system to axonal degeneration.* The simplest model of nerve fiber degeneration is Wallerian degeneration of the distal stump following transection of the nerves. Following a latent period [1–2 days in rats, 5–11 days in humans (58)], the axon of the distal stump abruptly breaks down. Shortly afterward the blood–nerve barrier breaks down, and macrophages enter the nerve from the circulation (59–61). These macrophages are not preceded or accompanied by significant numbers of polymorphonuclear leukocytes or lymphocytes. Many of these entering macrophages are MHC class II-, CD4-, and CR3-positive (59), and they become positive for tumor necrosis factor alpha (TNF-α) (54) and IL-1β (62,63). These activated macrophages enter the degenerating nerve fibers (59,60) and participate in removal of myelin and axonal debris (55). The foamy postphagocytic macrophages then lose their activation markers, including class II (59), and exit the nerve through both the endoneurial vessels and the perineurial vessels. This same sequence occurs in Wallerian-like degeneration in experimental and human axonal neuropathies (2,59,60).

3. *Contrasts with axonal degeneration in the CNS.* In the CNS, axonal degeneration follows much the same time course as in the peripheral nervous system (64), but all other aspects of the sequence are delayed or absent (55). The blood–tissue barrier remains intact, macrophages fail to enter, and axonal and myelin debris persist for long periods. Astrocytes respond with gliosis, and microglia gradually proliferate and give rise to macrophages locally.

4. *How does the neuropathy of AIDS contrast with otherwise comparable axonal neuropathies in HIV-seronegative individuals?* To examine the extent of lymphocytic and macrophage infiltration in the peripheral nerves, the dorsal root ganglia, and the dorsal columns in cases of PSN (54), peripheral nerves were studied immunocytochemically in 13 individuals with AIDS (12 autopsies and 1 sural nerve biopsy). These cases were selected because of the histologic quality of the frozen material; cases with severe freeze artifacts or other preparative problems were excluded. Of the selected cases, eight had clinically recognized neuropathy and three had severe neuropathic pain. The results were compared to five normal control cases of young adults who died suddenly and to six cases of predominantly sensory axonal neuropathies in HIV-seronegative individuals (two autopsies and four sural nerve biopsies).

T lymphocytes were uncommon within the endoneurium in all of the re-

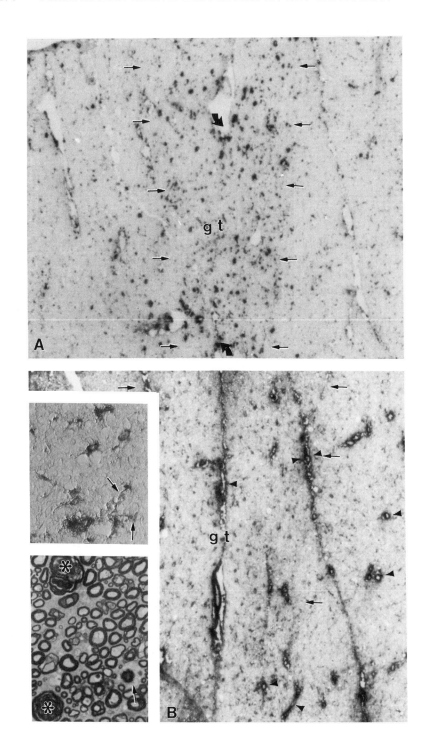

gions of the AIDS nerves examined; when they were present, they were typically in small clusters (54). The AIDS nerves differed from the controls and the HIV-seronegative nerves in the density of macrophages and their extent of activation. In the AIDS group, macrophages were abundant at all levels of the peripheral nerves. Their density was greatest in the sural nerve, intermediate in the peroneal nerve, and least in the lumbosacral plexus and spinal roots. In general, the degree of macrophage infiltration paralleled the degree of ongoing Wallerian-like degeneration in the nerves, as it did in the seronegative neuropathy group; in PSN, however, macrophage density was greater for a given degree of severity of Wallerian-like degeneration. There was also significant macrophage/microglial activation in the dorsal columns (Fig. 7). These responses of the microglial/macrophage system, if viewed simply as a response to myelinated fiber degeneration, were excessive in both these spinal cords (54).

The macrophages in the AIDS patients expressed several activation markers, including class II and TNF-α (54). The TNF-α-positive macrophages were usually within degenerating nerve fibers, and in the AIDS nerves were intensely stained. Some of the macrophages also stained positively for IL-1 and IL-6. The degree of class II expression was more prominent overall in the PSN nerves than in the seronegative neuropathies. In six of eight PSN nerves, MHC class II was also expressed on the endothelial cells of the endoneurial vessels; in two of these six nerves, Schwann cells of unmyelinated fibers and degenerating fibers were also positive (54).

We have recently used RNA PCR to examine cytokine transcripts in PSN nerves. We have recently used RNA PCR to examine cytokine transcripts in PSN nerves. In some cases with painful neuropathy, the relative levels of TNF-α mRNA were markedly elevated, and were in contrast to the relatively low levels of interleukin 1β (IL-1β) message (SL Wesselingh, DE Griffin, JD Glass, JC McArthur, and JW Griffin, *unpublished observations*). As

←——————————————————————————————————————

FIG. 7. Immunostaining of rostral gracile tracts (gt) from a patient with AIDS and PSN. **A:** This transverse section through the dorsal columns of the high thoracic spinal cord was immunostained for macrophages and activated microglia using the antibody EBM/11 and lightly counterstained. The gracile tracts are identified by arrows, and the midline is indicated by the dotted line. Note the increased density of the dark immunostained cells within the medial gracile tracts. ×80. **B:** This section from the same case as A was immunostained for IL-1 (examples are identified by small arrows). ×210. The gracile tracts are identified by the arrowheads, and the midline is indicated by the dotted line. Note that the blood vessels throughout the spinal cord are intensely stained for IL-1. Within the gracile tracts there is in addition staining of numerous other cells; as seen at higher power (×740) in the upper inset, some of these cells are stellate (processes identified by arrows), and are similar to the EBM/11-positive cells microglia in morphology. Similar cells within the same distribution were also positive for IL-6 and class II. The lower inset is a 1-μm plastic section from the medial gracile tracts of this same high thoracic spinal cord. The asterisks identify fibers undergoing Wallerian-like degeneration. The arrow identifies a foamy macrophage. ×1100.

noted below, these results are similar to those in the CNS of patients with AIDS dementia and vacuolar myelopathy.

The data reviewed above lead to two questions: First, what accounts for the macrophage recruitment and activation associated with axonal degeneration in nerve disease of any type? And second, why does the macrophage response appear to be particularly intense in PSN? With regard to the general problem of macrophage responses in axonal disease, the stimulus for this selective macrophage recruitment and activation is not known, but the pivotal event is clearly degeneration of the axon. Myelin breakdown may augment the extent of the response, but it is not required, as demonstrated by models in which only unmyelinated fibers degenerate (Lobato C, Shir Y, Oaklander RL, and Griffin JW, *unpublished observations*). The macrophage activation does not depend on IFN-γ: it occurs even though lymphocytes are not recruited into the nerve and IFN-γ is not present locally (G Stoll, *personal communication*). Neither anti-IFN-γ antibodies nor the SCID mouse phenotype (R George and J Griffin, *unpublished observations*) affects the process of macrophage infiltration and activation. Identifying this neuronal/axonal chemotropic and activating factor is a major challenge in cellular neurobiology.

With regard to the intense macrophage response in PSN, it may reflect the concomitant degeneration of both the myelinated and the unmyelinated fibers, a feature peculiar to PSN that is not seen in most axonal neuropathies (2). We favor an alternative interpretation: As indicated by the pattern of cytokine production, macrophages behave differently in diseases of the nervous system in the setting of AIDS, as compared to macrophages in similar diseases in seronegative individuals. This hypothesis is discussed in the final section.

SIMILARITIES AND CONTRASTS BETWEEN PSN AND AIDS DEMENTIA

AIDS dementia and the sensory neuropathy of AIDS both occur with sufficient frequency late in the course of AIDS to be often seen in the same individuals. Whether they have shared etiologies remains to be determined; a retrospective analysis by Dal Pan and McArthur *(unpublished observations)* suggested that their coincident occurrence did not exceed that expected by chance. Nevertheless, there are sufficient similarities in their neuropathology and immunopathology to warrant comment. In both, axonal loss is evident and, in AIDS dementia, is reflected in the reduction in cortical synaptic density (see Masliah et al., *this volume*). In both, there are pronounced changes in the macrophage/microglial cells; their numbers are increased and they express prominent activation markers. The pattern of cytokine expression in PSN and in AIDS dementia (65) is also similar, with increased TNF-α transcripts and relatively low levels of IL-1β transcripts being found in both. In addition, both have low levels of three lymphokines: IL-4, IL-10, and IFN-γ (65) (S Wesselingh, D Griffin, J Glass, J McArthur, and J Griffin, *unpublished observations*).

This pattern suggests that macrophages and microglia are being regulated abnormally by cytokines. An attractive explanation is that there is a deficiency of the macrophage "deactivating" cytokines IL-4, IL-10, or tumor growth factor-β. Because of the lymphopenia and the demonstrably low IL-4 and IL-10 in the AIDS dementia brains, these lymphokines are likely candidates to be the deficient factors. We suggest the following pathogenetic sequence for PSN:

1. Any of a variety of factors can trigger bland distal axonal degeneration in sensory neurons in individuals with AIDS. These factors might be specific to AIDS; for example, circulating gp120 neurotoxicity has been demonstrated *in vitro,* as summarized by Lipton *(this volume).* (Direct productive infection of the ganglia or peripheral nerves with HIV is not apt to be an important factor, because, in contrast to the CNS, HIV culture, *in situ* hybridization, and RNA PCR studies have been almost uniformly negative in the PNS.) Alternatively, the trigger could be nonspecific. For example, nutritional insufficiency, B_{12} deficiency, or a type of "critical care" neuropathy associated with systemic infection (66,67) have all been invoked. These factors are not likely to be the *sole* causes of PSN, because their pathology does not include the unmyelinated fiber loss seen in many cases of PSN (68,69).

2. Whatever the basis of the initial distal axonal degeneration, the "neuronal" stimulus for macrophage recruitment and activation is presumably elaborated, as in seronegative neuropathies (59), and macrophages infiltrate the affected regions of the PNS.

3. Deficient "deactivating" lymphokines might then lead to "hyper-responsive" macrophage behaviors, including excessive TNF-α production.

4. Macrophage stimulation of growth factor production by denervated Schwann cells might also be defective. For example, IL-1β is needed for nerve growth factor (NGF) production in transected nerves (62,63). NGF production might in turn contribute to the degeneration of NGF-dependent fibers, including the unmyelinated fibers, and to the failure of regenerative response.

In summary, there are parallels in both the cellular pathology and the immunopathology among the CNS disorders of AIDS (AIDS dementia and vacuolar myelopathy) and PSN. An outstanding difference is the near-absence of productive HIV infection in nerve. Thus, abnormalities in regulation of macrophage responses to nerve disease should be considered as potential contributors in both settings.

ACKNOWLEDGMENTS

Work from our laboratories was supported by NIH grants PO1-26643 and PO1-22849. We thank Drs. William Tyor, David Cornblath, and Richard Johnson.

REFERENCES

1. de la Monte SM, Gabuzda DH, Ho DD, et al. Peripheral neuropathy in the acquired immunodeficiency syndrome. *Ann Neurol* 1988;23:485–492.
2. Griffin JW, Crawford TO, Tyor WR, et al. Sensory neuropathy in AIDS. I. Neuropathology. *Brain* 1994 *(in press)*.
3. Cornford ME, Ho HW, Vinters HV. Correlation of neuromuscular pathology in acquired immune deficiency syndrome patients with cytomegalovirus infection and zidovudine treatment. *Acta Neuropathol* 1992;84:516–529.
4. Guillain G, Barré JA, Strohl A. Sur un syndrome de radiculonéurité avec hyperalbuminose du liquide céphalo-rachidien sans réaction cellulaire. Remarques sur les caractères cliniques et graphiques des reflexes tendineux. *Bull Soc Med Hop Paris* 1916;40:1462.
5. Asbury AK, Arnason BG, Karp HR, McFarlin DE. Criteria for diagnosis of Guillain–Barré syndrome. *Ann Neurol* 1978;3:565–566.
6. Asbury AK, Cornblath DR. Assessment of current diagnostic criteria for Guillain–Barré syndrome. *Ann Neurol* 1990;27(suppl):S21–S24.
7. Cornblath DR, Asbury AK, Albers JW, et al. Research criteria for diagnosis of chronic inflammatory demyelinating polyneuropathy (CIDP). *Neurology* 1991;41:617–618.
8. Asbury AK, Arnason BG, Adams RD. The inflammatory lesion in idiopathic polyneuritis. *Medicine* 1969;48:173–215.
9. Prineas JW. Acute idiopathic polyneuritis. An electron microscope study. *Lab Invest* 1972; 26:133–147.
10. Hartung H-P, Stoll G, Toyka KV. Immune reactions in the peripheral nervous system. In: Dyck PJ, Thomas PK, Griffin JW, Low PA, Poduslo JF, eds. *Peripheral neuropathy*. 3rd ed. Philadelphia: WB Saunders, 1993;418–444.
11. Griffin JW, Cornblath DR, Wesselingh SL, et al. Pathology of HIV-associated Guillain–Barré syndrome and chronic inflammatory demyelinating polyneuropathy. Submitted 1993.
12. Chavanet PY, Giroud M, Lancon J-P, et al. Altered peripheral nerve conduction in HIV-patients. *Cancer Detect Prev* 1988;12:249–255.
13. Cornblath DR, McArthur JC, Kennedy PGE, Witte AS, Griffin JW. Inflammatory demyelinating peripheral neuropathies associated with human T-cell lymphotropic virus type III infection. *Ann Neurol* 1987;21:32–40.
14. Leaf AN, Laubenstein LJ, Raphael B, Hochster H, Baez L, Karpatkin S. Thrombotic thrombocytopenic purpura associated with human immunodeficiency virus type 1 (HIV-1) infection. *Ann Intern Med* 1988;109:194–197.
15. Morris L, Distenfeld A, Amorosi E, Karpatkin S. Autoimmune thrombocytopenic purpura in homosexual men. *Ann Intern Med* 1982;96:714–717.
16. Walsh C, Krigel R, Lennette E, Karpatkin S. Thrombocytopenia in homosexual patients. *Ann Intern Med* 1985;103:542–545.
17. Prineas JW, McLeod JG. Chronic relapsing polyneuritis. *J Neurol Sci* 1976;27:427–458.
18. Prineas JW. Pathology of the Guillain–Barré syndrome. *Ann Neurol* 1981;9(suppl):6–19.
19. Cornblath DR, Griffin DE, Welch D, Griffin JW, McArthur JC. Quantitative analysis of endoneurial T-cells in human sural nerve biopsies. *J Neuroimmunol* 1990;26:113–118.
20. Sher A, Gazzinelli RT, Oswald IP, et al. Role of T-cell derived cytokines in the downregulation of immune responses in parasitic and retroviral infection. *Immunol Rev* 1992;127: 183–204.
21. Raphael SA, Price ML, Lischner HW, Griffin JW, Grover WD, Bagsra O. Inflammatory

demyelinating polyneuropathy in a child with systematic human immunodeficiency virus infection. *J Pediatr* 1991;118:242–245.

22. Arnason BGW. Acute inflammatory demyelinating polyradiculopathies. In: Dyck PJ, Thomas PK, Lambert EH, Bunge R, eds. *Peripheral Neuropathy*, vol II. Philadelphia: WB Saunders, 1984;2050:2100.

23. Feasby TE, Gilbert JJ, Brown WF, et al. An acute axonal form of Guillain–Barré polyneuropathy. *Brain* 1986;109:1115–1126.

24. McKhann GM, Cornblath DR, Ho TW, et al. Clinical and electrophysiological aspects of acute paralytic disease of children and young adults in northern China. *Lancet* 1991;338: 593–597.

25. McKhann GM, Cornblath DR, Griffin JW, et al. Acute motor axonal neuropathy: a frequent cause of acute flaccid paralysis in China. *Ann Neurol* 1993;33:333–342.

26. Ramos-Alvarez M, Bessudo L, Sabin A. Paralytic syndromes associated with noninflammatory cytoplasmic or nuclear neuronopathy: acute paralytic disease in Mexican children, neuropathologically distinguishable from Landry–Guillain–Barré syndrome. *JAMA* 1969; 207:1481–1492.

27. Lipkin WI, Parry G, Kiprov D, Abrams D. Inflammatory neuropathy in homosexual men with lymphadenopathy. *Neurology* 1985;35:1479–1483.

28. Miller RG, Parry G, Lang W, Lippert R, Kiprov D. AIDS-related inflammatory polyradiculoneuropathy: prediction of response to plasma exchange with electrophysiologic testing [Abstract]. *Muscle Nerve* 1985;8:626.

29. Behar R, Wiley C, McCutchan JA. Cytomegalovirus polyradiculoneuropathy in acquired immune deficiency syndrome. *Neurology* 1987;37:557–561.

30. Miller RG, Storey JR, Creco CM. Ganciclovir in the treatment of progressive AIDS-related polyradiculopathy. *Neurology* 1990;40:569–574.

31. Eidelberg D, Sotrel A, Vogel H, Walker P, Kleefield J, Crumpacker CS. Progressive polyradiculopathy in acquired deficiency syndrome. *Neurology* 1986;36:912–916.

32. Bishopric G, Bruner J, Butler J. Guillain–Barré syndrome with cytomegalovirus infection of peripheral nerves. *Arch Pathol Lab Med* 1985;109:1106–1108.

33. Mahieux F, Gray F, Fenelon G, et al. Acute myeloradiculitis due to cytomegalovirus as the initial manifestation of AIDS. *J Neurol Neurosurg Psychiatry* 1989;52:270–274.

34. Budzilovich G, Avitabile A, Niedt G, Aleksic S, Rosenblum M. Polyradiculopathy and sensory ganglionitis due to cytomegalovirus in acquired immune deficiency syndrome (AIDS). *Prog AIDS Pathol* 1989;1:143–157.

35. Said G, Lacroix C, Chemouilli P, et al. Cytomegalovirus neuropathy in acquired immunodeficiency syndrome: a clinical and pathological study. *Ann Neurol* 1991;29:139–146.

36. Cohen BA, McArthur JC, Grohman S, Patterson B, Glass JD. Neurologic prognosis of CMV polyradiculomyelopathy in AIDS. *Neurology* 1993;43:493–499.

37. Cornblath DR, Miller RG, Griffin JW, Greco C, Fuller GN, McArthur JC. Multifocal CMV polyneuropathy in AIDS. Submitted 1993.

38. Dalakas MC, Pezeshkpour GH. Neuromuscular diseases associated with human immunodeficiency virus infection. *Ann Neurol* 1988;23(suppl):S38–S48.

39. van Dorp WT, Vlieger A, Jiwa NM, et al. The polymerase chain reaction, a sensitive and rapid technique for detecting cytomegalovirus infection after renal transplantation. *Transplantation* 1992;54:661–664.

40. Wiley CA. Neuromuscular diseases of AIDS. *FASEB J* 1989;3:2503–2511.

41. Fuller GN, Jacobs JM, Guiloff RJ. Association of painful peripheral neuropathy in AIDS with cytomegalovirus infection. *Lancet* 1989;2:937–941.

42. Scaravilli F, Sinclair E, Arango J-C, Manji H, Lucas S, Harrison MJG. The pathology of the posterior root ganglia in AIDS and its relationship to the pallor of the gracile tract. *Acta Neuropathol* 1992;84:163–170.

43. Dyck PJ, Conn DL, Okazaki H. Necrotizing angiopathic neuropathy: three dimensional morphology of fiber degeneration related to sites of occluded vessels. *Mayo Clin Proc* 1972; 47:461–475.

44. Said G, Lacroix-Ciaudo C, Fujimura H, Blas C, Faux N. The peripheral neuropathy of necrotizing arteritis: a clinicopathological study. *Ann Neurol* 1988;23:461–465.

45. Yasuda H, Dyck PJ. Abnormalities of endoneurial microvessels and sural nerve pathology in diabetic neuropathy. *Neurology* 1987;37:20–28.

46. Cornblath DR, McArthur JC. Predominantly sensory neuropathy in patients with AIDS and AIDS-related complex. *Neurology* 1988;38:794–796.
47. So YT, Holtzman DM, Abrams DI, Olney RK. Peripheral neuropathy associated with acquired immunodeficiency syndrome: prevalence and clinical features from a population-based survey. *Arch Neurol* 1988;45:945–948.
48. Winer JB, Bang B, Clarke JR, et al. A study of neuropathy in HIV infection. *Q J Med* 1992;302:473–488.
49. Freeman R, Cohen JA. Autonomic failure and AIDS. In: Low PA, ed. *Clinical autonomic disorders: evaluation and management.* Boston: Little, Brown and Co, 1992;677–683.
50. Garcia-Erro MI, Sica REP, Losavio AS, Muchnik S, Arroyo H. Tools to differentiate immunologic and non-immunologic myasthenia gravis in infancy. *Neuropediatrics* 1988;19:92–95.
51. Dubinsky RM, Yarchoan R, Dalakas M, Broder S. Reversible axonal neuropathy from the treatment of AIDS and related disorders with 2',3'-dideoxycytidine (ddC). *Muscle Nerve* 1989;12:856–860.
52. Griffin JW, Cornblath DR. The ataxic neuropathies. In: Sluga E, Budka H, eds. *Sensory neuropathies.* Berlin: Springer-Verlag, 1993 *(in press).*
53. Rance N, McArthur JC, Cornblath DR, Landstrom D, Griffin JW, Price DL. Gracile tract degeneration in patients with sensory neuropathy and AIDS. *Neurology* 1988;38:265–271.
54. Griffin JW, Tyor WR, Glass JD, et al. Sensory neuropathy in AIDS. II. Immunopathology. *Brain* 1994 *(in press).*
55. Griffin JW, George R, Lobato C, Tyor WR, Li CY, Glass JD. Macrophage responses and myelin clearance during Wallerian degeneration: relevance to immune-mediated demyelination. *J Neuroimmunol* 1992;40:153–166.
56. Arvidson B. Cellular uptake of exogenous horseradish peroxidase in mouse peripheral nerve. *Acta Neuropathol* 1977;37:35–41.
57. Griffin JW, George R, Ho T. Macrophage systems in peripheral nerves. *J Neuropath Exp Neurol* 1993 *(in press).*
58. Chaudhry V, Glass JD, Griffin JW. Wallerian degeneration in peripheral nerve disease. In: Dyck PJ, ed. *Peripheral neuropathy: new concepts and treatments; Neurologic clinics,* vol 10, August 1992). Philadelphia: WB Saunder, 1992;613–627.
59. Stoll G, Griffin JW, Li CY, Trapp BD. Wallerian degeneration in the peripheral nervous system: participation of both Schwann cells and macrophages in myelin degradation. *J Neurocytol* 1989;18:671–683.
60. Griffin JW, Stoll G, Li CY, Tyor WR, Cornblath DR. Macrophage responses in inflammatory demyelinating neuropathies. *Ann Neurol* 1990;27(suppl):S64–S68.
61. Ignatius MJ, Shooter EM, Pitas RE, Mahley RW. Lipoprotein uptake by neuronal growth-cones *in vitro. Science* 1987;236:959–962.
62. Heumann R, Lindholm D, Bandtlow C, et al. Differential regulation of mRNA encoding nerve growth factor and its receptor in rat sciatic nerve during development, degeneration, and regeneration: role of macrophages. *Proc Natl Acad Sci USA* 1987;84:8735–8739.
63. Lindholm D, Heumann R, Hengerer B, Thoenen H. Interleukin-1 increases stability and transcription of mRNA encoding nerve growth factor in cultured rat fibroblasts. *J Biol Chem* 1988;263:16348–16351.
64. George R, Griffin J. The proximo-distal spread of Wallerian degeneration in the dorsal columns of the rat. Submitted for publication.
65. Wesselingh SL, Power C, Glass JD, et al. Intracerebral cytokine mRNA expression in AIDS. *Ann Neurol* 1993;33:576–582.
66. Bolton CF, Gilbert JJ, Hahn AK, Sibbald WJ. Polyneuropathy in critically ill patients. *J Neurol Neurosurg Psychiatry* 1984;47:1223–1231.
67. Zochodne DW, Bolton CF, Wells GA, et al. Critical illness polyneuropathy: a complication of sepsis and multiorgan failure. *Brain* 1987;110:819–842.
68. Behse F, Buchthal F, Carlsen F, Knappeis GG. Unmyelinated fibres and Schwann cells of sural nerve in neuropathy. *Brain* 1975;98:493–510.
69. Behse F, Buchthal F. Alcoholic neuropathy: clinical, electrophysiological, and biopsy findings. *Ann Neurol* 1977;2:95–110.

HIV, AIDS and the Brain, edited by
R. W. Price and S. W. Perry.
Raven Press, Ltd., New York © 1994.

10

Laboratory Basis of Novel Therapeutic Strategies to Prevent HIV-Related Neuronal Injury

Stuart A. Lipton

Laboratory of Cellular and Molecular Neuroscience, Department of Neurology, Children's Hospital; Departments of Neurology, Beth Israel Hospital, Brigham and Women's Hospital, and Massachusetts General Hospital; Program in Neuroscience, Harvard Medical School, Boston, MA 02115

Our laboratory has a long-standing interest in the relationship of neuronal viability/outgrowth to intracellular Ca^{2+} levels (reviewed in ref. 1). Glutamate, or a related excitatory amino acid (EAA), is the major excitatory neurotransmitter that controls the level of intracellular neuronal Ca^{2+} ($[Ca^{2+}]_i$). Escalating concentrations of glutamate have been measured *in vivo* following focal stroke and head injury (reviewed in refs. 2 and 3). As a result, there is an immediate elevation in $[Ca^{2+}]_i$ which precedes neurotoxicity by ~24 hr. Although the rise in $[Ca^{2+}]_i$ may not account by itself for the ensuing neuronal injury, several laboratories have now reported that prevention of the increase in $[Ca^{2+}]_i$ leads to the amelioration of anticipated neuronal cell death (reviewed in refs. 2 and 3). Two major routes of entry of Ca^{2+} occur via ion channels that are permeable to Ca^{2+} and can be summarized as follows:

1. Glutamate or related EAAs trigger voltage-dependent calcium channels (VDCCs) by depolarizing the cell membrane; the major VDCC subtype that is chronically activated by prolonged depolarizations is the L-type calcium channel (4).
2. Glutamate or related EAAs activate ligand-gated ion channels directly; the major glutamate receptor-operated channel stimulated under these conditions is the *N*-methyl-D-aspartate (NMDA) subtype (2).

We have shown that activation of these channel types can control neuronal plasticity during normal development, but, in excessive amounts, our laboratory and others have shown that this stimulation can lead to neuronal death (e.g., after a stroke) (1). Similar mechanisms may obtain in various neurodegenerative conditions. In fact, this mechanism may represent a final common pathway of neuronal injury, although not involved in the primary pathophysiology of a neurologic disorder. Most importantly, this pathway makes the disease process amenable to pharmacotherapy. This line of reasoning led us to think that this mechanism might be involved in acquired immunodeficiency syndrome (AIDS)-related neuronal injury.

NEURONAL LOSS IN AIDS BRAINS

A significant number of adults and children with AIDS eventually develop neurological manifestations, including dementia, myelopathy, and peripheral neuropathy; as many as 80 percent of infected children have neurological deficits presenting as delayed milestones. These deficits occur even in the absence of superinfection with opportunistic organisms or malignancy (5). Among the several neuropathological manifestations of AIDS in the brain is neuronal loss. In selected brains from AIDS patients, the groups of Budka (6), Wiley (7), Everall (8), and Sadun (9) have demonstrated the loss of 18–50 percent of cortical neurons and retinal ganglion cell neurons. The question remains, however, in at least a subject of patients with the disease, how can neurons be injured and yet not be infected?

gp120-INDUCED NEURONAL INJURY IS AMELIORATED BY CALCIUM CHANNEL ANTAGONISTS

Possibly at least partly accounting for the loss of neurons is the observation first made *in vitro* by Brenneman et al. (10) that picomolar concentrations of the envelope protein of human immunodeficiency virus type 1 (HIV-1), gp120, can induce neuronal injury in rodent hippocampal cultures. Subsequently, our group (11) demonstrated that in mixed cultures of neurons and glia, picomolar gp120 could increase $[Ca^{2+}]_i$ in rodent hippocampal neurons and retinal ganglion cells within a few minutes of application. Recently, similar findings were reported by Thayer's group (12), who were also able to resolve the increase in $[Ca^{2+}]_i$ into discrete oscillations by monitoring the calcium signal on a faster time scale. Within the next 24 hr, neuronal injury ensues (11). Both the early rise in $[Ca^{2+}]_i$ and the delayed neuronal injury could be prevented by antagonists of voltage-dependent calcium channels, including nimodipine (100 nM in 5 percent rat serum or approximately 4 nM free drug) (11). Other antagonists of the L-type of VDCC are also effective to some degree (ref. 13 and Table 1). Not only are rat retinal ganglion cells and cortical neurons *in vitro* partially protected by nimodipine and other voltage-dependent Ca^{2+} channel antagonists, but also in a rat pup animal model, stereotactic injection of gp120 into the cortex produces a lesion con-

TABLE 1. *Voltage-dependent calcium channel antagonists attenuate gp120-mediated neuronal injury* in vitro[a]

Amelioration[b] of gp120-induced neuronal injury by voltage-dependent calcium channel antagonists of the class:

Dihydropyridine[c]	Diphenylalkylamine piperazine derivative[d]	Phenylalkylamine[e]	Benzothiazepine[f]
$+ + + +$	$+ +$	$+$	$-$

[a] Adapted from Lipton (111).
[b] An increasing number of plus ($+$) signs indicates greater potency.
[c] Nimodipine and nifedipine (10–100 nM in 5 percent serum; ~4–40 nM free drug).
[d] Flunarizine (10 μM in 5 percent serum).
[e] Verapamil (100 μM in 5 percent serum).
[f] Diltiazem (1 μM in 5 percent serum).

sisting of cellular infiltrates of foamy macrophages and putative neuronal injury that is prevented by concomitant intraperitoneal administration of nimodipine (14). Because of these developments, the AIDS Clinical Trials Group (ACTG) of the NIH Division of AIDS has asked us to begin a clinical study to test the effects of nimodipine in adult patients with HIV-associated cognitive/motor complex (a subset of which have the more debilitating AIDS dementia complex).

Nevertheless, these developments do not tell us the mechanism of action of gp120 on neurons, which more recent evidence has led us to believe is an indirect action via macrophages/microglia (see below). For example, we noted that only neurons clustered in groups and presumably with synaptic contacts were vulnerable to gp120, and this fact suggested that cellular interactions were necessary to produce injury. Moreover, the HIV envelope protein does not appear to act directly on calcium channels; in whole-cell and single-channel patch clamp recordings, picomolar gp120 does not increase calcium current per se (VH-S Chen, M Plummer, P Hess, and SA Lipton, *unpublished findings*). It is possible that calcium channel antagonists ameliorate gp120-induced neuronal injury by reducing the overall intracellular Ca^{2+} burden of the neurons. After all, Ca^{2+} can accumulate in neurons during normal activity with each action potential fired, and nimodipine may be only indirectly beneficial by helping offset an increased calcium load due to another mechanism.

INVOLVEMENT OF THE NMDA RECEPTOR IN gp120-INDUCED NEURONAL INJURY

As outlined above, there is another prominent mode of Ca^{2+} entry via channels directly coupled to EAA/glutamate receptors. The type of glutamate receptor subtype that is primarily involved in this regard is named after NMDA, a glutamate analog that is a selective agonist of this receptor (however, NMDA does not occur naturally in the body). We reasoned that since gp120 causes an early rise in $[Ca^{2+}]_i$ and delayed toxicity, similar to glutamate acting at the NMDA receptor, perhaps glutamate or a closely related molecule was involved in HIV-related neuronal injury. Furthermore, it was well known that VDCC antagonists such as nimodipine could block some forms of glutamate neurotoxicity (15–17). Therefore, it was certainly possible that glutamate or a related NMDA agonist was somehow involved in gp120-induced neuronal damage. In addition, Heyes et al. (18,19) had found that cerebrospinal fluid (CSF) levels of quinolinate, a naturally occurring (albeit weak) NMDA agonist, was correlated with the degree of dementia in AIDS patients. To test the possibility that EAAs were involved, the following experiments were undertaken. NMDA antagonists were assessed for their ability to prevent gp120-induced neuronal injury. We found that MK-801 (dizocilpine), an open-channel blocker of the NMDA receptor-coupled ion channels, prevented gp120-induced neuronal injury (20,21).

D-2-Amino-5-phosphonovalerate (APV), a competitive antagonist at glutamate binding site of the NMDA receptor, was partially effective. In contrast, CNQX, a non-NMDA antagonist, did not protect from gp120-induced neuronal damage (20,21).

The simplest potential explanation for these findings is that gp120 might simulate an NMDA-evoked current, or somehow augment such currents. To examine this idea, we used the patch-clamp technique to determine if gp120 affected membrane currents. However, in whole-cell recordings, using both conventional and perforated-patch techniques, no effect of gp120 was observed, even in recordings lasting tens of minutes. Similarly, no enhancement of glutamate- or of NMDA-evoked currents was encountered (21). The next possible explanation that we considered is that endogenous levels of glutamate become toxic in the presence of gp120. To test this hypothesis, the enzyme glutamate-pyruvate transaminase (GPT) was used to degrade the endogenous glutamate. High-performance liquid chromatography (HPLC) analysis of amino acids was used to verify glutamate degradation. Under these conditions, the degradation of endogenous glutamate *in vitro* protected neurons from gp120-induced injury (20,21). Taken together, these data argue that concurrent activation of NMDA receptors are needed for neuronal injury by gp120 in AIDS. These experiments do not tell us, however, if the action of gp120 is mediated directly on neurons or indirectly via an intervening cell type, such as astrocytes or macrophages/microglia.

INDIRECT NEURONAL INJURY MEDIATED BY HIV-INFECTED OR gp120-STIMULATED MONOCYTIC CELLS

To determine cell types involved in neurotoxicity, the following experiment was performed. L-Leucine methyl ester was used to eliminate monocy-

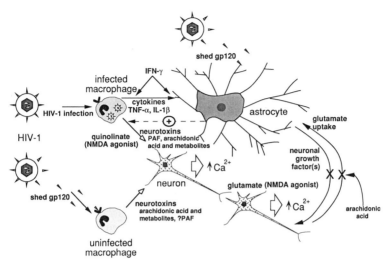

FIG. 1. Model summarizing evidence for at least one complete pathway of HIV-related neuronal injury. HIV-infected macrophages release factors that lead to neurotoxicity. These factors include PAF (platelet-activating factor), leukotriene B_4 (LTB$_4$), leukotriene D_4 (LTD$_4$), and lipoxin A_4 (LXA$_4$). Macrophages and astrocytes have mutual feedback loops in this system. The excitatory action of the macrophage factors appears to lead to an increase in neuronal Ca^{2+} and the consequent release of glutamate. In turn, glutamate overexcites neighboring neurons, leading to an increase in intracellular Ca^{2+}, neuronal injury, and subsequent further release of glutamate. This final common pathway of neurotoxic action can be blocked by NMDA antagonists. For certain neurons, this form of damage can also be ameliorated to some degree by calcium channel antagonists or non-NMDA antagonists. The major pathway of entry of HIV-1 into monocytoid cells is via gp120 binding to the cells; therefore, not surprisingly, gp120 (or a fragment thereof) appears capable of activating uninfected macrophages to release similar factors (the best evidence to date is for LTB$_4$ and LTD$_4$). Cytokines participate in this cellular network in several ways. For example, HIV infection or gp120 stimulation of macrophages enhances their production of TNF-α and IL-1β. The TNF-α and IL-1β produced by macrophages stimulate astrogliosis. TNF-α may also injure oligodendrocytes and increase voltage-dependent calcium currents in neurons. Interferon-γ (IFN-γ) induces macrophage/microgliosis and macrophage production of quinolinate and PAF; IFN-γ may also affect astrocytic cells in several ways, at least *in vitro* [e.g., by inducing expression of major histocompatibility (MHC) class II genes]. Many other cytokine loops also exist.

toid cells from cultures of mixed glia and neurons. Under these conditions, gp120 no longer injured neurons, suggesting that at least under our culture conditions, macrophages/microglial were necessary to mediate the neurotoxic effects of gp120 (22).

In conjunction with the data of other laboratories, these results suggest the following model of HIV-related neuronal injury (Fig. 1). HIV-infected macrophages (23,24) or gp120-stimulated macrophages (22; D Giulian, *personal communication*) release neurotoxic products. These neurotoxins include relatively small, heat-stable compounds, which have recently begun to be characterized by Gendelman and colleagues (25). They found that the products released by HIV-infected macrophages include the arachidonic acid metabolites leukotriene B_4 (LTB$_4$), leukotriene D_4 (LTD$_4$), lipoxin A_4 (LXA$_4$), and platelet-activating factor (PAF). Under their conditions, these substances are released only in the presence of astrocytes, implying some positive feedback loop between astrocytes and macrophages. HIV-infected macrophages also release the cytokines tumor necrosis factor alpha (TNF-α) and interleukin 1β (IL-1β), which have been shown to stimulate astrocyte proliferation (26,27)—another feature of HIV encephalitis. In addition, the cytokines present in conditioned medium from lipopolysaccharide (LPS)-treated astrocytes can stimulate HIV-1 gene expression in monocytic cells (28). Under certain *in vitro* conditions, TNF-α and IL-1 can be associated with the death of oligodendrocytes and, by implication, demyelination (see below and ref. 29).

Moreover, there are multiple, complex interactions and feedback loops affecting cytokine and arachidonic acid metabolite production by macrophages and astrocytes. For example, TNF-α enhances IL-1 production in macrophages (30). Arachidonic acid metabolites can influence the production of TNF-α and IL-1β in macrophages, and, in turn, TNF can amplify arachidonic acid metabolism, including the release of LTB4, in response to IL-1. PAF can enhance TNF and IL-1 production, and, in turn, PAF synthesis can be stimulated with TNF, IL1-β, or interferon gamma (IFN-γ) in human monocytes (31–36). Finally, the same arachidonic acid metabolites and cytokines released by HIV-infected macrophages appear to be produced by gp120-stimulated monocytic cells. For example, this HIV glycoprotein induces the release of LTB$_4$, LTD$_4$, TNF-α, and IL-1β from human monocytes (37–39). It remains to be shown definitively, however, that gp120-stimulated macrophages also release LXA$_4$ and PAF.

The cytokines TNF-α and IL1-β in the amounts produced by HIV-infected or gp120-stimulated macrophages do not appear to be neurotoxic in and of themselves (25). Could, however, the arachidonic acid metabolites emanating from HIV-infected or gp120-stimulated macrophages be involved in neurotoxicity? The arachidonic acid metabolites LTB$_4$, LTD$_4$, and LXA$_4$, as well as PAF, have excitatory effects on neurons (40–46), and this may represent at least one pathway whereby these arachidonic acid metabolites invoke EAA-induced neurotoxicity. In particular, PAF has recently been shown to increase intracellular neuronal Ca^{2+} and lead to enhanced neurotransmission, presumably by increasing the release of presynaptic glutamate (47,48). In collaboration with Gendelman's group, our laboratory has obtained preliminary evidence that the levels of LTB$_4$, LTD$_4$, and PAF found in cultures of HIV-infected monocytic cells (as reported in ref. 25) are toxic to cortical neurons *in vitro*. It is possible that TNF-α also contributes to this process by increasing voltage-dependent Ca^{2+} currents (49). Additional glutamate receptor activation may occur as a consequence of these events as neurons are injured and release their stores of glutamate onto neighboring neurons

(12,20,21,50). One line of evidence for this supposition lies in the finding, as detailed above, that enzymatic degradation of glutamate ameliorates gp120-induced neuronal injury in mixed neuronal–glial cultures (12,20,21).

Also, as alluded to above, another possible link between HIV-1 infection and EAA-induced neurotoxicity involves quinolinate, an endogenous NMDA agonist that is increased in the CSF of patients with the AIDS dementia complex (19). Quinolinate levels are known to be influenced by cytokines that are increased after HIV-1 infection. For example, it is known that IFN-γ is present in the brains of patients with AIDS (51), and human macrophages activated by IFN-γ release substantial amounts of quinolinate (52). In addition, under some conditions (e.g., following neuronal loss) quinolinate can also be produced by astrocytes (53,54).

POSSIBLE INVOLVEMENT OF ASTROCYTES, OLIGODENDROCYTES, AND OTHER HIV-1 PROTEINS IN NEURONAL INJURY

In at least some model systems, the presence of astrocytes is necessary for HIV-infected macrophages to release substantial amounts of their neurotoxic factors (25). In addition, astrocytes may be important in mediating HIV-related neuronal injury in other ways. For example, in murine hippocampal cultures Brenneman et al. (10) have found that gp120-induced neurotoxicity can be prevented by the presence of vasoactive intestinal polypeptide (VIP) or by a five-amino-acid substance with sequence homology to VIP, namely, peptide T. These workers have also found that VIP acts on astrocytes to increase oscillations in intracellular Ca^{2+} and to release factors necessary for normal neuronal outgrowth and survival (55). Thus, these results raise the possibility that gp120 may compete with endogenous VIP for a receptor, most likely on astrocytes, that is critical to normal neuronal function. This effect of gp120 is hypothesized to prevent the release of such astrocyte factors that are necessary to prevent neuronal injury and suggests that one pathway for neuronal damage is an indirect one that is mediated via astrocytes. Hence, neurotoxicity may in part be realized by interfering with the normal function of astrocytes and their release of neuronal growth factor(s) (56) (see Fig. 1).

The envelope protein gp120 has also been shown to bind to galactosyl ceramide (GalC), a molecule on the surface of oligodendrocytes, which are responsible for myelination in the CNS (57,58). Relatively high concentrations of gp120 (nanomolar) were necessary to observe this binding compared to the low (picomolar) concentrations of the coat protein that have been found to lead to neurotoxicity. Nonetheless, the findings concerning binding to GalC raise the possibility of participation of gp120 in myelin disruption and, therefore, a further indirect influence on the welfare of neurons. Future studies will be necessary to determine the significance of this potential pathway for cellular injury.

Recently, in addition to gp120, two other HIV-1 proteins have been reported to affect neurons or neuronal-like cells, raising the possibility of their involvement in HIV-related neuronal injury. The nuclear protein tat was shown to be toxic to glioma and neuroblastoma cell lines *in vitro* and to mice *in vivo* (59). The basic region of the peptide (amino acid residues 49–57) appears to act nonspecifically to increase the leakage conductance of the membrane, thus altering cell permeability. Further work will be necessary to attempt to relate these findings to the neuropathology encountered in the brains of patients with HIV-1-associated cognitive/motor complex. Another HIV-1 protein, Nef, has been shown to affect neuronal cell function. Nef shares sequence and structural features with scorpion toxin peptides; both recombinant Nef protein and a synthetic portion of scorpion peptide increase total K^+ current in chick dorsal root ganglion cells (60).

OVERSTIMULATION OF NMDA RECEPTORS, A FINAL COMMON PATHWAY

From the foregoing, there appear to be at least two sites of potential interaction of HIV-related neurotoxins with NMDA receptors (Fig. 1). First, quinolinate emanating from macrophages may directly stimulate neurons. Second, after excitation by quinolinate, arachidonic acid metabolites, and PAF, or after injury due to other toxic pathways, neurons would release glutamate onto second-order neurons. This "bad neighbor hypothesis" is in some ways similar to the damage thought to occur in the penumbra of a stroke: Glutamate released by injured neurons contributes to further injury to neighboring neurons.

Moreover, NMDA antagonists ameliorate HIV-related neuronal injury induced by either HIV-infected macrophages (23; H Gendelman, *personal communication*), or, as mentioned earlier, gp120-activated macrophages (20,21). Furthermore, in some cases calcium channel antagonists can attenuate this form of damage (11,13; L Pulliam, *personal communication*) (Table 2). In general, the pharmacology of neuroprotection from noxious agents depends upon the repertoire and diversity of ion channel types in a particular class of neurons (4). For example, neurons lacking NMDA receptors will obviously not be protected by NMDA antagonists. Conversely, if NMDA-receptor-associated channels are the predominant channel in a specific neuronal cell type whereby Ca^{2+} enters the cell, then the lethal effects of excessive stimulation by glutamate may be ameliorated with NMDA antagonists. Some non-NMDA-receptor-associated channels are directly permeable to Ca^{2+}, but most appear not to be (those containing the GluR2 receptor subunit). However, depolarization of neurons by stimulation of non-NMDA re-

TABLE 2. *Protective effects of calcium channel antagonists and NMDA antagonists against gp120-induced and HIV-infected macrophage-mediated neuronal injury* in vitro[a]

	Attenuation of neuronal injury by		
Insult	Ca^{2+} channel antagonists[b]	NMDA antagonists	Non-NMDA antagonists
gp120 glycoprotein or fragment	+	+	−
HIV-infected macrophage toxin(s)	+[c]	+	−

[a] Adapted from Lipton (111).

[b] Nimodipine or nifedipine (10–100 nM in 5 percent serum or ~4–40 nM free dihydropyridine).

[c] L. Pulliam *(personal communication)*—results in human brain cell aggregates [but see also the earlier work of D. Giulian et al. (23), who found no protective effective of high concentrations of calcium channel antagonists in chick ciliary and rat spinal cord neurons; nonetheless, it is possible that in these latter experiments the high concentration of calcium channel antagonist used was deleterious in and of itself or that these antagonists were not effective in the neuronal cell types tested].

ceptors will trigger VDCCs. If sufficient L-type calcium channels exist on a particular neuronal cell type, then the excessive influx of Ca^{2+} via these channels could lead to toxic consequences. Hence, in some cell types such as hippocampal pyramidal cells, cortical neurons, and retinal ganglion cells, there is evidence that calcium channel antagonists may attenuate damage due to activation of either NMDA or non-NMDA receptors (15–17).

Along similar lines of reasoning, the release of glutamate may be involved in the final common pathway of neuronal injury by HIV-infected macrophages or by gp120-stimulated macrophages. Thus, either NMDA or non-NMDA receptor activation may play a role in this form of toxicity depending on the exact repertoire of ion channels in a particular cell type. In fact, it has been suggested that non-NMDA receptors could also be important in contributing in the neurotoxic events triggered by gp120 (61,62). Nevertheless, the majority of findings to date suggest that NMDA receptor-mediated neuronal injury plays a predominant role in the pathogenesis of the neurological manifestations of AIDS in the CNS (50).

DEVELOPMENT OF CLINICALLY TOLERATED NMDA ANTAGONISTS FOR HIV-RELATED NEURONAL INJURY

NMDA receptors may be involved in HIV-related neurotoxicity at two separate sites, located (i) on the primary neuron injured by factors released from glial cells and (ii) on neurons that are secondarily affected (see above and Fig. 1). This fact has provided an impetus for our laboratory to begin a drug development program for clinically tolerated NMDA antagonists, as described below.

Sites of Action of Potential Clinically Tolerated NMDA Antagonists

Despite concerns about the potential complexity of EAA receptor pharmacology, we can consider currently available agents that appear to work on broad classes of these receptors. For the purposes of this review, we will concentrate mainly on NMDA antagonists that appear to be clinically tolerated and therefore can be considered for human trials.

There are several modulatory sites on the NMDA receptor-channel complex that could potentially be used to modify the activity of the receptor-operated ion channels and thus to prevent the excessive influx of Ca^{2+} (Fig. 2). The first site is the glutamate or NMDA binding site. An antagonist acting here would be competitive in nature; that is, it would compete for the site with an EAA. For both theoretical and practical reasons, a competitive inhibitor might not be as desirable an antagonist as one that is not competitive for the glutamate binding site. A competitive antagonist would perforce eliminate the normal, physiological activity of the NMDA receptor even before

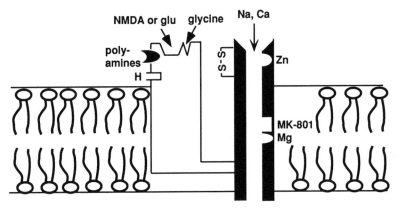

FIG. 2. Sites of potential antagonist action on the NMDA receptor-channel complex. Competitive antagonists can compete with NMDA or glutamate (glu) for binding to the agonist site. Several antagonists to the glycine co-agonist site have been described that are chlorinated and sulfated derivatives of kynurenic acid. These inhibitors do not compete with glutamate and hence are designated as noncompetitive. It is not yet known if any will prove to be tolerated clinically. H^+ effects are transmitted through another noncompetitive site; decreasing pH acts to down-regulate channel activity. Other sites for polyamines and Zn^{2+} can also be used to affect receptor-channel function. Sites that inhibit channel activity by binding Mg^{2+} or drugs such as MK-801, phencyclidine, and memantine are within the electric field of the channel and are only exposed when the channel is previously opened by agonist (termed uncompetitive antagonism). Finally, a redox modulatory site [probably a disulfide bond, or at least a long-lasting covalent modification of a thiol group, that can be converted to free sulfhydryl groups (S—S $\rightleftarrows$ 2-SH)] is affected by chemical reducing and oxidizing agents. Oxidation can favor the disulfide conformation (S—S) over free thiol (—SH) groups and thus down-regulate channel activity. Nitroso-compounds produce RS-NO (NO^+ equivalents) at the thiol group(s) of the NMDA receptor's redox site, also leading to down-regulation of channel activity.

it would affect potentially excessive levels of glutamate. Thus, cognition and memory, thought to be related to long-term potentiation (LTP), might be compromised as well as other important functions mediated by excitatory transmission in the brain. In any event, as part of the disease process, escalating levels of glutamate might be able to overcome or "out-compete" such an antagonist.

NMDA Open-Channel Blockers

In contrast, other modulatory sites should be able to inhibit the effects of high levels of glutamate in compromised areas of the brain while leaving relatively spared the effects of normal neurotransmission in other regions of the brain (63–65). For example, one site that appears to have this advantageous effect is located in the channel itself. There are drugs that only block the channel when it is open; that is, the antagonist can only gain access to the channel in the open state. On average, escalating levels of glutamate result in the channels remaining open for a greater fraction of time. Under these conditions, there is a better chance for an open-channel blocking drug to enter the channel and block it. The result of such a mechanism of action is that the untoward effects of greater (pathological) concentrations of glutamate are inhibited to a greater extent than lower (physiological) concentrations (65). Unfortunately, some of these open-channel blockers, which include phencyclidine (angel dust) and MK-801 (dizocilpine), have neuropsychiatric side effects and probably cannot be safely administered (66). Another concern with specific NMDA antagonists, such as phencyclidine and MK-801, is the development of reversible neuronal vacuolization (67). A problem with MK-801 is that once it enters an open channel, it leaves the channel only very slowly (half-time >1hr). In practical terms this means that the degree of blockade builds up after MK-801 administration because each molecule of the antagonist entering a channel effectively does not leave.

Several members of this open-channel blocking class of agents, however, are tolerated, such as ketamine and dextromethorphan or the related molecule dextrorphan (68–72). Unfortunately, it is not clear whether these particular drugs are sufficiently potent NMDA antagonists at clinically tolerated doses. Nevertheless, the fact that certain members of this open-channel blocker family are clinically tolerated appears to be associated with their rapid kinetics of interaction with the channel (the kinetic parameters are composed of the on-rate and off-rate for channel blockade) (65,73,74). Most importantly, the safe drugs, such as memantine (see ref. 75 and the discussion below), leave the channel promptly, with an off-rate ~5 sec at micromolar concentrations (65).

Mg^{2+} also blocks open NMDA channels, and this may be the basis for its antiepileptic and neuroprotective effects (76–78). These beneficial effects, however, may not be robust, probably because Mg^{2+} leaves the channel so quickly that it may not act effectively to offset toxic levels of glutamate. In addition, these charged channel-blocking drugs act to a lesser degree when neurons are depolarized (become more positively charged)—for example, under conditions of energy compromise.

In summary, an agent that remains in the channel for at least some period of time is necessary to block the effects of glutamate overstimulation. Of the known NMDA open-channel blockers, memantine is one candidate for clinical trials to combat neurological disorders, such as HIV-associated cognitive/motor complex, with a component of NMDA receptor-mediated neurotoxicity because memantine has been used clinically in Germany for over a dozen years in the treatment of Parkinson's disease and spasticity. Memantine is a congener of amantadine, the well-known antiviral and antiparkinsonian drug used in the United States. Amantadine, however, is considerably less potent on NMDA receptor-operated ion channels at clinically tolerated doses (65), probably precluding its use for these other neurological diseases. It may be no accident that memantine both inhibits NMDA receptor responses and alleviates parkinsonian symptoms; one theory of Parkinson's disease is that neurons die, at least in part, due to a form of NMDA receptor-mediated toxicity.

NMDA Redox Modulatory Site

Another modulatory site on the NMDA receptor-channel complex of possible clinical utility in the near future has been termed the *redox modulatory site*. This site consists of one or more sulfhydryl groups; these sulfhydryl groups may be in close approximation and form a disulfide bond under oxidizing conditions. Under chemical reducing conditions that favor the formation of free thiol (—SH) groups over a disulfide, the opening frequency of NMDA-receptor-associated channels increases (79,80), and thus there is a net increase in Ca^{2+} influx through the channels (81,82) and an increase in the extent of NMDA-receptor-mediated neurotoxicity (83,84). Conversely, redox reagents that mildly oxidize the NMDA receptor—for example, to reform disulfide bonds—might prove useful in combating the myriad of neurological maladies following a final common pathway of NMDA-receptor-mediated neuronal damage (85).

Indeed, several such redox reagents have recently been reported, including quite surprisingly the common nitroso-compound, nitroglycerin (86). One mechanism of nitroglycerin's action in this regard is mediated by a substance related to nitric oxide (NO·), but in a different oxidation state—for example, in the form of RS-NO (nitrosonium ion equivalents, NO^+) (87). Nitric oxide (NO·) itself can participate in reactions to form products that are toxic to nerve cells, such as peroxynitrite ($ONOO^-$) and its breakdown products including hydroxyl radical (HO·) (86,88–92). In other oxidation states, however, monoxides of nitrogen can interact with thiol groups, such as those comprising the redox modulatory site of the NMDA receptor, by *S*-nitrosation, which can be thought of as transfer of the NO group to a thiol (87,92). This action results in down-regulation of NMDA receptor activity and protects neurons from excessive stimulation of the receptor (86). Patients can be made tolerant to the cardiovascular effects of nitroglycerin within hours of continuous therapy. Under these conditions, our laboratory has shown in animal models that the extent of NMDA-receptor-mediated neurotoxicity can be markedly attenuated in the absence of behavioral side effects of the drug (93). Nevertheless, the exact dosing regimen must be carefully worked out before attempting to apply this technique to humans. Other promising reagents that appear to act either directly or indirectly on the NMDA redox modulatory site include oxidized glutathione (94–96) and the putative essential nutrient and redox co-factor, pyrroloquinoline quinone (PQQ) (97).

In addition, there are other important modulatory sites of the NMDA receptor, several of which are illustrated in Fig. 2. Antagonists of each of these sites could possibly be useful in the treatment or prevention of NMDA-receptor-mediated neurotoxicity. For the purposes of this review, I have chosen to highlight only two of these, namely, the ion channel and redox modulatory sites. The other modulatory sites may become therapeutically relevant, however, if clinically tolerated antagonists can be developed to interact with them. Intensive research efforts along these lines are now underway in both academic institutions and the pharmaceutical industry.

Since NMDA and non-NMDA receptor stimulation alike leads to neuronal depolarization and consequent activation of VDCCs, blockade of VDCCs might also ameliorate neurotoxicity, as discussed above. It has become apparent that different subpopulations of neurons have different repertoires of VDCCs, so it might be anticipated that an antagonist specific for a particular type of calcium channel may be effective only in certain regions of the brain or for certain cell types *(vide supra)* (4,98). Therefore, it will be important to develop antagonists specific for these various types of calcium channels, and many investigators are working in this area. Currently available in the clinics are central nervous system (CNS)-permeable antagonists of the L-type calcium channel, such as nimodipine. Other calcium channel antagonists that are permeable to the blood–brain barrier are also being tested in multicenter trials for entities other than the AIDS dementia complex (for a review see ref. 4).

EXCITATORY AMINO ACID ANTAGONIST TREATMENTS ON THE HORIZON

Among the aforementioned classes of NMDA antagonists, the pharmaceutical industry is currently sponsoring in humans Phase I studies for stroke using the open-channel blocker dextrorphan (Roche), and there is interest in testing the related compound dextromethorphan for amyotrophic lateral sclerosis (ALS). There is some evidence that these compounds also antagonize VDCCs as well as NMDA-receptor-operated channels, which might be a helpful dual property (99). The other current clinical trial is a Phase I and early Phase II study (for stroke) using the NMDA-competitive antagonist, CGS19755 (Ciba-Geigy). All of these trials to date have involved dose escalation and safety. Other companies are currently investigating both NMDA and non-NMDA antagonists, but for proprietary reasons information is scanty, and the indications do not as yet include the AIDS dementia complex. Based upon animal testing, it is quite possible that for various forms of glutamate-related neurotoxicity, a combination of agents may be the most effective—for example, combining calcium channel antagonists with NMDA antagonists (100–102).

Human clinical studies for indications other than the AIDS dementia complex are also in progress using agents that work downstream from EAA receptors. These include (a) gangliosides (GM1), which are being tested for improvement of outcome after stroke (103), and (b) the 21-aminosteroid, tirilazad mesylate.

Finally, a case can be made that the NMDA open-channel blocker, memantine (as well as its less potent congener, amantadine), has been in clinical use for years because it is known to ameliorate some of the symptoms of Parkinson's disease. Furthermore, it is now known that the level of memantine (2–12 μM) achieved in the human brain during this form of treatment (104) can afford protection from NMDA receptor-mediated neurotoxicity both *in vitro* and *in vivo* (65,105–108). Recently, our laboratory as well as another, independent group have reported that low micromolar levels of memantine can also protect neurons from damage induced by gp120 *in vitro* (109,110) and *in vivo* in an animal model (14). These preliminary findings raise the possibility that a clinically tolerated NMDA antagonist, memantine, might be useful in the treatment or prevention of the AIDS dementia complex. Therefore, it has been proposed to study the use of memantine as an adjunctive therapy with anti-retroviral drugs such as zidovudine or didanosine, and the AIDS Clinical Trials Group of the NIH is currently considering this option.

CONCLUSIONS

Although it is likely that a complex web of cell interactions leads to neuronal loss in AIDS, HIV-infected macrophages or gp120-stimulated macrophages release toxins whose action appears to be mediated by a final common pathway involving excessive stimulation of neurons by EAAs, such as glutamate and quinolinate. This represents one complete pathway to neuronal injury which is amenable to pharmacotherapy. A strong body of scientific evidence supports the premise that the mechanism for this form of HIV-related neuronal injury is similar to that currently thought to be responsible for a wide variety of acute and chronic neurological diseases (2,3,50). EAAs apparently exert this excitotoxic effect by engendering an excessive influx of Ca^{2+} into neurons. Currently, there is intensive investigation to discover clinically tolerated drugs to combat the neurotoxic effects associated with the excessive stimulation of glutamate receptors or the events triggered downstream to receptor activation. One therapeutic approach has been to use glutamate receptor antagonists, and although several promising drugs are already in hand, additional agents are needed. With the possibility of a final common pathophysiology for many disorders of the CNS (including, perhaps in part, the AIDS dementia complex), the future development of safe and effective EAA antagonists should become a high priority.

ACKNOWLEDGMENTS

I would like to thank my co-workers, Drs. E. B. Dreyer, N. J. Sucher, V. H.-S. Chen, P. K. Kaiser, M. Oyola, S. Lei, J. Pellegrini, D. Zhang, and Y.-B. Choi, for insightful discussions, and Dr. D. Leifer for comments on an earlier version of the manuscript. This work was supported by NIH grants HD29587, EY05477, EY09024, and NS07264, the American Foundation for AIDS Research, and an Established Investigator Award from the American Heart Association.

REFERENCES

1. Lipton SA, Kater SB. Neurotransmitter regulation of neuronal outgrowth, plasticity and survival. *Trends Neurosci* 1989;12:265–270.
2. Choi DW. Glutamate neurotoxicity and diseases of the nervous system. *Neuron* 1988;1: 623–634.
3. Meldrum B, Garthwaite J. Excitatory amino acid neurotoxicity and neurodegenerative disease. *Trends Pharmacol Sci* 1990;11:379–387.
4. Lipton SA. Calcium channel antagonists in the prevention of neurotoxicity. *Adv Pharmacol* 1991;22:271–291.
5. Price RW, Brew B, Sidtis J, Rosenblum M, Scheck AC, Clearly P. The brain and AIDS: central nervous system HIV-1 infection and AIDS dementia complex. *Science* 1988;239: 586–592.
6. Ketzler S, Weis S, Haug H, Budka H. Loss of neurons in frontal cortex in AIDS brains. *Acta Neuropathol (Berlin)* 1990;80:90–92.
7. Wiley CA, Masliah E, Morey M, et al. Neocortical damage during HIV infection. *Ann Neurol* 1991;29:651–657.
8. Everall IP, Luthbert PJ, Lantos PL. Neuronal loss in the frontal cortex in HIV infection. *Lancet* 1991;337:1119–1121.
9. Tenhula WN, Xu SZ, Madigan MC, Heller K, Freeman WR, Sadun AA. Morphometric comparisons of optic nerve axon loss in acquired immunodeficiency syndrome. *Am J Ophthalmol* 1992;113:14–20.
10. Brenneman DE, Westbrook GL, Fitzgerald SP, et al. Neuronal cell killing by the envelope

protein of HIV and its prevention by vasoactive intestinal peptide. *Nature* 1988;335: 639–642.

11. Dreyer EB, Kaiser PK, Offermann JT, Lipton SA. HIV-1 coat protein neurotoxicity prevented by calcium channel antagonists. *Science* 1990;248:364–367.

12. Lo T-M, Fallert CJ, Piser TM, Thayer SA. HIV-1 envelope protein evokes intracellular calcium oscillations in rat hippocampal neurons. *Brain Res* 1992;594:189–196.

13. Lipton SA. Calcium channel antagonists and human immunodeficiency virus coat protein-mediated neuronal injury. *Ann Neurol* 1991;30:110–114.

14. Lipton SA, Jensen FE. Memantine, a clinically-tolerated NMDA open-channel blocker, prevents HIV coat protein-induced neuronal injury *in vitro* and *in vivo*. *Soc Neurosci Abstr* 1992;18:757.

15. Abele AE, Scholz KP, Scholz WK, Miller RJ. Excitotoxicity induced by enhanced excitatory neurotransmission in cultured hippocampal pyramidal neurons. *Neuron* 1990;4: 413–419.

16. Weiss JH, Hartley DM, Koh J, Choi DW. The calcium channel blocker nifedipine attenuates slow excitatory amino acid neurotoxicity. *Science* 1990;247:1474–1477.

17. Sucher NJ, Lei SZ, Lipton SA. Calcium channel antagonists attenuate NMDA receptor-mediated neurotoxicity of retinal ganglion cells in culture. *Brain Res* 1991;551:297–302.

18. Heyes MP, Rubinow D, Lane C, Markey SP. Cerebrospinal fluid quinolinic acid concentrations are increased in acquired immune deficiency syndrome. *Ann Neurol* 1989;26: 275–277.

19. Heyes MP, Brew BJ, Martin A, et al. Quinolinic acid in cerebrospinal fluid and serum in HIV-1 infection: relationship to clinical and neurological status. *Ann Neurol* 1991;29: 202–209.

20. Lipton SA, Kaiser PK, Sucher NJ, Dreyer EB, Offermann JT. AIDS virus coat protein sensitizes neurons to NMDA receptor-mediated toxicity. *Soc Neurosci Abstr* 1990;16:289.

21. Lipton SA, Sucher NJ, Kaiser PK, Dreyer EB. Synergistic effects of HIV coat protein and NMDA receptor-mediated neurotoxicity. *Neuron* 1991;7:111–118.

22. Lipton SA. Requirement for macrophages in neuronal injury induced by HIV envelope protein gp120. *NeuroReport* 1992;3:913–915.

23. Giulian D, Vaca K, Noonan CA. Secretion of neurotoxins by mononuclear phagocytes infected with HIV-1. *Science* 1990;250:1593–1596.

24. Pulliam L, Herndler BG, Tang NM, McGrath MS. Human immunodeficiency virus-infected macrophages produce soluble factors that cause histological and neurochemical alterations in cultured human brains. *J Clin Invest* 1991;87:503–512.

25. Genis P, Jett M, Bernton EW, et al. Cytokines and arachidonic acid metabolites produced during human immunodeficiency virus (HIV)-infected macrophage–astroglia interactions: implications for the neuropathogenesis of HIV disease. *J Exp Med* 1992;176:1703–1718.

26. Selmaj KN, Farooq M, Norton T, Raine CS, Brosman CF. Proliferation of astrocytes *in vitro* in response to cytokines. *J Immunol* 1990;144:129–135.

27. Chung IY, Benveniste EN. Tumor necrosis factor-alpha production by astrocytes: induction by lipopolysaccharide, interferon-gamma and interleukin-1 beta. *J Immunol* 1990;144: 2999–3007.

28. Vitkovic L, Kalebic T, de Cunha A, Fauci AS. Astrocyte-conditioned medium stimulates HIV-1 expression in a chronically infected promonocyte clone. *J Neuroimmunol* 1990;30: 153–160.

29. Robbins DS, Shirazi T, Drysdale BE, Leiberman A, Shin HS, Shin ML. Production of cytotoxic factors for oligodendrocytes by stimulated astrocytes. *J Immunol* 1987;139: 2593–2597.

30. Morganati-Kossmann MC, Kossmann T, Wahl SM. Cytokines and neuropathology. *Trends Pharmacol Sci* 1992;13:286–290.

31. Conti P, Reale M, Barbacane RC, Bongrazia M, Panara MR, Fiore S. The combination of interleukin 1 plus tumor necrosis factor causes greater generation of LTB$_4$, thromboxanes and aggregation of human macrophages than these compounds alone. In: *Prostaglandins in clinical research: cardiovascular system*. New York: Alan R. Liss, 1989.

32. Dubois C, Bissonnette E, Rola-Pleszczynski M. Platelet-activating factor (PAF) enhances tumor necrosis factor production by alveolar macrophages: prevention by PAF receptor antagonists and lipoxygenase inhibitors. *J Immunol* 1989;143:964–970.

33. Poubelle PE, Gingras D, Demers C, et al. Platelet-activating factor (PAF-acether) enhances the concomitant production of tumour necrosis factor-alpha and interleukin-1 by subsets of human monocytes. *Immunology* 1991;72:181–187.
34. Pignol P, Sylvie H, Mencia-Huerta J-M, Rola-Pleszczynski M. Effect of platelet-activating factor (PAF-acether) and its specific receptor antagonist, BN 52021, on interleukin 1 (IL-1) release and synthesis by rat spleen adherent monocytes. *Prostaglandins* 1987;33:931–939.
35. Valone FH, Philip R, Debs RJ. Enhanced human monocyte cytotoxicity by platelet-activating factor. *Immunology* 1988;64:715–718.
36. Valone FH, Epstein LB. Biphasic platelet-activating factor synthesis by human monocytes stimulated with IL-β, tumor necrosis factor, or IFN-γ. *J Immunol* 1988;141:3945–3950.
37. Wahl LM, Corcoran ML, Pyle SW, Arthur LO, Harel-Bellan A, Farrar WL. Human immunodeficiency virus glycoprotein (gp120) induction of monocyte arachidonic acid metabolites and interleukin 1. *Proc Natl Acad Sci USA* 1989;86:621–625.
38. Merrill JE, Koyanagi Y, Chen ISY. Interleukin 1 and tumor necrosis factor α can be induced from mononuclear phagocytes by human immunodeficiency virus type 1 binding to the CD4 receptor. *J Virol* 1989;63:4404–4408.
39. Merrill JE, Chen ISY. HIV-1, macrophages, glial cells, and cytokines in AIDS nervous system disease. *FASEB J* 1991;5:2391–2397.
40. Palmer MR, Mathews WR, Hoffer BJ, Murphy RC. Electrophysiological responses of cerebellar Purkinje neurons to leukotriene D4 and B4. *J Pharmacol Exp Ther* 1981;219: 91–96.
41. Kornecki E, Ehrlich YH. Neuroregulatory and neuropathological actions of ether-phospholipid platelet-activating factor. *Science* 1988;240:1792–1794.
42. Kornecki E, Ehrlich YH. Calcium ion mobilization in neuronal cells induced by PAF. *Lipids* 1991;26:1243–1246.
43. Lindsberg PJ, Hallenbeck JM, Feurstein G. Platelet-activating factor in stroke and brain injury. *Ann Neurol* 1991;30:117–129.
44. Manzini S, Meini S. Involvement of capsaicin-sensitive nerves in the bronchomotor effects of arachidonic acid and melittin: a possible role for lipoxin A_4. *Br J Pharmacol* 1991;103: 1027–1032.
45. Manzini S, Meini S. Capsaicin desensitization selectively inhibits lipoxin A_4-induced contraction in guinea pig bronchus. *J Lipid Mediat* 1991;3:361–366.
46. Meini S, Evangelista S, Geppetti P, Szallasi A, Blumberg PM, Manzini S. Pharmacologic and neurochemical evidence for the activation of capsaicin-sensitive sensory nerves by lipoxin A_4 in guinea pig bronchus. *Am Rev Respir Dis* 1992;146:930–934.
47. Bito H, Nakamura M, Honda Z, et al. Platelet-activating factor (PAF) receptor in rat brain: PAF mobilizes intracellular Ca^{2+} in hippocampal neurons. *Neuron* 1992;9:285–294.
48. Clark GD, Happel LT, Zorumski CF, Bazan NG. Enhancement of hippocampal excitatory synaptic transmission by platelet-activating factor. *Neuron* 1992;9:1211–1216.
49. Soliven B, Albert J. Tumor necrosis factor modulates Ca^{2+} currents in cultured sympathetic neurons. *J Neurosci* 1992;12:2665–2671.
50. Lipton SA. Models of neuronal injury in AIDS: another role for the NMDA receptor? *Trends Neurosci* 1992;15:75–79.
51. Tyor WR, Glass JD, Griffin JW, et al. Cytokine expression in the brain during the acquired immunodeficiency syndrome. *Ann Neurol* 1992;31:349–360.
52. Heyes MP, Saito K, Markey SP. Human macrophages convert L-tryptophan to the neurotoxin quinolinic acid. *Biochem J* 1992;283:633–635.
53. Speciale C, Okuno E, Schwarz R. Increased quinolinic acid metabolism following neuronal degeneration in the rat hippocampus. *Brain Res* 1987;436:18–24.
54. Kohler C, Eriksson LG, Okuno E, Schwarz R. Localization of quinolinic acid metabolizing enzymes in the rat brain. Immunohistochemical studies using antibodies to 3-hydroxyanthranilic acid oxygenase and quinolinic acid phosphoribosyltransferase. *Neuroscience* 1988;27:49–76.
55. Brenneman DE, Nicol T, Warren D, Bowers LM. Vasoactive intestinal peptide: a neurotrophic releasing agent and an astroglial mitogen. *J Neurosci Res* 1990;25:386–394.
56. Giulian D, Vaca K, Corpuz M. Brain glia release factors with opposing actions upon neuronal survival. *J Neurosci* 1993;13:29–37.
57. Harouse JM, Bhat S, Spitalnik SL, et al. Inhibition of entry of HIV-1 in neural cell lines by antibodies against galactosyl ceramide. *Science* 1991;253:320–323.

58. Bhat S, Spitalnik SL, Gonzalez-Scarano F, Silberberg DH. Galactosyl ceramide or a deriv-ative is an essential component of the neural receptor for human immunodeficiency virus type 1 envelope glycoprotein gp120. *Proc Natl Acad Sci USA* 1991;88:7131–7134.
59. Sabatier J-M, Vives E, Mabrouk K, et al. Evidence for neurotoxic activity of *tat* from human immunodeficiency virus type 1. *J Virol* 1991;65:961–967.
60. Werner T, Ferroni S, Saermark T, et al. HIV-1 Nef protein exhibits structural and func-tional similarity to scorpion peptides interacting with K^+ channels. *AIDS* 1991;5: 1301–1308.
61. Dawson VL, Dawson TM, Uhl GR, Snyder SH. Nitric oxide mediates components of NMDA and gp120 neurotoxicities in primary striatal cultures. *Soc Neurosci Abstr* 1992; 18:756.
62. Dawson VL, Dawson TM, Uhl GR, Snyder SH. Human immunodeficiency virus-1 coat protein neurotoxicity mediated by nitric oxide in primary cortical cultures. *Proc Natl Acad Sci USA* 1993;90:3256–3259.
63. Karschin A, Aizenman E, Lipton SA. The interaction of agonists and noncompetitive antagonists at the excitatory amino acid receptors in rat retinal ganglion cells *in vitro. J Neurosci* 1988;2895–2906.
64. Levy DI, Lipton SA. Comparison of delayed administration of competitive and uncompeti-tive antagonists in preventing NMDA receptor-mediated neuronal death. *Neurology* 1990; 40:852–855.
65. Chen H-SV, Pellegrini JW, Aggarwal SK, et al. Open-channel block of NMDA responses by memantine: therapeutic advantage against NMDA receptor-mediated neurotoxicity. *J Neurosci* 1992;12:4427–4436.
66. Koek W, Woods JH, Winger GD. MK-801, a proposed non-competitive antagonist of excitatory amino acid neurotransmission produces phencyclidine-like behavioral effects in pigeons, rats and rhesus monkeys. *J Pharmacol Exp Ther* 1988;245:969–974.
67. Olney JW, Labruyere J, Price MT. Pathological changes induced in cerebrocortical neu-rons by phencyclidine and related drugs. *Science* 1989;244:1360–1362.
68. MacDonald JF, Miljkovic Z, Pennefather P. Use-dependent block of excitatory amino acid currents in cultured neurons by ketamine. *J Neurophysiol* 1987;58:251–266.
69. Davies SN, Alford ST, Coan EJ, Lester RA, Collingridge GL. Ketamine blocks an NMDA receptor-mediated component of synaptic transmission in rat hippocampus in a voltage-dependent manner. *Neurosci Lett* 1988;92:213–217.
70. O'Shaughnessy CT, Lodge D. N-Methyl-D-aspartate receptor-mediated increase in intra-cellular calcium is reduced by ketamine and phencyclidine. *Eur J Pharmacol* 1988;153: 201–209.
71. Choi DW. Dextrorphan and dextromethorphan attenuate glutamate neurotoxicity. *Brain Res* 1987;403:333–336.
72. Choi DW, Peters S, Viseskul V. Dextrorphan and levorphanol selectively block N-methyl-D-aspartate receptor-mediated neurotoxicity on cortical neurons. *J Pharmacol Exp Ther* 1987;242:713–720.
73. Rogawski MA, Porter RJ. Antiepileptic drugs: pharmacological mechanisms and clinical efficacy with consideration of promising developmental stage compounds. *Pharmacol Rev* 1990;42:223–286.
74. Jones SM, Rogawski MA. The anticonvulsant (±)-5-aminocarbonyl-10,11-dihydro-5H-di-benzo[a,d]cyclohepten-5,10-imine (ADCI) selectively blocks NMDA-activated current in cultured rat hippocampal neurons: kinetic analysis and comparison with dizocilpine. *Mol Pharmacol* 1993 *(in press)*.
75. Bormann J. Memantine is a potent blocker of N-methyl-D-aspartate (NMDA) receptor channels. *Eur J Pharmacol* 1989;166:591–592.
76. Goldman RS, Finkbeiner SM. Therapeutic use of magnesium sulfate in selected cases of cerebral ischemia and seizure. *N Engl J Med* 1988;319:1224–1225.
77. Wolf G, Keilhoff G, Fischer S, Hass P. Subcutaneously applied magnesium protects relia-bly against quinolinate-induced N-methyl-D-aspartate (NMDA)-mediated neurodegenera-tion and convulsions in rats: are there therapeutical implications. *Neurosci Lett* 1990;117: 207–211.
78. Wolf G, Fischer S, Hass P, Abicht K, Keilhoff G. Magnesium sulphate subcutaneously injected protects against kainate-induced convulsions and neurodegeneration: *in vivo* study on the rat hippocampus. *Neuroscience* 1991;43:31–34.

79. Aizenman E, Lipton SA, Loring RH. Selective modulation of NMDA responses by reduction and oxidation. *Neuron* 1989;2:1257–1263.
80. Tang LH, Aizenman E. Modulation of *N*-methyl-D-aspartate receptors by redox and alkylating reagents in rat cortical neurones *in vitro*. *J Physiol* 1993;4:65:303–323.
81. Sucher NJ, Wong LA, Lipton SA. Redox modulation of NMDA receptor-mediated Ca^{2+} flux in mammalian central neurons. *NeuroReport* 1990;1:29–32.
82. Reynolds IJ, Rush EA, Aizenman E. Reduction of NMDA receptors with dithiothreitol increases [^{3}H]-MK-801 binding and NMDA-induced Ca^{2+} fluxes. *Br J Pharmacol* 1990; 101:178–182.
83. Levy DI, Sucher NJ, Lipton SA. Redox modulation of NMDA receptor-mediated toxicity in mammalian central neurons. *Neurosci Lett* 1990;110:291–296.
84. Aizenman E, Hartnett KA. The action of CGS-19755 on the redox enhancement of NMDA toxicity in rat cortical neurons *in vitro*. *Brain Res* 1992;585:28–34.
85. Aizenman E, Hartnett KA, Reynolds IJ. Oxygen free radicals regulate NMDA receptor function via a redox modulatory site. *Neuron* 1990;5:841–846.
86. Lei SZ, Pan ZH, Aggarwal SK, et al. Effect of nitric oxide production on the redox modulatory site of the NMDA receptor-channel complex. *Neuron* 1992;8:1087–1099.
87. Stamler JS, Singel DJ, Loscalzo J. Biochemistry of nitric oxide and its redox activated forms. *Science* 1992;258:1898–1902.
88. Beckman JS, Beckman TW, Chen J, Marshall PA, Freeman BA. Apparent hydroxyl radical production by peroxynitrite: implications for endothelial injury from nitric oxide and superoxide. *Proc Natl Acad Sci USA* 1990;87:1620–1624.
89. Radi R, Beckman JS, Bush KM, Freeman BA. Peroxynitrite oxidation of sulfhydryls. The cytotoxic potential of superoxide and nitric oxide. *J Biol Chem* 1991;266:4244–4250.
90. Dawson VL, Dawson TM, London ED, Bredt DS, Snyder SH. Nitric oxide mediates glutamate neurotoxicity in primary cortical cultures. *Proc Natl Acad Sci USA* 1991;88: 6368–6371.
91. Dawson TM, Dawson VL, Snyder SH. A novel neuronal messenger molecule in brain: the free radical, nitric oxide. *Ann Neurol* 1992;32:297–311.
92. Lipton SA, Choi Y-B, Pan Z-H, Lei SZ, Chen VH-S, Sucher NJ, Loscalzo J, Singel DJ, Stamler JS. A redox-based mechanism for the neuroprotective and neurodestructive effects of nitric oxide and related nitroso-compounds. *Nature* 1993;364:626–632.
93. Manchester KS, Jensen FE, Warach S, Lipton SA. Chronic administration of nitroglycerin decreases cerebral infarct size. *Neurology* 1993;43:A365.
94. Levy DI, Sucher NJ, Lipton SA. Glutathione prevents *N*-methyl-D-aspartate receptor-mediated neurotoxicity. *NeuroReport* 1991;2:345–347.
95. Sucher NJ, Lipton SA. Redox modulatory site of the NMDA receptor-channel complex: regulation by oxidized glutathione. *J Neurosci Res* 1991;30:582–591.
96. Gilbert KR, Aizenman E, Reynolds IJ. Oxidized glutathione modulates *N*-methyl-D-aspartate- and depolarization-induced increases in intracellular Ca^{2+} in cultured rat forebrain neurons. *Neurosci Lett* 1991;133:11–14.
97. Aizenman E, Hartnett KA, Zhong C, Gallop PM, Rosenberg PA. Interaction of the putative essential nutrient pyrroloquinoline quinone with the *N*-methyl-D-aspartate receptor redox modulatory site. *J Neurosci* 1992;12:2362–2369.
98. Regan LJ, Sah DWY, Bean BP. Ca^{2+} channels in rat central and peripheral neurons: high-threshold current resistant to dihydropyridine blockers and ω-conotoxin. *Neuron* 1991;6: 269–280.
99. Carpenter CL, Marks SS, Watson DL, Greenberg DA. Dextromethorphan and dextrorphan as calcium channel antagonists. *Brain Res* 1988;439:372–375.
100. Uematsu D, Araki N, Greenberg JH, Sladky J, Reivich M. Combined therapy with MK-801 and nimodipine for protection of ischemic brain damage. *Neurology* 1991;41:88–94.
101. Rod MR, Auer RN. Combination therapy with nimodipine and dizocilpine in a rat model of transient forebrain ischemia. *Stroke* 1992;23:725–732.
102. Hewitt K, Corbett D. Combined treatment with MK-801 and nicardipine reduces global ischemic damage in the gerbil. *Stroke* 1992;23:82–86.
103. Rocca WA, Dorsey FC, Grigoletto F, et al. Design and baseline results of the monosialoganglioside early stroke trial. *Stroke* 1992;23:519–526.
104. Wesemann W, Sturn G, Fünfgeld EW. Distribution and metabolism of the potential antiparkinson drug memantine in the human. *J Neural Transm [Suppl]* 1980;16:143–148.

105. Seif el Nasr M, B P, Rossberg C, Mennel H-D, Krieglstein J. Neuroprotective effect of memantine demonstrated *in vivo* and *in vitro*. *Eur J Pharmacol* 1990;185:19–24.
106. Erdö SL, Schäfer M. Memantine is highly potent in protecting cortical cultures against excitotoxic cell death evoked by glutamate and N-methyl-D-aspartate. *Eur J Pharmacol* 1991;198:215–217.
107. Keilhoff G, Wolf G. Memantine prevents quinolinic acid-induced hippocampal damage. *Eur J Pharmacol* 1992;219:451–454.
108. Osborne NN, Quack G. Memantine stimulates inositol phosphates production in neurones and nullifies N-methyl-D-aspartate-induced destruction of retinal neurones. *Neurochem Int* 1992;21:329–336.
109. Lipton SA. Memantine prevents HIV coat protein-induced neuronal injury *in vitro*. *Neurology* 1992;42:1403–1405.
110. Müller WEG, Schröder HC, Ushijima H, Dapper J, Bormann J. gp120 of HIV-1 induces apoptosis in rat cortical cell cultures: prevention by memantine. *Eur J Pharmacol* 1992; 226:209–214.
111. Lipton SA. Amelioration of HIV-1-related neuronal injury by Ca^{2+} channel antagonists and N-methyl-D-aspartate (NMDA) antagonists. In: Weis S, Hippius, eds. *HIV-1 infection of the central nervous system*. Seattle, WA: Hogrefe & Huber, 1992;251–260.

HIV, AIDS and the Brain, edited by
R. W. Price and S. W. Perry.
Raven Press, Ltd., New York © 1994.

11

Cytokine Expression and Pathogenesis in AIDS Brain

* Ljubisa Vitkovic, † Anna da Cunha, and ‡ William R. Tyor

* Division of Neuroscience and Behavioral Science and † Laboratory of Cell
Biology, National Institute of Mental Health, National Institutes of Health,
Rockville, MD 20857; and ‡ Department of Neurology, Medical University of
South Carolina, Charleston, SC 29425

The clinical and pathological features of human immunodeficiency virus (HIV)-associated dementia have been well characterized (1–6). However, the relationship between the clinical manifestations of HIV-associated dementia and these pathological findings is not completely understood (7,8). The reason for this has been due to, at least in part, a lack of knowledge of the cellular and molecular details of the neuropathogenesis of HIV infection, such as how HIV gets to the brain, which precise factors control its expression there, and ultimately what are pathophysiological effects of HIV expression on the functions of brain cells (9).

The most constant findings of HIV encephalitis are HIV-infected macrophages/microglia (in a form of multinucleated giant cells and microglial nodules, respectively) (10–14), astrocytosis, and diffuse myelin pallor (5). However, these features are not always present in patients who die with HIV-associated dementia (7,8), although HIV-infected macrophages/microglia and astrocytosis usually are found (primarily in the basal ganglia and white matter) (5,14). Neuronal abnormalities and loss have been described (15–17), but, since HIV probably does not infect neurons or oligodendrocytes, investigators have postulated that a soluble factor or factors must be present that are toxic in some way to neurons and/or glial cells. Thus, the neuropathogenesis of HIV infection could be mediated directly, by the viral products (18–21) and/or indirectly. The indirect mechanism may be mediated by products secreted by HIV-infected macrophages/microglia (22–24), other glial cells responding to the infection (25,26), and/or soluble factors crossing the blood–brain barrier either from cerebrospinal fluid (CSF) or from circulation.

Findings of HIV-containing macrophages/microglia surrounded by reactive astrocytes (13) led to a hypothesis that elevated expression of HIV in the brain (in symptomatic HIV-positive individuals) may be due, at least in part, to a cytokine-mediated interaction between astrocytes and chronically infected monocyte/macrophages (25,26). HIV replication/expression in these cells has been shown *in vitro* to be up-regulated by interleukin-1 (IL-1), interleukin-6 (IL-6), tumor necrosis factor alpha (TNF-α), and four other cytokines (27). HIV expression can be stimulated and/or suppressed by transforming growth factor β1 (TGF-β1) and interferon gamma (IFN-γ), depending on the cell type and initial state of the virus (provirus, latent, replicating) (27). Thus, cytokines may have bifunctional effects on HIV replication. Cytokines are produced by various cell types resident in the brain (28–34) and could, therefore, if present in the AIDS brain, modulate HIV expression by both autocrine and paracrine mechanisms (27). Concentrations of several cytokines were found elevated in CSF of HIV-infected individuals, suggesting that some of these molecules may play an important role as regulators of virus expression also in CSF (23,35,36). Published data implicating cytokines in AIDS-associated nervous system dysfunction have been reviewed in numerous publications and most recently by Merrill (37). Thus, we review here primarily the most recent data from our laboratories.

Cytokine expression in the brain is regionally determined. For example, IL-1 immunoreactivity is present in neurons of human hypothalamus and in glia of the frontal cortex (30,34). IL-1β mRNA also is regionally distributed in rat brain (38). TGF-β1 is constitutively expressed in choroid plexus and meninges but apparently not in the parenchyma (33,34,39). Thus, we focused our investigations of expression and function of these molecules on frontal cortex and subcortical white matter, where cognitive and motor impairments observed in acquired immunodeficiency syndrome (AIDS) patients likely originate. The cytokines described here have also been detected in brain tissues from individuals who died with a variety of other CNS and non-CNS diseases (29,34). However, the unique aspects of cytokine expression in AIDS brain described here, together with an abundance of other important *in vivo* and *in vitro* data from experimental systems, strongly suggest that cytokines IL-1, TGF-β1, and TNF-α likely control three important stages in the neuropathogenesis of HIV infection: (i) entry of HIV into brain parenchyma probably early upon systemic infection, during meningitis and/or choroid plexitis with viremia (40); (ii) up- or down-regulation of HIV expression (replication or expression of only some HIV genes) in the brain; and (iii) the most frequent neuropathologic response to HIV infection, namely, astrocytosis and myelin pallor (41).

INTERLEUKIN 1

IL-1 mRNA and protein are constitutively expressed in human and rodent brains where they are generally low and unevenly distributed (28,30,38,42).

IL-1 mRNA and immunoreactive product (IRP) are abundant in normal hypothalamus, low in frontal cortex, and undetectable in granular cell perikarya (38,42). However, IL-1 IRP is high in the preoptic area of the hypothalamus, where it may play a role in regulation of body temperature (30,43). Increasing IL-1 in cerebral ventricles or in the hypothalamic tissue itself elicits fever in experimental animals (43). IL-1 increase in the brain likely elicits a local cellular response because of the presence of high-affinity receptors for IL-1 (44–47). A likely cellular response is a cascade of cytokines, because IL-1 can stimulate production of itself and several other cytokines such as TGF-β1 (33,34), IL-6, and TNF-α (48,49), probably in all cell types in the brain.

IL-1 (α and β) was immunocytochemically detected in frozen tissues from the frontal cortex and white matter of HIV-negative and HIV-positive autopsy cases (35,50; Fig. 1B). IL-1β mRNA was also detected by polymerase chain reaction (PCR) in brain tissues of the same individuals (51), thus indicating that the IL-1β protein detected by immunocytochemistry is generated within the CNS. IL-1 immunoreactivity was detected on endothelium, cells that morphologically appear to be macrophages, and stellate parenchymal cells (Fig. 1B) that proved to be microglia by double immunofluorescent labeling (50). IL-1 immunoreactivity appeared to permeate the frozen tissues, suggesting that IL-1 may have diffused away from producing cells and, if active, acted on cells that initially were not making IL-1 (Fig. 1B). In addition, IL-1 immunoreactivity was also detected in astrocytes and oligodendrocytes, but not in neurons, as judged by double labeling for cytokines and cell markers (34). In addition, each isoform of IL-1 alone was also detected and its expression partially characterized in these cells (34). However, not all cells of any one kind in a 1 mm^3 of tissue contained IL-1 immunoreactivity (34). Intensity of staining of frozen tissues with antibodies against IL-1 visually graded from 0 to 4 was higher in tissues from individuals who died with AIDS compared to HIV-negative individuals who died without disease. The increase was statistically significant (50) and confirmed by measuring density of IL-1-immunoreactive cells (52) and morphometrically quantifying IL-1 immunoreactivity (34). However, the increase in density of IL-1 was observed in brain tissues of individuals who died with a variety of CNS and non-CNS diseases and, thus, apparently was not specific for HIV infection (34). This change, therefore, represents a general response of the brain to pathogenic stimuli originating within or outside the CNS. The elevation of IL-1 was observed not only in the presence but also in the absence of pathologic changes in the CNS. All patients who died without CNS disease and who had elevated IL-1 in cerebral cortex died with fever. Thus, IL-1 increase appeared to be associated with fever (52), which is a cardinal manifestation of many diseases (43). Thus, the elevation of IL-1 in the brain may be one of the earliest responses of a body to infection by HIV if it is associated with the first persistent fever occurring after HIV seroconversion and accompanying viremia (7,9).

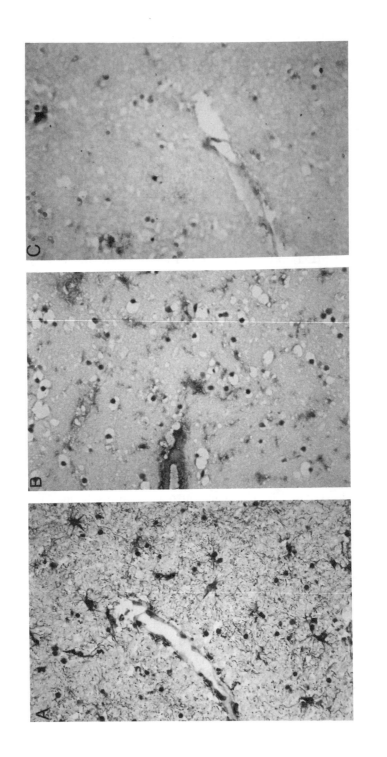

Detection of IL-1 in the CSF of patients with AIDS and HIV-associated dementia has been inconsistent. IL-1β was detected in the CSF of 58 percent of patients with HIV infection (35), and IL-1α was elevated in the CSF of 60 percent of patients with HIV-associated dementia (36). IL-1 has also been measured in the CSF of patients with a variety of neurological disorders and was found to be elevated in 15 percent of patients with meningococcal meningitis (53). However, Weller et al. (54) did not detect IL-1β in the CSF of patients with HIV infection or variety of other neurological diseases involving inflammatory cells, including multiple sclerosis, Guillain–Barré syndrome, chronic inflammatory demyelinating polyradiculopathy, and viral encephalitis (54). We have not consistently detected IL-1β in the CSF of HIV-infected patients, either demented or without dementia (50). These results indicate that levels of IL-1 in the CSF do not necessarily correlate with levels in the brain parenchyma. The parenchyma and CSF represent two connected compartments that are not in equilibrium regarding solutes (55). Thus, the concentrations of solutes in the CSF may qualitatively rather than quantitatively reflect concentrations in parenchyma.

TRANSFORMING GROWTH FACTOR β1

TGF-β1 mRNA is constitutively synthesized in normal rat (33) and human (35,51) brains, but the protein is not detectable (33,34,52; Fig. 3A). Steady-state TGF-β1 mRNA level increases twofold during development of cerebral cortex in rat and during proliferation and differentiation of astrocytes in primary culture (33). This response is not accompanied by the appearance of detectable TGF-β1 protein either *in vivo* or *in vitro*. However, both intracellular immunoreactive TGF-β1 and extracellular TGF-β1 activity are detectable upon stimulation of astrocytes *in vitro* with IL-1. The extracellular TGF-β1 increases with time of exposure to, and with concentration of, IL-1. In contrast, the amount of TGF-β1 mRNA remains unchanged during stimulation of astrocytes with IL-1 (33). These results suggest that the production of TGF-β1 in astrocytes in regulated at both mRNA and protein

←——————————————————————————————

FIG. 1. IL-1 and TGF-β1 immunoreactivities and reactive astrocytosis are present in the same region of frontal cortex from AIDS brain. **A:** A representative, frozen tissue section was fixed in methanol, stained with an antibody against glial fibrillary acidic protein, an astrocytic marker (Dako, Santa Barbara, CA; 1:1000 v/v), and counterstained with cresyl violet. The antibody–antigen complex was detected with an ABC kit (Vector, Burlingame, CA). **B:** Section from the same block of tissue as the one in A, fixed in ethanol, stained with antibodies against IL-1 (α and β) (Endogen, Boston, MA; 1:100 v/v) using the ABC kit and counterstained with hematoxylin to reveal nuclei. Note the precipitate of the peroxidase reaction product on vascular endothelium and in the parenchyma. **C:** Another section adjacent to that shown in A stained with an antibody against TGF-β as previously described (32). The data are representative of five independent experiments. Magnification ×400.

levels. The former may occur during astrocytic development, and the latter may occur during astrocytic response to injury in association with elevation of IL-1 (33). IL-1 stimulates production of TGF-β1 immunoreactivity in cells and TGF-β1 activity in culture fluids of all glial cells, astrocytes, microglial cells, and oligodendrocytes derived from the neonatal rat brain and grown in cell type-enriched cultures (34) and in microglia derived postmortem from normal human brain tissues (52). TGF-β1 production *in vitro* varies with the cell type and isoform of IL-1. Oligodendrocytes produce the greatest amount of TGF-β1, whereas astrocytes produce the least. IL-1α stimulates production in all glial cell types, whereas IL-1β does not. IL-α also stimulates TGF-β1 production in human microglial cells in time- and dose-dependent manners (52). Interestingly in this context, IL-1α and not IL-1β production by monocytes correlates with their activation (56); in monocytes, α rather than β isoform stimulates TGF-β production (L Wakefield, *personal communication*).

TGF-β1 mRNA was detected in brain tissues from individuals who died with AIDS, by both *in situ* hybridization (34,52) and PCR (51). Lack of increase in concentration of TGF-β1 mRNA in brain tissues containing elevated IL-1 (51) is consistent with the post-transcriptional regulation of the TGF-β1 gene by IL-1 in astrocytes, described above. This indicates that only measuring cytokine mRNA levels, a common current practice, may not be informative about the corresponding protein levels.

In vivo TGF-β1 immunoreactivity is present in human tissues from cerebral frontal cortex and subcortical white matter only when IL-1 is elevated in the same tissues (34,52). TGF-β1 immunoreactivity is present in tissue sections adjacent to those in which IL-1 immunoreactivity is seen, indicating that these cytokines are present in the same tissues (Fig. 1). In addition, distributions of parenchymal cells immunoreactive for the two cytokines are also similar to each other. The amount of TGF-β1 is correlated with the amount of IL-1 as determined by morphometry, and the correlation is statistically significant (34). Double labeling of cells for their phenotypic markers and expression of TGF-β1 indicate that all glial cell types, but not neurons, express TGF-β1 in these tissues. IL-1α and IL-β immunoreactivities are also present in all three glial cell types. The cells containing immunoreactivities of both cytokines are also detected (34). These results indicate that TGF-β1 may be induced in all glial cell types of the frontal cortex by IL-1 via both autocrine and paracrine mechanisms.

TGF-β1 immunoreactive cells are scattered throughout the tissues we examined from individuals who died with AIDS ($n = 12$) (Fig. 1C) and a variety of other CNS and non-CNS ($n = 21$) diseases (34). This indicates that TGF-β1 expression in the brain is not a priori specific to any particular disease process, in contrast to a previous suggestion (32), but rather a general response of brain to disease. However, superimposed on this pattern were foci of TGF-β1 immunoreactive cells in rare tissues from individuals who died with AIDS and contained the morphological hallmarks of HIV infection (i.e., multinucleated giant cells and microglial nodules). The foci of TGF-β1 immunoreactivity were centered in and around multinucleated giant cells coinciding with the foci of IL-1 immunoreactivity (52). The focal distribution of cytokine-producing cells was not, however, observed in brain tissues from another patient who died with AIDS which contained hypertrophied, cytomegalic cells, a pathological hallmark of infection by cytomegalovirus (CMV) (Fig. 2A,B). CMV infection of brain has been reported in up to 33 percent of cases with HIV encephalitis, and CMV has been proposed a cofactor of HIV infection (57,59). TGF-β1 immunoreactive cells were scattered throughout this tissue in a pattern resembling that observed in a variety of other CNS and non-CNS diseases (Fig. 2C). This suggests that the presence of any virus-infected cells in cerebral frontal cortex was insufficient for the focal distribution of IL-1- and TGF-β1 immunoreactive cells. These observations indicate that the focal pattern of cytokine-containing cells observed in HIV-infected tissue may not be common to all viruses. The density of these cells was much lower than the density of inflammatory cells permeating the infected area (Fig. 2). Few, if any, inflammatory cells contained TGF-β1 immunoreactivity in this tissue. Does the focal distribution exist in other, nonviral, opportunistic infections of AIDS? One such rare infection is with the fungus, aspergillus (60). To determine the pattern of distribution of the immunoreactive cells due to this fungus in the absence of HIV infection, we stained aspergillus-containing tissue from an HIV-negative individual, with antibodies against TGF-β1. TGF-β1 immunoreactivity was detected and the immunoreactive cells were focused in the area of fungal infection (Fig. 3). The scattered pattern appeared absent (data not shown), and TGF-β1 immunoreactive cells were apparently immunocytes that invaded the infected area rather than resident brain cells (Fig. 3). This pattern contrasts the previously described patterns of TGF-β1 expression with respect to both the identity of the cytokine-producing cells and their distribution in tissue. These observations suggest, although they do not prove, that the focal distribution of IL-1- and TGF-β1-immunoreactive glial cells surrounding HIV-infected macrophages/microglia is related to HIV infection. Furthermore, this pattern is consistent with the hypothesis that activated glial cells interact with HIV-infected cells via cytokines capable of regulating HIV expression in the infected cells.

HIV-infected macrophages/microglia are surrounded by reactive astrocytes (13). Mild to severe gliosis is seen in all brain tissues from individuals who died with AIDS (5,6,9,40). It consists of morphologically and metabolically altered astrocytes and microglial cells. Astrocytosis is a common neurocellular manifestation of brain pathology in individuals with a variety of diseases. It is comprised of astrocytic hyperplasia (an increase in number of astrocytes) and astrocytic hypertrophy (an increase in size of astrocytes) (61). The precise cause(s) of astrocytosis is (are) unknown. We morphometri-

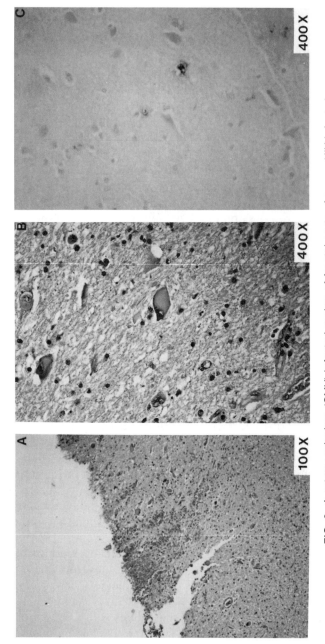

FIG. 2. A cytomegalovirus (CMV)-infected region of frontal cortex from an HIV-infected individual contains TGF-β immunoreactive cells scattered throughout parenchyma as in CMV-free tissues. Photomicrographs of hematoxylin-and-eosin-stained tissue section depict an encephalitic area **(A)** containing cytomegalic cells **(B)**. Tissue section from the same block as the sections shown in A and B, stained with antibodies against TGF-β (32), depicts immunoreactive cell pattern similar to that shown in Fig. 1C **(C)**. Data are representative of three independent stainings of the same tissue.

210

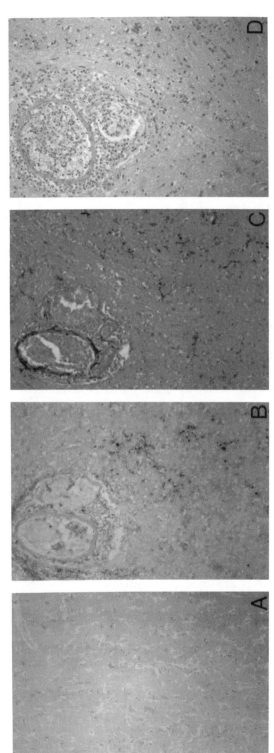

FIG. 3. TGF-β-immunoreactive cells concentrated in a region of aspergillosis. Tissue from frontal cortex of an individual who committed suicide (control) stained with antibodies to TGF-β (32) displays no immunoreactive cells **(A)**, indicating that TGF-β either is not expressed or is below detection. The result is representative of five independent experiments. Serial sections of tissue from frontal cortex of an individual who died with a glioma and aspergillosis stained with antibodies against TGF-β **(B)**, methenamine silver to reveal the fungus **(C)**, and hematoxylin and eosin **(D)**. TGF-β-immunoreactive cells were seen only in the region containing fungus and inflammatory cells. The results are representative of two independent stainings of this tissue. Approximate magnification ×400.

cally measured the relative extent of astrocytosis in brains of 22 individuals who died with seven different diseases. The relative amounts of IL-1 and TGF-β1 immunoreactive products (IRPs) were measured in serial sections. The relative increase in number and size of astrocytes correlated with the relative increase in IL-1 and TGF-β1 IRPs, respectively, but not vice versa. These correlations were statistically significant (63). Furthermore, these cytokines and astrocytosis were colocalized in all examined tissues. Because the change in number and size of astrocytes constitutes the response of astrocytes to HIV infection, these cytokines likely mediate the most frequent pathological change in AIDS brain.

INTERLEUKIN 6

IL-6 is produced by a large number of cell types, including macrophages/microglia, astrocytes, and endothelial cells (62). Human astrocytes in primary culture and several human astrocytoma cell lines constitutively express IL-6 (26). This expression is stimulated severalfold by lipopolysaccharide (LPS) (26) and IL-1 (49). IL-6 was identified by several independent criteria as a principal stimulant of HIV expression in latently infected promonocytic cells exposed to a medium conditioned by growth of activated human astrocytes (26). This is consistent with ability of IL-6 to activate HIV replication in these cells (27).

We found IL-6 immunoreactivity (50) and mRNA (51) in AIDS and HIV-negative autopsy brains. The immunoreactivity was visualized on endothelium and stellate cells (Fig. 4) that appeared to be microglia, but not on astrocytes (50). The discrepancy regarding IL-6 production by human astrocytes *in vitro* (26) and *in vivo* (50) illustrates the need to cautiously interpret data obtained *in vitro* until they are verified *in vivo* or *in situ*. Interestingly, IL-6+ microglia-like cells tended to be present only in AIDS cases (Fig. 4B). Grading of anti-IL-6 staining of tissues and measuring mRNA by semiquantitative PCR did not reveal statistically significant differences between AIDS and HIV-negative cases at the level of antigen (50) or mRNA (51), respectively.

Although IL-6 can be elevated in the CSF of patients with meningococcal meningitis (48), relapsing multiple sclerosis, and Guillain–Barré syndrome (54), it is not elevated in HIV infection (35,50). The latter result is in agreement with semiquantitative results obtained in parenchyma. However, it disagrees with the increase in density of microglial cells observed in brains of patients with AIDS (6). If all microglia produce IL-6, then there ought to be an increase in IL-6 at least in the parenchyma. It is possible that IL-6 was high in inflammatory sites within the brain but was measured late in the CSF when the patients have recovered from meningitis.

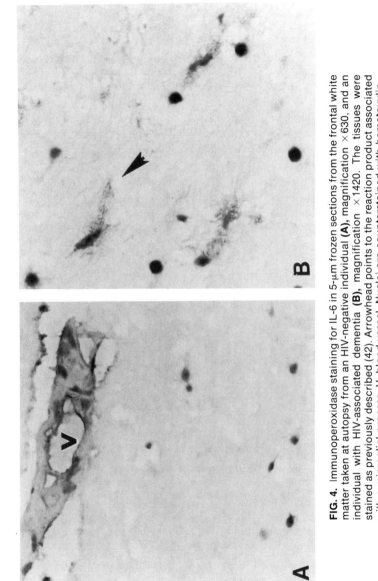

FIG. 4. Immunoperoxidase staining for IL-6 in 5-μm frozen sections from the frontal white matter taken at autopsy from an HIV-negative individual **(A)**, magnification ×630, and an individual with HIV-associated dementia **(B)**, magnification ×1420. The tissues were stained as previously described (42). Arrowhead points to the reaction product associated with a microglial process. V, blood vessel. Nuclei are counterstained with hematoxylin.

TUMOR NECROSIS FACTOR ALPHA

TNF-α derived from nonstimulated and LPS-stimulated rat astrocytes in primary culture, like IL-6, also activated HIV expression in latently infected promonocytic cells *in vitro* (25). This is consistent with the ability of TNF-α to stimulate HIV replication in these cells (27). These results first documented the possibility that astrocytes are indeed capable of up-regulating HIV expression in monocytes/macrophages. However, human astrocytes, in contrast to their rat counterparts, do not constitutively secrete TNF-α (26). In addition, when stimulated with IL-1 (or LPS), they only transiently secrete TNF-α, which is rapidly degraded 3 hours after stimulation (26,49). These results suggest that human astrocytes may differ from their rat counterparts regarding production of some cytokines.

We have immunocytochemically stained brain tissues from AIDS and HIV-negative individuals for TNF-α. TNF-α immunoreactivity was occasionally found on endothelium in both AIDS and HIV-negative cases (50; Fig. 5). TNF-α antigen was detected in homogenates of AIDS brain tissue (WR Tyor, et al., *unpublished observations*). TNF-α mRNA was detected in subcortical white matter of HIV-infected and noninfected individuals who died without disease. These results indicate that TNF-α protein is produced in human brain. TNF-α-positive microglia also were observed only in AIDS cases and frequently were quite numerous (Fig. 5B). TNF-α immunoreactivity was not occasionally observed in astrocytes as demonstrated by double immunofluorescent staining (50). This is consistent with data obtained *in vitro*. However, immunocytochemical staining for TNF-α in the brain has been reported in astrocytes, in addition to macrophages, in inflammatory CNS diseases such as multiple sclerosis and subacute sclerosing panencephalitis (29,54,64).

When we graded the staining for TNF-α in HIV-negative and AIDS cases, we found a statistically significant increase in staining of tissues from AIDS cases compared to controls (50). Semiquantitative PCR measurements of TNF-α mRNA from frozen brain tissues also revealed a statistically significant increase in HIV-positive compared to HIV-negative cases. In addition, HIV-positive demented individuals had greater amounts of TNF-α mRNA in their brains compared to HIV-positive nondemented individuals, and the increase was statistically significant (51). Furthermore, individuals who were more severely demented prior to death tended to have higher TNF-α mRNA levels than did those with mild dementia. Preliminary data of TNF-α measured by enzymed-linked immunosorbent assay (ELISA) in brain homogenate confirm the TNF-α mRNA findings (WR Tyor et al., *unpublished observations*). These results indicate that TNF-α is specifically increased in AIDS brain and that the magnitude of the increase is associated with the severity of dementia.

Results of measuring TNF-α in CSF of AIDS patients have been conflict-

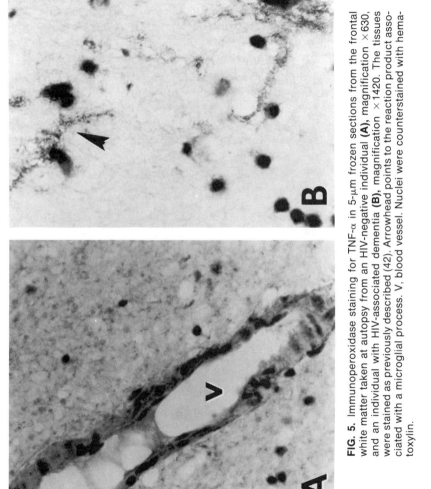

FIG. 5. Immunoperoxidase staining for TNF-α in 5-µm frozen sections from the frontal white matter taken at autopsy from an HIV-negative individual (**A**), magnification ×630, and an individual with HIV-associated dementia (**B**), magnification ×1420. The tissues were stained as previously described (42). Arrowhead points to the reaction product associated with a microglial process. V, blood vessel. Nuclei were counterstained with hematoxylin.

ing. Two studies did, and another two did not, find elevation of TNF-α in CSF of HIV-infected patients (35,36,54,65). We studied 70 HIV-negative and HIV-positive nondemented and demented patients and found slightly elevated levels of TNF-α in the CSF of patients with HIV infection compared to HIV-negative patients (WR Tyor et al., *unpublished observations*). However, there was no difference between HIV-positive nondemented and demented patients. In contrast, Perrella et al. (36) and Grimaldi et al. (66) reported increased TNF-α levels in the CSF of demented versus nondemented HIV-positive patients. The discrepancy between these results may be due to the differences in quantification of TNF-α, sampling time during disease progression, and so on. TNF-α is elevated in the CSF in bacterial meningitis (53,54), in metastatic melanoma (53), and occasionally in viral encephalitis (54). Thus, changes in TNF-α levels in the CNS, just as the type of cells producing TNF-α in the parenchyma, may be related to etiology of various CNS diseases.

DISCUSSION

The evidence presented here indicates that amounts of at least three cytokines—IL-1, TGF-β1, and TNF-α—are increased in cerebral cortices of individuals who died with AIDS. These changes were specific for these cytokines in that the amount of another cytokine, IL-6, apparently was unchanged. Present data are insufficient to discern a precise role for IL-6 in the neuropathogenesis of HIV infection in frontal cortex. In the initial stages of disease process, IL-6 may stimulate B cells to secrete immunoglobulin G (IgG) and to proliferate, contributing to the presence of oligoclonal bands and intrathecal levels of IgG seen in the CSF of patients with AIDS (1–3). Constitutive overproduction of IL-6 transgene in astrocytes of a developing murine brain causes astrocytosis (67). Astrocytosis is found early in the AIDS brain (68). This model is expected to clarify the role of IL-6, if any, in neuropathogenesis.

IL-1, TGF-β1, and TNF-α were either elevated or induced in endothelial cells and astrocytes comprising the blood-brain barrier (BBB). IL-1- and TGF-β1-producing astrocytes (and other cells) likely surround HIV-producing macrophages/microglia consistent with the hypothesis that noninfected cells in the brain stimulate HIV expression via cytokines they secrete. IL-1 and TGF-β1 levels correlate with changes in astrocytes characteristic of astrocytosis. Amounts of TNF-α correlate with the extent of dementia. These observations, together with abundant data from a variety of experimental *in vivo* and *in vitro* systems partly summarized below, indicate that cytokines mediate the three stages of HIV neuropathogenesis. Although the data presented here derive from an endpoint of the complex disease process (i.e., post mortem), a cascade of events can be postulated. Elevation in concentration of IL-1 in the hypothalamus [where IL-1 regulates body temperature (43)] and in circulation is associated with the first persistent fever signaling infection of a body with HIV. Precise causes of elevation of IL-1 in various regions of the brain are unknown but likely are region-specific. IL-1 made by the hypothalamic interneurons may be released into brain regions innervated by these neurons, thereby locally stimulating production of itself and other cytokines. Circulating IL-1 may penetrate parenchyma in the region of vasculosum lamina terminalis and, if active, could stimulate its own production in endothelial cells (64,69,70) and possibly astrocytes at the BBB. IL-1 produced intrathecally in the CSF could enter parenchyma from CSF in the region of circumventricular organs via inflammatory cells that have been seen in the ependymal cell layer lining the ventricles (68). Inflammatory cells in the meninges and choroid plexus may contribute to increasing concentration of IL-1 in CSF. Alternative possibility is that the initial elevation of IL-1 in the brain is related to early invasion of the CNS by HIV-infected monocytes/macrophages which in turn stimulate the initial secretion of IL-1 by astrocytes, endothelial cells, and microglial cells. Increase in local concentration of IL-1 may spread throughout parenchyma by paracrine stimulation of its own production in neighboring cells and/or diffusion. Thus, increase in IL-1 may be one of the earliest changes in the brain after HIV infection and a principal pathogenic stimulus in the AIDS brain. IL-1 alters the BBB by inducing other cytokines and adhesion molecules. IL-1 likely stimulates the expressions of adhesion molecules VCAM-1, ELAM-1, and GMP120 on endothelial cells (71,72) and possibly ICAM-1 in astrocytes (72), facilitating interactions between circulating monocytes/macrophages and cells comprising the BBB. These molecules have been detected in brains from HIV-infected humans and SIV-infected monkeys (73). These interactions undoubtedly facilitate entry of circulating, chronically HIV-infected monocytes/macrophages into brain parenchyma. The entry of these cells is also facilitated by the induction of TGF-β1 in astrocytes of the BBB (34) because TGF-β1 is a potent attractant for monocytes (74). Secretion of this molecule in nanogram quantities into the circulation likely would provide a necessary signal attracting monocytes/macrophages, including those that are latently infected with HIV, into parenchyma. If constitutive synthesis of TGF-β1 in meninges and choroid plexus also increases and if the molecule is secreted, then it, too, would draw monocytes/macrophages into those areas. Elevation of IL-1 causes induction of TGF-β1 in all three glial cell types (33,34) and probably TNF-α in microglial cells (75). Elaboration of these cytokines (IL-1, TGF-β1, and TNF-α) by endothelial cells, macrophages/microglia, and astrocytes activates HIV replication (26,27), and a vicious cycle ensues. There is increased viral load as HIV infection progresses. IL-1, TNF-α, and IL-6 may induce the proliferation of astrocytes, thereby adding to the ever-increasing pool of cytokine-producing cells within the CNS during HIV infection. The end result is increased numbers of activated macrophages/microglia, astrocytes, and endothelial cells (50), all producing cytokines that stimulate further cytokine production, recruitment of macrophages, proliferation of microglia and astrocytes, and increased HIV replication. Cytokines may also act by stimulating cellular metabolism with the generation of neurotoxic metabolites (76–78). TGF-β1 inhibits glutamine synthetase production in astrocytes (79), the sole producers of glutamine, the substrate for glutamate synthesis. TGF-β1 can, in addition to attracting monocytes, exert multiple effects dependent on microenvironment and type of cell it interacts with (33,34).

In AIDS brains, endothelial cells frequently are found to be immunoreactive for IL-1, IL-6, TNF-α, TNF-β, IFN-γ, TNF-α, and MHC class I and II molecules (50) whose expression is related to inflammatory events. TNF-α induces MHC class I [which is produced in a larger number of endothelial cells of AIDS patients (50)] and MHC class II expression [which is produced in microglial cells in addition to endothelial cells in AIDS brain (50)]. TNF-α production is likely stimulated by IL-1.

The heterogeneity of cytokine-producing cells in the frontal cortex (34) suggests that cytokine production is uniquely regulated in each cell. Thus, details of the IL-1-initiated cascade depend on the presence of appropriate receptors on individual cells, whether or not the produced cytokines are biologically active, and on an interaction of cytokines with other effectors simultaneously acting on the same cell (such as growth/trophic factors, neurotransmitters, hormones, etc.). Extent of activation of resident brain cells by cytokines produced by noninfected and HIV-infected cells will vary temporally and spatially.

TNF-α, *in vitro*, is cytotoxic to oligodendrocytes (80,81) and can alter the function of cultured neurons (76). TNF-α can induce HIV expression in monocytes/macrophages by autocrine and paracrine mechanisms (27) and by astrocyte proliferation (82) and swelling (83). Thus, TNF-α likely performs multiple pathophysiological roles in the neuropathogenesis of HIV infection, including dementia.

ACKNOWLEDGMENTS

Results contributed by LV and AdC were obtained in the Laboratory of Immunoregulation, National Institute of Allergy and Infectious Diseases, National Institutes of Health. The authors are grateful to A. S. Fauci, D. Griffin, and R. Johnson for support and advice, and to Jane J. Jefferson and Lena Bezman for technical assistance. AdC is a Pediatric AIDS Foundation Scholar.

REFERENCES

1. Janssen RS, Cornblath DR, Epstein LG, et al. (American Academy of Neurology AIDS Task Force) Nomenclature and research case definitions for neurologic manifesta-

tions of human immunodeficiency virus-type 1 (HIV-1) infection. *Neurology* 1991;41: 778–785.
2. Navia BA, Jordan BD, Price RW. The AIDS dementia complex. I. Clinical features. *Ann Neurol* 1986;19:517–524.
3. McArthur J. Neurologic disease associated with HIV-1 infection. In: Johnson RT, ed. *Current therapy in neurologic disease—3.* New York: BC Decker, 1990;124–129.
4. Navia BA, Cho E, Petito CK, Price RW. The AIDS dementia complex. II. Neuropathology. *Ann Neurol* 1986;19:525–535.
5. Budka H. Neuropathology of human immunodeficiency virus infection. *Brain Pathol* 1991; 1:163–175.
6. Kure K, Llena JF, Lyman WD, et al. Human immunodeficiency virus-1 infection of the nervous system: an autopsy study of 268 adult, pediatric and fetal brains. *Hum Pathol* 1991; 22:700–710.
7. Rosenblum M. Infection of the central nervous system by the human immunodeficiency virus-type 1: morphology and relation to syndrome of progressive encephalopathy and myelopathy in patients with AIDS. *Pathol Ann* 1990;25:117–169.
8. Glass JD, Wesselingh S, Selnes OA, McArthur JC. Clinical–neuropathological correlation in HIV-associated dementia. *Neurology* 1993 *(in press).*
9. Price RW, Brew B, Sidtis J, Rosenblum M, Scheck AC, Cleary P. The brain in AIDS: central nervous system HIV-1 infection and AIDS dementia complex. *Science* 1988;239: 586–591.
10. Pumarola-Sune T, Navia BA, Cordon-Cardo C, et al. HIV antigen in the brains of patients with the AIDS dementia complex. *Ann Neurol* 1987;21:490–496.
11. Wiley CA, Schrier RD, Nelson JA, et al. Cellular localization of human immunodeficiency virus infection within the brains of acquired immunodeficiency syndrome patients. *Proc Natl Acad Sci USA* 1986;83:7089–7093.
12. Koenig S, Gendelman HE, Orenstein JM, et al. Detection of AIDS virus in macrophages in brain tissue from AIDS patients with encephalopathy. *Science* 1986;233:1089–1093.
13. Gabuzda DH, Ho DD, de la Monte SM, et al. Immunohistochemical identification of HTLV-III antigen in brains of patients with AIDS. *Ann Neurol* 1986;20:289–295.
14. Kure K, Weidenheim KM, Lyman WD, Dickson DW. Morphology and distribution of HIV-1 gp41-positive microglia in subacute AIDS encephalitis. *Acta Neuropathol* 1990;80: 393–400.
15. Wiley CA, Masliah E, Morey M, et al. Neocortical damage during HIV infection. *Ann Neurol* 1991;29:651–657.
16. Everall IP, Luthert PJ, Lantos PL. Neuronal loss in the frontal cortex in HIV infection. *Lancet* 1991;337:1119–1121.
17. Masliah E, Morey M, DeTeresa R, et al. Cortical dendritic pathology in human immunodeficiency virus encephalitis. *Lab Invest* 1992;66:285–291.
18. Dreyer EB, Kaiser PK, Offermann JT, Lipton SA. HIV-1 coat protein neurotoxicity prevented by calcium channel antagonists. *Science* 1990;248:364–367.
19. Kaiser PK, Offermann JT, Lipton SA. Neuronal injury due to HIV-1 envelope protein is blocked by anti-gp120 antibodies but not by anti-CD4 antibodies. *Neurology* 1990;40: 1757–1761.
20. Sabatier J, Vives E, Mabrook K, et al. Evidence for neurotoxic activity of tat from human immunodeficiency virus type 1. *J Virol* 1991;65:961–967.
21. Werner T, Ferroni S, Saermark T, et al. HIV-1 nef protein exhibits structural and functional similarity to scorpion peptides interacting with K⁺ channels. *AIDS J* 1991;5:1301–1308.
22. Heyes MP, Brew BJ, Martin A, et al. Quinolinic acid in cerebrospinal fluid and serum in HIV-1 infection: relationship to clinical and neurological status. *Ann Neurol* 1991;29: 202–209.
23. Griffin DE, McArthur JC, Cornblath DR. Neopterin and interferon-γ in serum and cerebrospinal of patients with HIV-associated neurologic disease. *Neurol* 1991;41:69–74.
24. Giulian D, Vaca K, Noonan CA. Secretion of neurotoxins by mononuclear phagocytes infected with HIV-1. *Science* 1990;250:1593–1596.
25. Vitkovic L, Kalebic T, da Cunha A, Fauci AS. Astrocyte-conditioned medium stimulates HIV-1 expression in a chronically infected promonocyte clone. *J Neuroimmunol* 1990;30: 153–160.

26. Vitkovic L, Wood G, Major EO, Fauci AS. Human astrocytes stimulate HIV-1 expression in a chronically infected promonocyte clone via interleukin-6. *AIDS Res Hum Retroviruses* 1991;7:723–727.
27. Poli G, Fauci AS. The role of monocyte/macrophages and cytokines in the pathogenesis of HIV infection. *Pathobiology* 1992;60:246–251.
28. Hofman FM, von Hanwehr RI, Dinarello CA, Mizel SB, Hinton D, Merrill JE. Immunoregulatory molecules and IL-2 receptors identified in multiple sclerosis brain. *J Immunol* 1986; 136:3239–3245.
29. Hoffman FH, Hinton DR, Johnson K, Merrill JE. Tumor necrosis factor identified in multiple sclerosis brain. *J Exp Med* 1989;170:607–612.
30. Breder CD, Dinarello CA, Saper CB. Interleukin-1 immunoreactive innervation of the human hypothalamus. *Science* 1988;240:321–324.
31. Wesselingh SL, Gough NM, Finla-Jones JJ, McDonald PJ. Detection of cytokine mRNA in astrocyte cultures using the polymerase chain reaction. *Lymphokine Res* 1990;9:177–178.
32. Wahl SM, Allen JB, McCartney-Francis N, et al. Macrophage- and astrocyte-derived transforming growth factor β as a mediator of central nervous system dysfunction in acquired immune deficiency syndrome. *J Exp Med* 1991;173:981–991.
33. da Cunha A, Vitkovic L. Transforming growth factor-beta 1 (TGF-β1) expression and regulation in rat cortical astrocytes. *J Neuroimmunol* 1992;36:157–169.
34. da Cunha A, Jefferson JJ, Jackson RW, Vitkovic L. Glial cell-specific mechanisms of TGF-β1 induction by IL-1 in cerebral cortex. *J Neuroimmunol* 1993;42:71–86.
35. Gallo P, Frei K, Rordorf C, et al. Human immunodeficiency virus typ-1 (HIV-1) infection of central nervous system: an evaluation of cytokines in cerebrospinal fluid. *J Neurommunol* 1989;23:109–116.
36. Perrella O, Carrieri PB, Guarnaccia D, Soscia M. Cerebrospinal fluid cytokines in AIDS dementia complex. *J Neurol* 1992;239:387–388.
37. Merrill JE. Cytokines and retroviruses. *Clinical Immunol Immunopathol* 1992;64:23–27.
38. Higgins GA, Olschowka JA. Induction of interleukin-1β mRNA in adult rat brain. *Mol Brain Res* 1991;9:143–148.
39. Unsicker K, Flanders KC, Cissel PS, Lafyates R, Sporn MS. Transforming growth factor beta isoforms in the adult rat peripheral central nervous system. *Neuroscience* 1991;44: 613–625.
40. Black PH. HTLV-IIIb, AIDS and the brain. *N Engl J Med* 1985;313:1538–1540.
41. Schmidbauer M, Huemer M, Cristina S, Tabattoni GR, Budka H. Morphological spectrum, distribution and clinical correlation of white matter lesions in AIDS brains. *Neuropathol Applied Neurobiol* 1992;18:489–501.
42. Lechan RM, Toni R, Clark BD, et al. Immunoreactive interleukin-1B localization in the rat forebrain. *Brain Res* 1990;514:135–140.
43. Dinarello CA. The role of cytokines in the pathogenesis of fever. In: Mackoviak PA, ed. *Fever basic mechanism and management*. New York: Raven Press, 1991;123–147.
44. Katsura G, Gotschall PE, Arimura A. Identification of high-affinity receptor for interleukin-1 beta in rat brain. *Biochem Biophy Res Commun* 1988;156:61–67.
45. Tako T, Tracey DE, Mitchell WM, de Souza EB. Interleukin-1 receptors in mouse brain: characterization and neuronal localization. *Endocrinology* 1990;127:3070–3078.
46. Haour FG, Ban EM, Millon GM, Baran D, Fillon GM. Brain interleukin-1 receptors: characterization and modulation after lipopolysaccharide injection. *Prog Neuroendocrinimmunol* 1990;3:196–204.
47. Cunningham ET, Wada E, Carter DB, et al. Localization of interleukin-1 receptor messenger RNA in murine hippocampus. *Endocrinology* 1991;128:2666–2668.
48. Dinarello CA. Role of interleukin-1 in infectious diseases. *Immunol Rev* 1992;127:119–146.
49. Vitkovic L, Chatham JJ, da Cunha A. Distinct expressions of cytokines in human astrocytes *in vitro*. *Trans Am Soc Neurochem* 1992;23:211.
50. Tyor WR, Glass JD, Griffin JW, et al. Cytokine expression in the brain during AIDS. *Ann Neurol* 1992;31:349–360.
51. Wesselingh SL, Power C, Glass JD, et al. Intracerebral cytokine mRNA expression in AIDS dementia. *Ann Neurol* 1993;33:576–589.
52. da Cunha A, Jefferson JJ, Tyor WR, et al. Correlative IL-1 and TGF-beta increases in human brain independent of AIDS and other disease etiologies. *Proc Natl Acad Sci USA* 1993 *(in press)*.

53. Waage A, Halstensen A, Shalaby R, et al. Local production of tumor necrosis factor-α, interleukin-1, and interleukin-6 in meningococcal meningitis. *J Exp Med* 1989;170: 1859–1867.
54. Weller M, Stevens A, Sommer N, et al. Comparative analysis of cytokines patterns in immunological, infectious, and other neurological disorders. *J Neurol Sci* 1991;104:215–221.
55. Pardridge WM. *Peptide drug delivery to the brain.* New York: Raven Press, 1991;108–114.
56. Beuscher HU, Rausch U-P, Otternse IG, Rollinghoff M. Transition from interleukin-1β (IL-1β) to IL-1α production during maturation of inflammatory macrophages *in vivo. J Exp Med* 1992;175:1793–1797.
57. Wiley CA, Nelson JA. Role of human immunodeficiency virus and cytomegalovirus in AIDS encephalitis. *J Pathology* 1988;133:10–88.
58. Schmidbauer M. Cytomegalovirus (CMV) disease of the brain in AIDS and connatal infection: a comparative study by histology, immunocytochemistry and *in situ* DNA hybridization. *Acta Neuropathol* 1989;79:286–293.
59. Fiala M, Cone LA, Christopher R, Kermani V, Gornbein JA. Human immunodeficiency virus type 1 antigenemia is enhanced in patients with disseminated cytomegalovirus infection and deficient T lymphocytes. *Res Immunol* 1991;142:815–819.
60. Houff SA. Neuroimmunology of human immunodeficiency virus infection. In: Rosenblum ML, et al., eds. AIDS and the nervous system. New York: Raven Press, 1988;347–375 (see p. 360).
61. da Cunha, Jefferson JJ, Tyor WR, et al. Gliosis in human brain: relationship to size but not other properties of astrocytes. *Brain Res* 1993;600:161–165.
62. Van Snick J. Interleukin-6: an overview. *Annu Rev Immunol* 1990;8:253–278.
63. da Cunha A, Jefferson JJ, Tyor WR, et al. Submitted for publication.
64. Selmaj KW, Raine CS, Cannella B, Brosran CF. Identification of lymphotoxin and tumor necrosis factor in multiple sclerosis lesions. *J Clin Invest* 1991;87:949–954.
65. Howells GH, Chantry D, Feldman M. Interleukin-1 (IL-1) and tumor necrosis factor synergise in the induction of IL-1 synthesis by human vascular endothelial cells. *Immunol Lett* 1988;19:169–174.
66. Grimaldi LME, Martino GV, Franciotta DM, et al. Elevated alpha-tumor necrosis factor levels in spinal fluid from HIV-1 infected patients with central nervous system involvement. *Ann Neurol* 1991;29:21–25.
67. Campbell IL, Oldstone MBA, Mucke L. Neurologic disease induced in transgenic mice by the astrocyte-specific expression of interleukin-6. *Soc Neurosci Abstr* 1992;18:482.
68. Gray F, Leses M-C, Keohane C, et al. Early brain changes in HIV infection: neuropathological study of 11 HIV seropositive non-AIDS cases. *J Neuropathol Exp Neurol* 1992;51: 177–185.
69. Shingu M, Nobunaga M, Ezaki I, Yoshioka K. Recombinant human IL-1β and TNF-α stimulate production of IL-1α and IL-1β by vascular smooth muscle cells and IL-1α by vascular endothelial cells. *Life Sci* 1991;49:241–246.
70. Mantovani A, Dejana E. Cytokines as communication signals between leukocytes and endothelial cells. *Immunol Today* 1989;10:370–375.
71. Springer TA. Adhesion receptors of the immune system. *Nature* 1990;346:425–434.
72. Frohman EM, Frohman TC, Dustin ML, et al. The induction of ICAM-1 on human fetal astrocytes by interferon-gamma, tumor necrosis factor-alpha, lymphotoxin, and interleukin-1: relevance to intracellular antigen presentation. *J Neuroimmunol* 1989;23:117–124.
73. Sassevile VG, Mcever RP, Newman W, Ringler DJ. Vcam-1 expression in brain and detection in CSF in SIV-induced AIDS encephalopathy. *FASEB J* 1992;6:1327.
74. Wahl S, Hunt DA, Wakefield LM, et al. Transforming growth factor type β induces monocyte chemotaxis and growth factor production. *Proc Natl Acad Sci USA* 1987;84:5788–5792.
75. Philip R, Epstein LB. TNF as immunomodulator and mediator of monocyte cytotoxicity induced by itself, gamma interferon and interleukin-1. *Nature* 1986;323:86–89.
76. Soliven B, Albert J. Tumor necrosis factor modulates Ca^{2+} currents in cultured sympathetic neurons. *J Neurosci* 1992;12:2665–2671.
77. Zbinder G. Toxicity of interferons and interleukins in the CNS. In: Frederickson RCA, McGaugh JL, Felten DL, eds. *Peripheral signaling of the brain.* Toronto: Hogrete & Huber, 1991:193–201.
78. Genis P, Jett M, Bernton EW, et al. Cytokines and arachidonic metabolites produced during

human immunodeficiency virus (HIV)-infected macrophage-astroglia interactions: implications for the neuropathogenesis of HIV disease. *J Exp Med* 1992;176:1703–1718.

79. Toru-Delbauffe D, Baghdassarian-Chalaye D, Gavaret JM, et al. Effects of transforming growth factor beta 1 on astroglial cells in culture. *J Neurochem* 1990;54:1056–1061.

80. Robbins DS, Shirayi Y, Drysdale B, et al. Production of cytotoxic factor for oligodendrocytes by stimulated astrocytes. *J Immunol* 1987;139:2593–2597.

81. Selmaj KW, Raine CS. Tumor necrosis factor mediates myelin and oligodendrocyte damage *in vitro. Ann Neurol* 1988;23:339–346.

82. Selmaj KW, Farooq M, Norton WT, et al. Proliferation of astrocytes *in vitro* in response to cytokines: a primary role for tumor necrosis factor. *J Immunol* 1990;144:129–135.

83. Bender AS, Rivera IV, Norenberg NP. Tumor necrosis factor-alpha induces astrocyte swelling. *Trans Am Soc Neurochem* 1992;23:113.

HIV, AIDS and the Brain, edited by
R. W. Price and S. W. Perry.
Raven Press, Ltd., New York © 1994.

12

HIV-Related Depression

Samuel W. Perry III

*Department of Psychiatry, Cornell University Medical College,
The New York Hospital, New York, NY 10021*

In early 1986, after the effects of the acquired immunodeficiency syndrome (AIDS) epidemic became more appreciated, the National Academy of Sciences and the Institute of Medicine established a committee to assess the extent of the problems and to propose an appropriate national response. As the psychiatrist on the committee, I recall how members were impressed with advances that had already been made in characterizing the etiologic virus, but members were dismayed that so little systematic data were available in regards to the psychological and behavioral effects of HIV infection. Accordingly, high on the agenda was the committee's recommendation to improve our understanding in these areas (1).

It is reassuring to note that within a relatively short time, mental health researchers have responded to this clarion call. As one example, investigators have been examining human immunodeficiency virus (HIV)-related depression—its frequency among infected and high-risk adults, variables that predict depression in these populations, the risks of suicide, and the effectiveness of psychosocial and pharmacological antidepressant treatments. This chapter summarizes our progress to date.

FREQUENCY OF DEPRESSION AMONG HIV-INFECTED ADULTS

During the early years of the AIDS epidemic, numerous articles reported high rates of "depression" among adults with HIV infection (2). These reports, based on either clinical impression or chart reviews, reflected a general impression that depression was an inevitable consequence of living with a stigmatizing and ultimately fatal infection.

More recent studies with standardized self-report measures have tended to modify this view (3). In a sample of 257 HIV-positive gay and bisexual men participating in the San Francisco-based Center for AIDS Prevention (CAPS), Hays et al. (4) found that about 20 percent had scores that are associated with clinical depression. Perry et al. (5) examined a more sociode-mographically diverse sample of 106 HIV-positive men and women 1 year after HIV testing with counseling and found that 32 percent had scores in the depressed range.

Standardized diagnostic interviews provide a more accurate measure of clinical depression, but require time and expense for training and for sustaining adequate inter-rater reliability. Furthermore, these interviews, generally lasting an hour or longer, are less convenient and more burdensome for subjects than are self-report questionnaires. For these reasons, few studies have used diagnostic clinical ratings. Among those studies that have, rates of depression have been lower than by self-report. In a small San Diego sample of 45 HIV-positive gay men, Atkinson et al. (6) found that 11 percent had current depressive disorder. Perry et al. (7) found a similar rate among 105 HIV-positive men and women during the first year after voluntary HIV testing. An even lower rate of current depression was found in a longitudinal neuropsychiatric study at Columbia University, where 8 out of 124 (6 percent) HIV-positive gay men had depression at entry (8). Perhaps even more surprising, in collaboration with the Gay Men's Health Crisis in New York City, Rabkin et al. (9) assessed 53 gay men who had an AIDS-defining diagnosis for at least 3 years and found that only 6 percent met diagnostic criteria for a current depressive disorder.

Although these and other studies represent a first-step toward determining the incidence and prevalence of HIV-related depression, one must be cautious in generalizing their results. As suggested by the underrepresentation of minorities, injection drug users and women, selection bias no doubt plays a role in most reported samples. Rates of current depression may prove to be higher in populations less likely to participate in longitudinal studies. On the other hand, because depressive symptoms overlap with both normal sadness and somatic manifestations of HIV, rates of clinical depression in any sample may actually be lower than rates determined by measures that have not yet been standardized for physically ill populations. An individual late in the course of HIV infection should not be labeled as having depressive symptoms merely because of reported loss in weight, appetite, concentration, libido, and energy.

In summary, available data indicate that while low-grade depressive symptoms are common among HIV-positive adults, depressive disorders are the exception and not the rule. This tentative conclusion is consistent with studies of other fatal illnesses, such as cancer (10). Furthermore, this conclusion is supported both by Rabkin et al. (11), who found that a sample of 124 HIV-positive gay men maintained reasonable hopefulness over time, and by Joseph et al. (12), who found in a sample of 436 gay and bisexual men that psychiatric symptoms did not increase over 3 years. The clinical point is that physicians should not assume that severe depressive symptoms in an

HIV-infected adult are understandable and justified. Depressive disorder is never "normal." Rather, it is an indication for evaluation and treatment.

RISK FACTORS FOR HIV-RELATED DEPRESSION

Investigators are examining what factors place an individual at increased risk for developing a depressive disorder during the prolonged period of HIV infection. To date, most published studies have been retrospective or cross-sectional, but some prospective studies are underway. The choice of examined predictor variables has been largely guided by the non-HIV literature.

Psychiatric Risk Factors for Depression

A few studies suggest that at-risk groups may have elevated rates of life-time depression—that is, a history of depressive disorders before acquiring HIV infection. Williams et al. (8) found that among 124 HIV-positive gay men enrolled in the Columbia University neuropsychiatric study, 40 (32 percent) at entry had a lifetime history of one or more depressive disorders. Perry et al. (13) found a similar rate (43 percent) among 207 at-risk adults seeking HIV testing. These rates are about seven times higher than rates found in the general population. Perhaps more striking, Rabkin et al. (14) found that among 87 HIV-positive adults seeking treatment for depression, 78 percent had a history of prior depression.

In addition to a history of depression, another psychiatric risk factor appears to be the presence of a personality disorder. Jacobsberg et al. (15) administered Loranger's Personality Disorder Evaluation (PDE) to at-risk adults before voluntary HIV testing. Depression scores after serological notification were significantly higher among those who met criteria for any personality disorder.

Psychological Risk Factors for Depression

Several studies have found that lower perceived social support is associated with higher depressive scores. Using a brief 12-item measure, Hays et al. (4) found that among 257 HIV-positive gay men in the CAPS study, lower social support was correlated with self-reported depressive symptoms over 1 year ($r = -.28$ to $-.37$). In the New York City study of responses to HIV testing, Fishman et al. (16) found that a more extensive measure of social support had even higher correlations with depressive symptoms over 2 years after HIV-positive notification ($r = -.38$ to $-.52$).

Concerns were raised early in the epidemic that bereavement over partners and friends who had died of AIDS might increase the risk of depression among those who are HIV-infected. It appears, however, that grief and depression can be distinguished. Whereas Martin et al. (17) did find an association between loss of loved ones and self-reported "demoralization," more recently Neugebauer et al. (18) reported no relationship between depressive symptoms and loss of loved ones.

Medical Risk Factors for Depression

Consistent with non-HIV studies, the expectation has been that depressive symptoms would increase over time as HIV-positive adults developed more severe physical symptoms. Two prospective studies have supported this expectation. Hays et al. (4) in the San Francisco CAPS study found significant but relatively weak correlations between self-reported depressive symptoms and the number of HIV physical symptoms ($r = .19$ to $.25$). Because the array of HIV physical symptoms can vary widely in their medical implications, Perry et al. (7) developed a scale that assessed the severity of HIV illness. Using this scale, they found somewhat higher correlations between severity of HIV symptoms and severity of depressive symptoms ($r = .35$ to $.50$), though again most subjects with HIV physical symptoms did not have a score associated with clinical depression.

Ever since reports that HIV affects subcortical areas early in the course of infection, investigators have been trying to determine if these early central nervous system (CNS) effects may induce clinically significant mental changes (19). To date, the weight of the evidence is that even in the presence of impairment on neuropsychological tests, most HIV-positive adults do not develop an organic mood disorder prior to the development of severe physical illness. It is true that among HIV-positive adults who did not have AIDS, Krikorian and Wrobel (20) found moderate correlations between neuropsychological impairment and depressive scores; however, among similar samples, Yakov Stern et al. (21) found only weak correlations in a Columbia University study and Robert Stern et al. (22) found no such correlations in a North Carolina study.

Knowledge as a Risk Factor for Depression

Although clinicians have understandably been wary about notifying HIV-positive patients about their "T cell" counts, Perry et al. (7) found no relationship between notification of CD4 cell number and depressive scores. These results are again consistent with non-HIV studies that have found that notification of a potentially fatal illness in the absence of severe physical symptoms does not generally cause a clinical depression (10).

Conversely, the lay literature and a few non-HIV psychoimmune studies have raised the concern that depression may accelerate HIV disease. While the final word is still out, several prospective studies have not found that psychosocial stressors, including depressive symptoms, predict decrease in CD4 cell count or other enumerative lymphocyte markers of HIV disease progression (7,23,24).

An even greater clinical and public health issue has been the concern that HIV-positive notification would lead to profound depression. The fear has been that despite the established efficacy of early medical interventions, many at-risk individuals would avoid HIV testing because they could not cope with the knowledge of an incurable and stigmatizing infection. Available evidence indicates that this is not generally the case. In the prospective CAPS study, Hays et al. (4) reported that neither HIV status nor knowledge of one's status was significantly associated with depression. Similarly, Perry et al. (5) found that during the first year after voluntary HIV testing with counseling, knowledge of HIV infection did not increase depressive symptoms as measured both by self-report with the Beck Depression Inventory (BDI) and by clinical assessment with the Hamilton Depression Rating Scale (HDRS). In fact, as shown in Figs. 1 and 2, severity of depressive symptoms on average was not significantly different after HIV testing with counseling than was severity among followed at-risk subjects who were HIV-negative. Presented differently, Fig. 3 illustrates the relatively small percentage of HIV-positive subjects who were above cutoff scores associated with either moderate or severe depression.

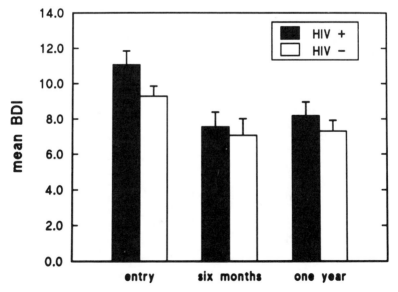

FIG. 1. Self-reported depressive symptoms before and after HIV testing among 103 HIV-positive and 203 HIV-negative adults.

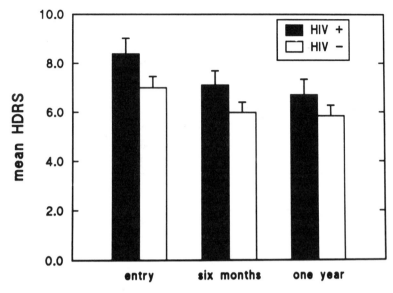

FIG. 2. Clinically rated depressive symptoms before and after HIV testing among 101 HIV-positive and 201 HIV-negative adults.

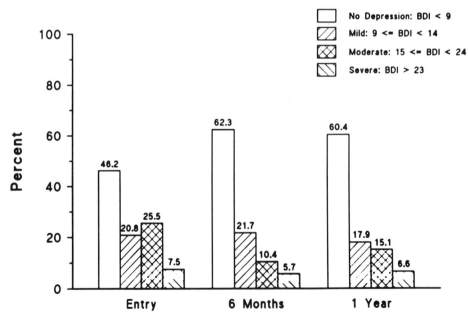

FIG. 3. Rates of self-reported depression before and after HIV testing among 106 HIV-positive subjects.

In summary, studies to date suggest that HIV-related depression is most strongly predicted by a history of prior depression, the presence of an Axis II personality disorder, and low perceived social support. Severity of HIV physical symptoms is a moderate predictor. Although perhaps counterintuitive, weak predictors for depressive symptoms include bereavement, early neuropsychological impairment, knowledge of "T cell" count, and even knowledge of HIV infection. These tentative conclusions support the clinical maxim that in terms of developing depression, it may be less important what illness the person has and more important what person has the illness.

SUICIDAL BEHAVIOR AND HIV

Related to the development of depression has been concerns about the increased risk of suicide among HIV-infected populations. These concerns were heightened when Marzuk et al. (25) reported a 36-fold increased relative risk for suicide among middle-aged men with AIDS. This conclusion was based on a study conducted in collaboration with the New York City medical examiner's office in which 12 men with AIDS were found to have committed suicide in 1985. A follow-up study by the same team of investigators found 30 suicides among men with AIDS in 1986–1987, which again was calculated to represent a 36-fold increased relative risk (26).

Using different methods, other investigators have found roughly similar rates of increased risk. Kizer et al. (27) examined death certificates in California and, on the basis of 13 suicides in middle-aged men with AIDS, calculated that the increased relative risk was 17-fold. Brown and Rundell (28) examined the records of U.S. Air Force personnel. Two of 711 men completed suicide within several months after HIV-positive notification, a rate calculated to represent a 37-fold increased risk. More recently, Buehler et al. (29) examined death certificates throughout the United States. Although they found 33 completed suicides in adults with AIDS, they concluded that the epidemic was not having a profound impact on suicide mortality either nationally or in any particular geographical area.

While these studies are reasonable attempts, there are numerous problems in trying to discern precisely how much the HIV epidemic has affected rates of suicide. Suicide is such a rare event that prospective studies are not feasible, and even retrospective studies must deal with relatively small numbers. Other problems include (a) deciding on the numerator and denominator in making epidemiological calculations, (b) estimating the ascertainment bias due to underreporting of suicide, and (c) distinguishing active suicide from passive resignation, such as when a terminally ill patient refuses yet another hospitalization. And even if an active suicide in an individual with HIV infection is revealed, it is not always clear whether the primary contributing factor was related to HIV or to some other factor, such as lifelong psychiatric illness or drug abuse. In comparison with the relatively small number of reported AIDS-related suicides, rates of suicide attempts (30) and suicidal ideation (31,32) among HIV-infected adults have been considerably higher. For example, in the Los Angeles Multicenter AIDS Cohort Study (MACS), Schneider et al. (31) found that self-reported suicidal ideation was present in 27 percent of 778 gay and bisexual men, about half of whom were HIV-positive. Interestingly, however, these investigators found that in attempting to distinguish those with suicidal ideation from those without, only 1.2 percent of the variance could be explained by HIV stressors, including knowledge of HIV status. Using the suicide item on the BDI, similar results have been found among adults before and after voluntary HIV testing (32). As shown in Fig. 4, rates of suicidal ideation among 106 HIV-positive adults actually decreased over 1 year after serological notification and were not significantly different than rates among 223 at-risk HIV-negative subjects (Fig. 5). One can also note from the figures that whereas rates of suicidal thoughts remained relatively high among both serology groups, rates of suicidal wishes or intent remained low.

Because of the inherent methodological problems in studying suicidal behaviors and ideation, caution is warranted in interpreting available data, especially since prospective studies have not yet followed large cohorts with adequate representation of subjects with more severe HIV-related diseases.

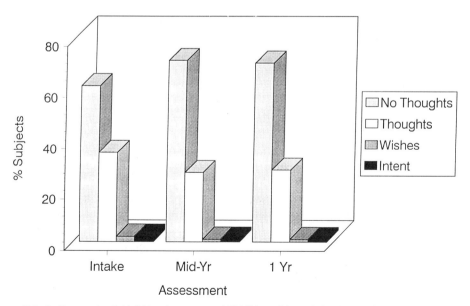

FIG. 4. Rates of suicidal ideation among 106 HIV-positive adults during the first year after HIV testing.

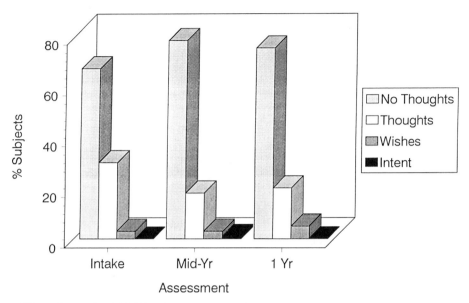

FIG. 5. Rates of suicidal ideation among 223 HIV-negative adults during the first year after HIV testing.

Nevertheless, a couple of tentative conclusions can reasonably be made. First, from a public health perspective, the presence of AIDS may statistically increase rates of completed suicide, but this event is still relatively rare compared to the other devastating effects of this fatal disease. Second, from a clinical perspective, because suicidal ideation appears not to be related to HIV status but rather to concomitant depression (32), the presence of such thoughts in HIV-positive patients should not routinely be considered "normal" but rather as a signal to evaluate and, if indicated, to treat for a depressive disorder.

TREATMENTS OF HIV-RELATED DEPRESSION

Considering that antidepressant treatments are widely administered to patients with medical illnesses, it may seem a bit disturbing that so few controlled antidepressant trials have been conducted with this population (33–35). Part of the reason is the numerous methodological problems. The assessment of depression in the physically ill is difficult because the psychological symptoms may overlap with the normal sadness associated with having a disease and because the somatic symptoms of depression may overlap with the systemic effects of the physical illness or its treatment (loss of weight, appetite, energy, sleep, libido, and concentration). Other research problems include the hesitancy to push maximum dosages of antidepressants in the physically ill because of the drugs' potential cardiotoxic or hypotensive side effects or because of concerns about possible unknown drug–drug interactions. Furthermore, when new physical symptoms do occur, one is unsure whether they are side effects of the antidepressant or due to the medical illness or its treatment. And finally, it is often difficult to determine whether a positive response is due to the antidepressant or to recovery from the medical illness and, conversely, whether a negative response is due to a failure of the antidepressant or to a worsening of the underlying physical problems.

Despite these methodological difficulties, a few controlled antidepressant studies among HIV-infected adults have been completed or are in progress. These include the use of tricyclics, serotonin reuptake inhibitors, psychostimulants, electroconvulsive therapy, and manualized psychotherapies.

Tricyclic Antidepressants

Fernandez et al. (36) compared desipramine with amitrityline over 1 year in 28 subjects with relatively advanced HIV disease [19 with AIDS-related complex (ARC) and 9 with AIDS]. These investigators found that both drugs were similarly effective, but subjects with ARC usually had a better antidepressant response.

Manning et al. (37) compared imipramine with placebo in a double-blind, randomized 6-week trial. Subjects were in various stages of HIV infection, but were excluded at entry if they had dementia. Of the 40 completers, 67 percent of subjects on the active drug had a good response compared with 47 percent who received the placebo. Whereas statistically imipramine had a slight edge, also encouraging was how well the drug was tolerated at a mean peak dose of 225 mg/day.

Rabkin et al. (14) conducted a controlled trial of imipramine that was similar in design. Among the 64 HIV-positive subjects who completed the 6-week trial, 69 percent responded to imipramine whereas 23 percent responded to placebo, a significant effect. The lower response rate to placebo may have been partly due to recruiting subjects with higher entry depression scores than in the study by Manning et al. (37). Otherwise the results were basically the same: Response to imipramine occurred even among those subjects with total CD4 cell less than 200 mm^3, and the drug was well tolerated at therapeutic levels (mean peak dosage 225 mg/day).

Consistent with their earlier report (38), Rabkin et al. (14) also found that regardless of treatment condition or antidepressant response, CD4 cell counts increased nonsignificantly in all groups. Furthermore, when the 20 imipramine responders were maintained openly on medication for an average of 20 weeks, mean change in total CD4 cell count between baseline (319/mm^3) and endpoint (320/mm^3) was negligible. These findings may help allay the concern among physicians and their HIV-positive patients about the possible immunosuppressive effects of tricyclic antidepressants.

Serotonin Reuptake Inhibitors

Although fluoxetine is now the most widely prescribed antidepressant medication, no controlled trials have yet been published regarding its efficacy among HIV-infected adults. Levine et al. (39) did report that eight HIV-positive depressed subjects responded to an open trial of fluoxetine 20–40 mg/day as evidenced by a remarkable drop in mean depression scores on the HDRS (23 at baseline, 6 after 1 month, and 2 after 3 months). None of the subjects had AIDS, but all were taking zidovudine.

Perhaps more compelling, in conjunction with the imipramine study described above (14), Rabkin et al. *(personal communication)* conducted an open trial of fluoxetine among 35 depressed HIV-positive men who comprised an interesting group: 12 imipramine nonresponders, 8 placebo nonresponders, 7 dropouts due to imipramine side effects, 5 imipramine responders who disliked imipramine's side effects despite improved mood, and 3 imipramine responders who relapsed and whose side effects precluded raising imipramine dosage. Considering that this was a rather problematic sample, it is noteworthy that 49 percent had a good response to fluoxetine after 6 weeks at 20–40 mg/day *(personal communication)*.

Of additional note, the investigators of both fluoxetine studies reported that side effects were generally not severe. No subjects in the study by Levine et al. lost weight or discontinued the medication because of the mild anxiety, insomnia, and gastrointestinal discomfort often associated with drug induction. In the fluoxetine study by Rabkin et al., 3 of the 35 subjects did discontinue the drug: one man after taking just a single capsule, and two others after 6 weeks because the medication made them feel "wired" (a term sometime used to describe the activation syndrome associated with the drug).

Psychostimulants

Prior to the HIV epidemic, both dextroamphetamine and methylphenidate were reported to improve mood, energy, and alertness in the physically ill (40). Following this lead, Fernandez and colleagues (41–43) began systematically documenting the efficacy of psychostimulants in HIV-positive adults, especially those with more severe physical illnesses and with the lethargy and apathy often seen in the later stages of disease. Among the total of 30 or so cases reported by this group, individually adjusted dosages of methylphenidate have ranged between 10 and 90 mg/day while those of dextroamphetamine have ranged between 5 and 60 mg/day (the impression being that the latter drug is slightly more activating but also more potentially agitating).

Based on these encouraging reports by Fernandez and his colleagues, Rabkin and her group added dextroamphetamine in dosages of 5–15 mg/day among the subjects who had not responded to fluoxetine alone (see above). All the previous partial or nonresponders improved, perhaps because the combination of drugs was more effective or perhaps because of the passage of more time (fluoxetine often takes more than 6 weeks to reach maximum effect).

In an even more challenging pilot study, Rabkin and Rabkin (*personal communication*) treated with dextroamphetamine seven depressed men suffering from the severe anergy of very late HIV illness. The patients' mean baseline total CD4 cell count was only 10 mm^3 (range: 5–30 mm^3), and all were on multiple medications. With a starting daily dose of 5 mg in divided doses, every third day dextroamphetamine was increased in 5-mg increments as tolerated and needed. Mean final dose was 20 mg/day (range: 5–40 mg). One of the subjects dropped out after the first day, feeling too revved up; but the other six had marked improvement in energy and mood within 2 weeks. Reassuring was the fact that no relapses were reported up to 13 months or until death (to date, four of the seven have died). Indeed, one subject insisted upon continuing dextroamphetamine during this final morphine drip to help him be more alert when he was awake.

The above case reports as well as others (44,45) reflect an increased willingness not only to administer psychostimulants to very ill hospitalized patients with AIDS, but also to maintain HIV-infected outpatients on these drugs for prolonged periods to sustain improvement in energy, mood, and alertness. Nevertheless, physicians may be wary about prescribing controlled substances that are associated with tolerance and psychological dependence, especially when the patient has a current or past history of drug abuse. In this regard, an ongoing study by Fernandez and Levy (46) may prove helpful. They are comparing methylphenidate 30 mg/day with desipramine 150 mg/day in a 6-week randomized trial. Among the first 25 depressed HIV-positive subjects, this research team reports that both treatments have been similarly effective in improving mood *and* energy and alertness. Of some note, desipramine even in rather modest dosages was so energizing and stimulating that the "blinded" investigators could not distinguish the two drugs. This "nonaddicting" tricyclic antidepressant may therefore be a reasonable alternative to a psychostimulant when concerns about potential abuse are present.

Electroconvulsive Therapy (ECT)

For the patient whose severe depression does not respond to medication, the question is then raised about ECT. Accumulating clinical experience indicates that this modality is both safe and effective for HIV-infected depressed populations (with the usual proviso about the absence of a space-occupying lesion in the brain). For example, Schaerf et al. (47) reported that four HIV-positive patients (three with delusional depressions) had a sustained response to 6–12 treatments with unilateral ECT without evidence of cognitive deficits.

Antidepressant Psychotherapies

Early in the epidemic, clinicians described multiple psychosocial stressors associated with HIV infection, including: stigmatization; uncertainty; deaths of lovers, family, and friends; and, of course, attenuation of one's own expected life span (2). When these stressors were combined with biomedical stressors, such as fatigue, cognitive decline, and drug side effects, HIV-infected patients were thought to be particularly vulnerable to depression. As noted at the beginning of this chapter, it now appears that depressive disorders do not occur nearly so often as was initially feared. Nevertheless, there is no doubt that individual or group therapy can be extraordinarily helpful in offering support and advice and thereby reducing isolation, bewilderment, distress, despair (48–51) and possibly risk behaviors (52).

The antidepressant effects of specific psychotherapies for HIV-infected adults have not yet been extensively studied. Perry et al. (53) administered a six-session individual stress-prevention training (SPT) program to adults after HIV testing. They found that among HIV-positive subjects randomly assigned to an SPT program, this brief weekly manualized treatment reduced depression scores more than pre/post-test counseling alone. Having established that a treatment based on cognitive-behavioral therapy (CBT) could be effective, this same team of investigators (54) then conducted an open trial of a treatment based on another model, interpersonal psychotherapy (IPT). After a mean of 16 weekly IPT sessions, 20 of 23 HIV-positive depressed men and women markedly improved. With the efficacy of imipramine, CBT, and IPT tentatively shown, this same team has now launched a more ambitious randomized 4-month trial that is comparing these three modalities with less intensive supportive therapy.

SUMMARY

While there is still much to be learned about depression in the context of HIV illness, studies over the past decade are generally reassuring. True, low-grade depressive symptoms are frequent among both HIV-positive and at-risk HIV-negative adults, but depressive disorders are the exception and not the rule, occurring in about 1 of 10 individuals. Similar to non-HIV populations, these depressive disorders are more likely to occur among those

HIV-infected adults with severe personality problems, with a history of previous depressions, and with limited current social support. Although rates of depression may slightly increase with development of more severe physical symptoms, even then the clinician should not consider the presence of a depressive disorder as understandable, justified, and therefore "normal." Rather, depressive symptoms accompanied by suicidal ideation are signals for further evaluation and treatment.

When antidepressant treatment is indicated, the weight of current evidence suggests that standard therapies can be safely and effectively prescribed for HIV-infected adults. For outpatients without severe physical illness, antidepressant medications are generally well tolerated in recommended dosages and do not increase immunosuppression. For those with more severe physical impairment, the adage for geriatric populations is applicable: "Start low and go slow." If lethargy and cognitive slowing is a major component of the depression, especially among those in later stages of disease, then psychostimulants may be helpful. When concerns about drug abuse preclude such a prescription, an activating antidepressant may be just as helpful to improve both mood and energy. For severe or refractory depressions, such as delusional affective disorders, ECT has been safely given to HIV-infected patients. And finally, accumulated clinical experience and a couple of systematic studies suggest that psychotherapy, alone or in combination with antidepressant drug therapy, can be remarkably beneficial.

In sum, data support the fact that we have much to offer our depressed HIV-infected patients. Our task is to make sure that we identify their depressions when present and counter their feelings of hopelessness by ensuring that effective antidepressant treatments are provided.

ACKNOWLEDGMENTS

Preparation of this chapter was supported by the National Institute of Mental Health grants MH4277 and MH46250. The author is grateful for the assistance of Kelly McKinney, M.A.

REFERENCES

1. Runck B. *Coping with AIDS: psychological and social considerations in helping people with HTLV-III infection,* Rockville, MD: NIMH Office of Scientific Information, 1986.
2. Faulstich ME. Psychiatric aspects of AIDS. *Am J Psychiatry* 1987;144:551–556.
3. Ostrow DG, Monjan A, Joseph JG et al. HIV related symptoms and psychological functioning in a cohort of homosexual men. *Am J Psychiatry* 1989;146:737–742.
4. Hays RB, Turner H, Coates TJ. Social support, AIDS-related symptoms, and depression among gay men. *J Consult Clin Psychol* 1992;60:463–469.
5. Perry S, Jacobsberg L, Card C, Ashman T, Frances A, Fishman B. Severity of psychiatric symptoms after HIV testing. *Am J Psychiatry* 1993;150:50.
6. Atkinson JH, Grant I, Kennedy CJ, Richman DD, Spector SA, McCutchan A. Prevalence of psychiatric disorders among men infected with HIV. *Arch Gen Psychiatry* 1988;45:859–864.

7. Perry S, Fishman B, Jacobsberg L, Frances A. Relationships over one year between lymphocyte subsets and psychosocial variables among adults infected by HIV. *Arch Gen Psychiatry* 1992;49:396–401.
8. Williams JBW, Rabkin JG, Remien RH, Gorman JM, Ehrhardt AA. Multidisciplinary baseline assessment of homosexual men with and without human immunodeficiency virus infection, II: standardized clinical assessment of current and lifetime psychopathology. *Arch Gen Psychiatry* 1991;48:124–130.
9. Rabkin JG, Remien R, Katoff L, Williams JH. Resilience in adversity among long-term survivors of AIDS. *Hosp Community Psychiatry* 1993;44:162–167.
10. Derogatis LR, Morrow GR, Fetting J, et al. The prevalence of psychiatric disorders among cancer patients. *JAMA* 1983;249:751–757.
11. Rabkin JG, Williams JBW, Neugebauer R, Remien RH, Goetz R. Maintenance of hope in HIV-spectrum homosexual men. *Am J Psychiatry* 1990;147:1322–1326.
12. Joseph JG, Caumartin DG, Tal M, et al. Psychological functioning in a cohort of gay men at risk for AIDS. *J Nerv Ment Dis* 1990;178:607–615.
13. Perry S, Jacobsberg L, Fishman B, Frances A, Bobo J, Jacobsberg BK. Psychiatric diagnosis before serological testing for HIV. *Am J Psychiatry* 1990;147:89–93.
14. Rabkin JG, Rabkin R, Harrison W. Imipramine effects on mood and immune status in depressed patients with HIV illness: preliminary findings. Presented at the National Institute of Mental Health-sponsored meeting, "Neurobehavioral Findings in AIDS Research," Washington, DC, 1991.
15. Jacobsberg L, Perry S, Fishman B, Frances A, Ryan J, Fogel K. Psychiatric diagnoses among volunteers for HIV testing. V International Conference on AIDS, Montreal, June 1989.
16. Fishman B, Perry S, Jacobsberg L., Frances A. Psychological factors predicting distress after HIV testing. V International Conference on AIDS, Montreal, June, 1989.
17. Martin JL. Psychological consequences of AIDS-related bereavement among gay men. *J Consult Clin Psychol* 1988;56:856–862.
18. Neugebauer R, Rabkin JG, Williams JBW, Remien RH, Goetz R, Gorman JM. Bereavement reactions among homosexual men experiencing multiple losses in the AIDS epidemic. *Am J Psychiatry* 1992;149:1374–1379.
19. Perry S. Organic mental disorders caused by HIV: update on early diagnosis and treatment. *Am J Psychiatry* 1990;147:696–710.
20. Krikorian R, Wrobel AJ. Cognitive impairment in HIV infection. *AIDS* 1991;5:1501–1507.
21. Stern Y, Marder K, Bell K, et al. Multidisciplinary baseline assessment of homosexual men with and without human immunodeficiency virus infection, III: neurological and neuropsychological findings. *Arch Gen Psychiatry* 1991;48:131–138.
22. Stern RA, Singer NG, Silva SG, et al. Neurobehavioral functioning in a nonconfounded group of asymptomatic HIV-seropositive homosexual men. *Am J Psychiatry* 1992;149:1099–1102.
23. Rabkin JG, Williams JBW, Remien RH, Goetz R, Kertzner R, Gorman JM. Depression, distress, lymphocyte subsets, and human immunodeficiency virus symptoms on two occasions in HIV-positive homosexual men. *Arch Gen Psychiatry* 1991;48:111–119.
24. Kessler RC, Foster C, Joseph J, et al. Stressful life events and symptom onset in HIV infection. *Am J Psychiatry* 1991;148:733–738.
25. Marzuk PM, Tierney H, Tardiff K, et al. Increased risk of suicide in persons with AIDS. *JAMA* 1988;259:1333–1337.
26. Marzuk PM. Suicidal behavior and HIV illness. *Int Rev Psychiatry* 1991;3:365–371.
27. Kizer KW, Green M, Perkins CI, Doebbert G, Hughes MJ. AIDS suicide in California. *JAMA* 1988;260:1881.
28. Brown G, Rundell J. Suicidal tendencies in women with human immunodeficiency virus infection. *Am J Psychiatry* 1989;146:556–557.
29. Buehler J, Devine O, Berkelman R, Chevarley F. Impact of human immunodeficiency virus epidemic on mortality trends in young men, United States. *Am J Public Health* 1990;80:1080–1086.
30. Rundell J, Thomason J, Zajac R, Beatty R. Psychiatric diagnoses and attempted suicide in HIV infected USAF personnel. Presented at the IVth International Conference on AIDS, Stockholm, 1988, Abstract 8595.
31. Schneider SG, Taylor SE, Kemeny ME, Hammen C. AIDS-related factors predictive of

suicidal ideation of low and high intent among gay and bisexual men. *Suicide Life Threat Behav* 1991;21:313–328.

32. Perry S, Jacobsberg L, Fishman B. Suicidal ideation and HIV testing. *JAMA* 1990;263: 679–682.
33. Roose SP, Glassman AH, Giardina EG, et al. Nortriptyline in depressed patients with left ventricular impairment. *JAMA* 1986;256(23):3253–3257.
34. Parikh RM, Robinson RG, Lipsey JR, Starkstein SE, Fedoroff JP. The impact of poststroke depression on recovery in activities of daily living over a 2-year follow-up. *Arch Neurol* 1990;47:785–789.
35. Popkin MK, Callies AL, MacKenzie TB. The outcome of antidepressant use in the medically ill. *Arch Gen Psychiatry* 1985;42:1160–1163.
36. Fernandez F, Levy JK, Mansell PWA. Response to antidepressant therapy in depressed persons with advanced HIV infection. Presented at the Vth International Conference on AIDS, Abstract WBP 191, Montreal, 1989.
37. Manning D, Jacobsberg L, Erhart S, et al. The efficacy of imipramine in the treatment of HIV-related depression. Presented at the VIth International Conference on AIDS, Abstract ThB 32, San Francisco, 1990.
38. Rabkin JG, Harrison WM. Effect of imipramine on depression and immune status in a sample of men with HIV infection. *Am J Psychiatry* 1990;147:495–497.
39. Levine SH, Anderson D, Bystritsky A, Baron D. A report of eight HIV-seropositive patients with major depression responding to fluoxetine. *AIDS* 1990;3:1074–1077.
40. Chairello RJ, Cole JO. The use of psychostimulants in general psychiatry: a reconsideration. *Arch Gen Psychiatry* 1987;44:286–295.
41. Fernandez F, Adams F, Levy JK, Holmes VF, Neidhart M, Mansell PWA. Cognitive impairment due to AIDS-related complex and its response to psychostimulants. *Psychosomatics* 1988;29:38–46.
42. Holmes VF, Fernandez F, Levy JK. Psychostimulant response in AIDS-related complex patients. *J Clin Psychiatry* 1989;50(1):5–8.
43. Fernandez F, Levy JK, Galizzi H. Response of HIV-related depression to psychostimulants: case reports. *Hosp Community Psychiatry* 1988;39:628–631.
44. Walling VR, Pfefferbaum B. The use of methylphenidate in a depressed adolescent with AIDS. *J Dev Behav Pediatr* 1990;11:195–197.
45. White JC, Christensen JF, Singer CM. Methylphenidate as a treatment for depression in acquired immunodeficiency syndrome: an n-of-1 trial. *J Clin Psychiatry* 1992;53:153–156.
46. Fernandez F, Levy JK. Treatment of depression in HIV patients with the dopamine agonist methylphenidate. Presented at the meeting of Neuroscience and HIV Infection: Basic and Clinical Frontiers, Amsterdam, 1992.
47. Schaerf FW, Miller RR, Lipsey JR, et al. ECT for major depression in four patients with human immunodeficiency virus. *Am J Psychiatry* 1989;146:782–784.
48. Perry S, Markowitz J. Psychiatric interventions for AIDS-spectrum disorders. *Hosp Community Psychiatry* 1986;37:1001–1006.
49. Schaffner B. Psychotherapy with HIV infected persons. In: Goldfinger SM, ed. *New directions in psychiatry and mental health services.* San Francisco: Jossey-Bass, 1990.
50. Coates T, McKusick L, Stites D, Kuno R. Stress management training reduced number of sexual partners but did not improve functioning in men infected with HIV. *Am J Public Health* 1989;79:885–887.
51. Beckett A, Rutan JS. Treating persons with ARC and AIDS in group psychotherapy. *Int J Group Psychother* 1990;40:19–29.
52. Kelly JA, St. Lawrence JS, Hood HV, Brasfield TL. Behavioral intervention to reduce AIDS risk activities. *J Consult Clin Psychol* 1989;57:60–67.
53. Perry S, Fishman B, Jacobsberg L, Young J, Frances A. Effectiveness of psychoeducational interventions in reducing emotional distress after human immunodeficiency virus antibody testing. *Arch Gen Psychiatry* 1991;48:143–147.
54. Markowitz JC, Klerman GL, Perry SW. Interpersonal psychotherapy of depressed HIV-seropositive patients. *Hosp Community Psychiatry* 1992;43:885–890.

HIV, AIDS and the Brain, edited by
R. W. Price and S. W. Perry.
Raven Press, Ltd., New York © 1994.

13

Evaluation and Treatment of Psychiatric Disorders Associated with HIV Infection

Glenn Treisman, Marc Fishman, Constantine Lyketsos, and
Paul R. McHugh

*Department of Psychiatry and Behavioral Science, Johns Hopkins University
School of Medicine, Johns Hopkins Hospital, Baltimore, MD 21287*

A remarkable phenomenon occurred among psychiatric services when they were confronted with the beginnings of the acquired immunodeficiency syndrome (AIDS) epidemic. The thought of the emotional problems of young people caught up in a devastating, stigmatizing, and relentlessly fatal illness provoked assumptions about what psychiatrists would find among such patients and what they could do for them.

Psychiatrists divided into two groups. One group thought that any emotional condition to be found amongst human immunodeficiency syndrome (HIV)-infected people would be appropriate psychological reactions to the patient's life situation. Thus, except for some palliative gestures, such individuals would be therapeutically inaccessible. In fact, with the expanding epidemic, a ''bottomless pit'' for psychiatric resources seemed to loom in front of these individuals. This stance of therapeutic nihilism based on an empathic posture led to the avoidance of the clinics and the patients by this group of psychiatrists.

A second group, who in fact agreed with the fundamental assumptions of the first, nonetheless saw their roles as psychiatrists to be expressing a sense of human loyalty and solidarity with the victims of the AIDS epidemic. These therapists threw themselves into intense personalized interactions in an attempt to alleviate what distress they could for the people in this tragic situation. They often found their energies quickly exhausted by their efforts to comply with all the demands of their patients. After some months they began to report that they themselves felt ''burned out'' and either had to decide to leave the service completely or needed frequent respites in order to manage the demands that they felt were imposed upon them.

This situation among psychiatric services was an example of how an empathic stance based upon a hypothesis and interpretation that *preceded* observation acted to the detriment of effective action. When faced with these problems and these responses at the Johns Hopkins Hospital, the director of the department persuaded an energetic and distinguished young resident to visit the clinic with him in order to see exactly what could be found amongst those patients and only then decide what services they required and what the department of psychiatry might do about it.

In this report, two studies that evolved from that enterprise are presented. First are the results of a psychiatric evaluation of a consecutive series of patients on their admission to the HIV clinic. This study was an effort to seek the nature and prevalence of psychiatric disorder at the first visit to an HIV clinic. The second study is an assessment of the particular psychiatric disorders and their treatment response in a series of patients that were referred to the psychiatric services in the clinic.

The major point that we believe these data reveal is that HIV patients, like all other groups of patients that eventually seek psychiatric help, have within their number a diversity of psychiatric disorders and that the treatments and the prognosis vary with the nature of these disorders and can be matched to them. Although the HIV epidemic continues, psychiatric services to patients can be effectively and appropriately provided.

STUDY 1

Method

Fifty consecutive patients were evaluated with the Johns Hopkins standard psychiatric interview on their initial evaluation for medical intake into the Moore Clinic. This is an infectious diseases clinic specializing in the treatment of HIV-infected patients at the Johns Hopkins Hospital. Each patient received a complete psychiatric history and Mental Status Examination and a DSM-IIIR diagnosis. No patients declined to participate, and all patients evaluated were offered a follow-up for psychiatric illness. All examinations were carried out by one of the authors. In addition, a screening tool was administered by a a trained social worker in the Moore Clinic prior to psychiatric evaluation.

Results

Fifty-four percent of the patients examined had a primary psychiatric diagnosis other than substance abuse. The diagnoses are shown in Table 1. It is interesting to note that 20 percent of patients had a DSM-IIIR diagnosis of major depression while 18 percent of patients had a diagnosis of adjustment disorder (all types).

TABLE 1. *Psychiatric diagnoses in a pilot study of new HIV clinic intakes[a]*

Primary diagnosis	
Major depressive episode	10 (20)
Adjustment disorder, all types	9 (18)
Dementia	4 (8)
Organic mood disorder	2 (4)
Bipolar mood disorder, mixed	1 (2)
Life circumstance problem	1 (2)
Total	27 (54)

[a] Number in parentheses are percentages of total sample.

TABLE 2. *Cognitive impairment in patients during pilot screening study*

Primary diagnosis of demetia	4 (8%)
Psychiatric diagnosis with dementia	2 (4%)
Mental retardation	3 (6%)
Total	9 (18%)

Table 2 shows that 18 percent of patients had some cognitive impairment at the time of entry into the clinic. The diagnosis of mental retardation, shown for 6 percent, was made only in patients when reliable data about early developmental milestones in childhood were available. Patients with all other forms of dementia are shown in the table. Diagnosis of dementia was made only in patients in which cognitive impairment other than that caused by depression or delirium were ruled out. Table 3 shows that 74 percent of patients had either current or prior history of a substance use disorder. As shown in Table 4, many patients had primary psychiatric diag-

TABLE 3. *Psychiatric diagnoses in a pilot study of new HIV clinic intakes[a]*

Substance use disorders	
Current substance use disorder	22 (44)
Prior substance use disorder	15 (30)
Total	37 (74)

[a] Number in parentheses are percentages of total sample.

TABLE 4. *Primary psychiatric disorder with comorbid substance use disorder*

	n	Percent
Current substance use disorders	12	(24)
Prior substance use disorder	8	(16)
Total	20	(40)

TABLE 5. *Compliance with next scheduled visit: effect of psychiatric evaluation on patient compliance*

Attendance rates at first visit following intake:		
Clinic baseline	1151/2125	54%
Patients receiving psychiatric evaluation	37/50	74%[a]

[a] $p < 0.01$.

noses as well as substance abuse diagnoses (the so-called triply diagnosed patient); it also shows the details of those patients with prior or current substance use disorder as well as another axis-I psychiatric disorder. Although not shown, patients presenting for this series were equally divided among CDC stages II, III, and IV. Risk factors for HIV were known in only two-thirds of cases. Of those with known risk factors, approximately half were intravenous drug users and approximately half were male homosexuals. In the remaining third, HIV infection was most likely heterosexually transmitted.

Because of concerns about patient noncompliance given the burden of a psychiatric interview, next visit compliance was determined for all 50 patients in the study. This was compared with 2125 patients similarly evaluated without a psychiatric interview in the standard manner of the clinic. There was a significant increase in next visit compliance among those patients evaluated psychiatrically compared to the clinic baseline as shown in Table 5.

Discussion

This study revealed that right at the time of first visit to an HIV medical clinic, a majority of patients have at least one psychiatric disorder. It also shows that these disorders are very diverse, ranging from lifelong problems (such as mental retardation), to conditions that arise in response to the HIV infection, such as depression and dementia.

This high a prevalence of psychiatric disorders is similar to that reported by other authors (1–4). Similar estimates of major depression have also been reported from comparable settings (5,6). It was reassuring to discover that our enterprise did not discourage patients from returning but perhaps may even have encouraged them to see that the physicians and other therapists were interested in them.

STUDY 2

Study 2 is a cumulative report of the treatment outcome and diagnoses of referred patients during a 17-month period with a particular focus on affective disorders. All patients in the study were evaluated with a standard psychiatric evaluation from Johns Hopkins by one of the treating clinicians from our service. All patients received a DSM-IIIR diagnostic formulation, and standard psychiatric treatment recommendations were made based on diagnosis. Follow-up data was gathered whenever available, and therapeutic response was recorded in a simplified manner by treating clinicians with scores being given as unimproved, improved, or completely well. High inter-rater reliability for this simplified system was achieved by frequent inter-rater discussion and reevaluation. All records were available to treating clinicians, and there was no blind as to diagnosis. All data shown are for outpatient treatment, and patients were seen in all stages of infection.

Method of Treatment

For patients meeting DSM-IIIR criteria for major depression, treatment was initiated with either tricyclic antidepressants or fluoxetine in standard clinical doses. When patients failed treatment because of either medication intolerance or lack of response, second- and third-line agents were used, and agents from all classes of antidepressants were used in this study. Results shown represent last available response to treatment at time of study closure, and represent extensive treatment efforts on behalf of some patients. No patients in the study required inpatient electroconvulsive therapy.

Results

Table 6 reveals that during the 17-month period of the study, 162 patients were referred from the 1001 patients currently cared for in the Moore Clinic for psychiatric evaluation. Of that number, 110 patients received psychiatric evaluation and 52 received a diagnosis other than major depression while 58 received a diagnosis of major depression. Of the 52 patients who received a diagnosis other than major depression, 45 have a primary axis-I psychiatric diagnosis other than substance abuse. All patients receiving a diagnosis of major depression were offered treatment; and of those who elected to receive

TABLE 6. *HIV-positive outpatients referred to psychiatrists over a 17-month period*

1001 patients in AIDS clinic	
162 patients referred (15%)	
110 patients were evaluated	
52 patients without major depression	58 patients with major depression
(45 had a diagnosis)	(58/110)

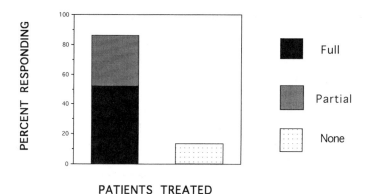

FIG. 1. Treatment outcome in all 44 patients. Patients were included if they took medications for 2 weeks even if they were noncompliant or refused treatment thereafter. Patients were rated by clinicians as follows: 1, completely well and at baseline; 2, better but not completely well; or 3, unimproved. Patients were treated with clinically indicated antidepressants and were switched to a new drug if they could not tolerate treatment or if they failed treatment.

treatment, the overall response is shown in Figure 1. The bar graph reveals that 85 percent of all patients receiving treatment for any length of time had some improvement on antidepressants. Approximately 50 percent of patients receiving antidepressant therapy had complete return to baseline. Fifteen percent of patients received no benefit from treatment, although this group included patients who elected to discontinue treatment after only one visit. Figure 2 shows a stratification of patients by either comorbid diagnosis or by compliance. In summary, 85 percent of patients improved regardless of axis-II disorder, substance use, or dementia. It is worthy of note, however, that patients with intercurrent substance abuse, axis-II disorder, and dementia had a decreasing complete response to antidepressant therapy.

Table 7 shows demographics of patients in the Moore Clinic, those receiving a diagnosis of major depression, and those having other psychiatric diagnosis. Although patients with major depression were slightly older, there was no other statistically significant difference between groups. Looking at Table 8 as well, one can see that family history of psychiatric disorder, family history of substance abuse, or personal history of previous psychiatric disorder or hospitalization does not predict a distinction between those patients receiving a diagnosis of major depression and those patients with other psychiatric diagnoses. It is worthy of note that there is a high percentage of these difficulties in both groups of patients.

The estimated prevalence of manic episodes in the clinic was 1.4 percent during the 17 months covered by this study. Although the rate of mania in HIV-infected patients could not be shown to be elevated from background, 8 percent of patients who had AIDS had manic episodes during the period

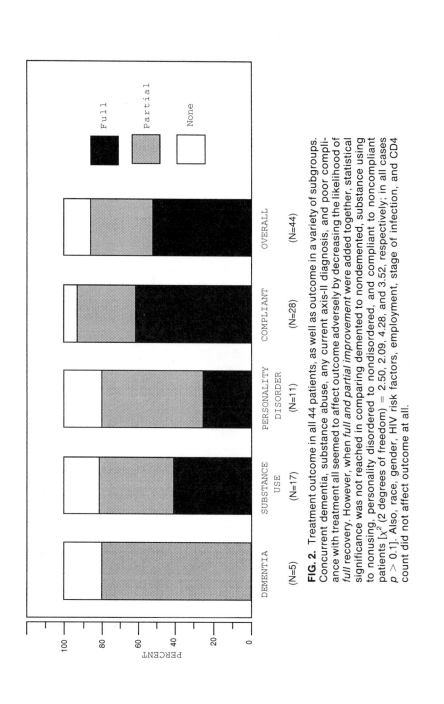

FIG. 2. Treatment outcome in all 44 patients, as well as outcome in a variety of subgroups. Concurrent dementia, substance abuse, any current axis-II diagnosis, and poor compliance with treatment all seemed to affect outcome adversely by decreasing the likelihood of *full recovery*. However, when *full and partial improvement* were added together, statistical significance was not reached in comparing demented to nondemented, substance using to nonusing, personality disordered to nondisordered, and compliant to noncompliant patients [χ^2 (2 degrees of freedom) = 2.50, 2.09, 4.28, and 3.52, respectively; in all cases $p > 0.1$]. Also, race, gender, HIV risk factors, employment, stage of infection, and CD4 count did not affect outcome at all.

TABLE 7. *Demographics of all Moore Clinic patients, nondepressed psychiatric patients, and depressed psychiatric patients*

Parameter	All patients in Moore Clinic ($N = 1001$)	No diagnosis of major depression ($N = 52$)	Diagnosis of major depression ($N = 58$)
Age (mean/SD[a])	32.9/10.8	35.2/6.9	37.2/7.2
Sex (% male)	69.5	75.2	78.6
Race (% black)	76.4	65.3	56.9
Employment (%)	Unknown	15.3	22.4
Risk factors (%)			
Homosexual	26.3	34.6	36.2
Intravenous drugs	43.6	38.8	34.4
Other	30.1	27.0	29.4

[a] SD, standard deviation.

TABLE 8. *Psychiatric history of depressed and nondepressed psychiatric patients*

Parameter	Diagnosis of major depression ($N = 58$)	No diagnosis of major depression ($N = 52$)
Psychiatric history in family (%)		
Yes	41	32.7
No	32.7	44.2
Unknown	24.1	21.2
Family substance abuse history (%)		
Yes	43.1	46.1
No	31.0	26.9
Unknown	25.8	25.0
Substance abuse prior to HIV (%)		
Yes	24.1	36.5
No	10.3	23.0
Unknown	65.5	38.5
Other axis I prior to HIV (%)		
Yes	37.9	36.5
No	50.0	53.8
Unknown	12.0	7.7
Axis II prior to HIV (%)		
Yes	15.5	30.8
No	65.5	55.8
Unknown	19.0	11.5
Prior psychiatric admissions (%)		
Yes	20.7	26.9
No	72.4	63.5
Unknown	6.9	7.8
Axis II now (%)		
Yes	27.6	32.6
No	63.8	53.8
Unknown	8.6	11.5
Substance abuse now (%)		
Yes	41.3	46.1
No	55.2	50.0
Unknown	3.4	3.9

TABLE 9. *Comparison between those with low risk for mania (personal and family history negative for bipolar illness) and those with high risk for mania (personal or family history positive for bipolar illness)[a]*

Parameter	Low risk ($N = 7$) (negative history)	High risk ($N = 7$) (positive history)
Age	Mean 33.6 SD 5.4	Mean 35.1 SD 9.0
Gender	7 men	5 men
HIV risk factor	4 homosexuals 2 IVDUs	3 homosexuals 4 IVDUs
HIV stage at diagnosis of mania	0 asymptomatic 7 AIDS	5 asymptomatic 2 AIDS
CD4 count at diagnosis of mania	6 less than 100 0 more than 100	2 less than 100 3 more than 100
Dementia at diagnosis of mania	6 patients	No patients
Mini-mental score at diagnosis of mania	Mean 21 SD 5.62	Mean 26 SD 1.41
Brain image at diagnosis of mania	4 abnormal 3 normal	0 abnormal 2 normal

[a] The groups were similar in terms of demographics and risk factors for HIV infection [for age comparisons, t (12) = 0.395, $p > 0.5$; for gender and risk factor comparisons, $p > 0.5$ by Fisher's exact test]. In contrast, more patients in the low-risk had AIDS ($p = 0.01$ by Fisher's exact), and more patients in the low-risk group had CD4 counts below 100 ($p = 0.06$ by Fisher's exact). SD, standard deviation; IVDUs, intravenous drug users.

of the study. Patients with mania could be stratified into two groups, as shown in Table 9. This table shows patients stratified into a group in which there was no personal or family history of mania (low risk) and a group with either a family history of manic depressive illness or an episode of mania prior to the diagnosis of HIV. As can be seen, those patients with a low prior risk for mania all developed mania late in the course of their HIV infection, after their T cells had dropped below 100, and after formal diagnosis of AIDS. In addition, all had developed HIV dementia at the time of the diagnosis of mania. In the other group, patients developed mania any time in the course of their HIV illness, only two had T cells below 100, and none had developed dementia at the time of the diagnosis.

Discussion

These results of a survey of patients referred to psychiatrists by the clinicians of an HIV clinic reveal that among a diverse group of different psychiatric conditions in referred patients, a large number suffer from affective disorder.

The patients with depression are not distinguished from the other patients by any obvious risk factors, although the importance of such risk factors may be obscured by the high prevalence of family history and previous psychiatric history found in all patients in our clinic. The depressions seem to occur at almost any stage in the HIV infection.

In contrast, the manic patients can be differentiated in that the patients who have mania and lack previous psychiatric disorder or a family history of disorder seem to develop their mania late in the course of their HIV infection close to the time of the appearance of HIV encephalopathy. Patients with family histories and previous histories of mania develop mania at almost any phase of the HIV infection (7).

A relatively simple method of assessing therapeutic response to these patients reveals that they do well on antidepressant medication. These responses, though, were the outcome of extensive clinical efforts and the deployment of a full range of antidepressants. It included cognitive behavioral and rehabilitational psychotherapy where appropriate. These results are comparable to findings of other investigators (8–10) and represent a refutation of the view that the affective disorders of patients with HIV infection are relatively refractory to treatment.

The treatment of mania was also successful, particularly amongst those individuals who were not demented. Amongst the demented patients, lithium was problematic because it produced delirium. Patients had to be treated with low-dose neuroleptics and often remained chronically manic at that stage of their life.

GENERAL DISCUSSION

This is a report on two studies carried out in the course of offering diagnosis and treatment of psychiatric disorders to people attending an HIV clinic. Logically, it has the strengths of such studies in that the patients were actively investigated by physicians enthusiastically working to care for them. Their energies were directed towards finding an appropriate diagnosis and treatment to achieve the goals of a clinic. Lacking in this study is the extensive deployment of standardized instruments and double-blind controls for therapeutic conclusions.

However, for the purposes of this report, the results are extremely encouraging and speak to the issues that had previously inhibited the development of psychiatric enterprises in HIV clinics. It is clear from these results that the patients have a diversity of psychiatric conditions, and learning about these conditions and differentiating them from one another encourages specific treatment matching to the conditions. The therapies offered to these patients were quite successful. With results such as these, no longer should there be a reluctance of psychiatrists to become involved in the care of patients with HIV conditions, nor should there be any encouragement to offer simply a general paliative psychotherapy to all patients defined as emotionally or otherwise psychiatrically disturbed.

Further implications, though, can be drawn from these data. The success of the therapeutic treatments of both depression and mania means that patients with these conditions should be identified early and brought to the attention of psychiatrists or other people who are prepared to treat them. The first study demonstrates that some 20 percent of patients that come to this clinic suffer from major depression at the time of initial evaluation, and we can assume that we will need to extend our services given the magnitude of the epidemic. A psychiatric screening should be part and parcel of every medical admission to an HIV clinic. From that screening appropriate referrals should be made.

Because these results match data from other studies, we are even more secure in our conclusions. We also presume that there may well be relationships between these conditions and the engaging in risky behavior both in relationship to the initiation of HIV infection and in passing it to others. In particular, the diagnosis of mania raises this issue even as it tends to confirm that the affective conditions we are talking about represent those of a neurobiological kind.

PERSPECTIVE FOR THE FUTURE

The importance of more data acquired in a still more systematic fashion can be appreciated once the implications of these data are understood. There is some suggestion in the literature that our 50 percent prevalence estimate may represent an increasing amount of psychiatric disorder in the HIV-infected population. People without psychiatric conditions may be able to modify their behavior so as to avoid exposure to HIV infection, now that risk factors are known.

Finally, these data support that we have in HIV infection still another example in which a subcortical condition is provocative of affective disorder. HIV depression and mania seems to be symptomatic affective disorders and can be included amongst the other conditions such as Huntington's disease (11), stroke (12), and Parkinsonism as subcortical brain diseases with symptomatic affective disorder.

REFERENCES

1. Atkinson JH, Grant I, Kennedy CJ, Richman DD, Spector SA, McCutchan JA. Prevalence of psychiatric disorders among men infected with human immunodeficiency virus. *Arch Gen Psychiatry* 1988;45:859–864.
2. Chuang HT, Jason GW, Pajurkova EM, Gill JM. Psychiatric morbidity in patients with HIV infection. *Can J Psychiatry* 1992;37:109–115.
3. Gorman JM, Kertner R, Todak G, Goetz RR, Williams JB, Rabkin J, Meyer-Bahlburg HF, Mayeux R, Stern Y, Lange M, Spitzer DJR, Ehrhardt AA. Multidisciplinary baseline assessment of homosexual men with and without human immunodeficiency virus infection. *Arch Gen Psychiatry* 1991;48:120–123.

4. Perry S, Jacobsberg LB, Fishman B, Frances A, Bobo J, Jacobsberg BK. Psychiatric diagnosis before serological testing for the human immunodeficiency virus. *Am J Psychiatry* 1990;147(1):89–93.
5. Seth R, Granville-Grossman K, Goldmeier D, Lynch S. Psychiatric illnesses in patients with HIV infection and AIDS referred to the liaison psychiatrist. *Br J Psychiatry* 1991;159: 347–350.
6. Sno HN, Storosum JG, Swinkels JA. HIV Infection: psychiatric findings in The Netherlands. *Br J Psychiatry* 1989;155:814–817.
7. Lyketsos CG, Hanson AL, Fishman M, Rosenblatt A, McHugh PR, Treisman GJ. Manic episode early and late in the course of HIV infection. *Am J Psychiatry* 1993;150:326–327.
8. Fernandez F, Levy JK, Neidhart M. Cognitive impairment due to AIDS-related complex and its response to psychostimulants. *Psychosomatics* 1988;29(1):38–46.
9. Hintz S, Kuck J, Peterkin JJ, Volk DM, Zisook S. Depression in the context of human immunodeficiency virus infection: implications for treatment. *J Clin Psychiatry* 1990;51(12): 497–501.
10. Rabkin JG, Harrison WM. Effect of imipramine on depression and immune status in a sample of men with HIV infection. *Am J Psychiatry* 1990;147(4):495–497.
11. Folstein SE. *Huntington's disease: a disorder of families.* Baltimore: The Johns Hopkins University Press, 1989.
12. Starkstein SE, Robinson RG. Affective disorders and cerebral vascular disease. *Br J Psychiatry* 1989;154:170–182.

HIV, AIDS and the Brain, edited by
R. W. Price and S. W. Perry.
Raven Press, Ltd., New York © 1994.

14

HIV Dementia

Incidence and Risk Factors

*Justin C. McArthur, *Ola A. Selnes, *Jonathan D. Glass,
†Donald R. Hoover, and †Helena Bacellar

*Department of Neurology, Johns Hopkins University School of Medicine, Johns
Hopkins Hospital, Baltimore, MD 21287; and †Johns Hopkins School of Hygiene
and Public Health, Baltimore, MD 21205

Neurological disorders associated with human immunodeficiency virus (HIV) infection occur in 30–60 percent of individuals with advanced HIV disease. These can be subdivided into opportunistic processes affecting the central nervous system (CNS), a consequence of HIV disruption of cellular immunity, and a range of neurological disorders which have been directly associated with HIV infection, including dementia, myelopathy, peripheral neuropathy, and myopathy. Each adds to the morbidity of HIV disease and may shorten survival or complicate the management of patients with AIDS. The number of patients who develop HIV-related neurologic disease is not trivial; projections are for 65,000 new cases of dementia, myelopathy, or neuropathy annually (1). This presentation will focus on HIV-associated dementia complex (HIV dementia), which has been estimated to affect up to 60 percent of all individuals in the late stages of HIV disease (2,3) and has been an acquired immunodeficiency syndrome (AIDS)-defining condition since 1987 (4). While HIV-associated dementia can develop concurrently with other HIV-associated neurological disorders such as myelopathy and neuropathy, it appears that these are all discrete disorders with different manifestations and potentially different pathogenetic mechanisms. Thus, the concept of lumping all of these disorders together as "neuro-AIDS" is simplistic.

DEFINITIONS

HIV-associated dementia was originally described a decade ago and termed "subacute encephalitis" (5). In the years before identification of HIV as the causative agent of AIDS, this progressive dementia was thought to be a consequence of a CNS opportunistic infection, probably cytomegalovirus (CMV). In 1986, Navia et al. (6) defined the syndrome with a detailed retrospective study of 70 cases and coined the term *AIDS dementia complex*. This terminology indicates the association with AIDS, as well as the predominance of cognitive impairment and dementia in the syndrome, but the additional term "complex" indicates the frequency of motor deficits and myelopathy. In 1991, the American Academy of Neurology AIDS Task Force developed terminology and definitional criteria for AIDS dementia, myelopathy, and neuropathy, as well as for the less severe forms of cognitive impairment (7). Table 1 lists the criteria for dementia and cognitive impairment.

TABLE 1. *Definitional criteria for HIV-1-associated dementia complex and cognitive impairment (7)*

Probable (must have **each** of the following)
1. a. Acquired abnormality in at least two of the following cognitive abilities (present for at least 1 month): attention/concentration, speed of processing of information, abstraction/reasoning, visuospatial skills, memory/learning, and speech/language. The decline should be verified by reliable history and mental status examination. In all cases, when possible, history should be obtained from an informant, and examination should be supplemented by neuropsychological testing.
   b. Cognitive dysfunction causing impairment of work or activities of daily living (objectively verifiable or by report of a key informant). This impairment should not be attributable solely to severe systemic illness.
2. At least **one** of the following:
   a. Acquired abnormality in motor function or performance verified by clinical examination (e.g., slowed rapid movements, abnormal gait, limb incoordination, hyperreflexia, hypertonia, or weakness), neurophychological tests (e.g., fine motor speed, manual dexterity, perceptual motor skills), or both.
   b. Decline in motivation or emotional control or change in social behavior. This may be characterized by any of the following: change in personality with apathy, inertia, irritability, emotional lability, or new onset of impaired judgment, characterized by social inappropriate behavior or disinhibition.
3. Absence or clouding of consciousness during a period long enough to establish the presence of criterion 1, above.
4. Evidence of another etiology—including active CNS opportunistic infection or malignancy, psychiatric disorders (e.g., depressive disorder), active alcohol or substance use, or acute or chronic substance withdrawal—must be sought from history, physical and psychiatric examination, and appropriate laboratory and radiologic investigation (e.g., lumbar puncture, neuroimaging). If another potential etiology (e.g., major depression) is present, it is *not* the cause of the above cognitive, motor, or behavioral symptoms and signs.
Possible (must have **one** of the following)
1. Other potential etiology present (must have **each** of the following):
   a. Same as criteria 1, 2, and 3 in **Probable.**
   b. Other potential etiology is present, but the cause of criterion 1 above is uncertain.
2. Incomplete clinical evaluation (must have **each** of the following):
   a. Same as criteria 1, 2, and 3 in **Probable.**
   b. Etiology cannot be determined (appropriate laboratory or radiologic investigations not performed).

HIV DEMENTIA: CLINICAL, LABORATORY, AND PATHOLOGIC FEATURES

Clinical Features

The clinical features of HIV dementia are reviewed briefly below, principally because diagnosis depends on the recognition of certain features and the exclusion of other neurological disorders. For more detailed description, see ref. 6. In adults, the clinical manifestations of HIV dementia suggest predominantly subcortical involvement (6). A typical presentation includes (a) apathy and inertia, (b) memory loss and cognitive slowing, (c) depressive symptoms, and (d) withdrawal from usual activities. The early symptoms are often subtle and may be confused with psychiatric complaints or even overlooked. Occasionally, agitation or mania may be the initial manifestation. HIV dementia appears to be a subcortical dementia characterized primarily by (a) memory loss selective for impaired retrieval, (b) impaired manipulation of acquired knowledge, (c) personality changes characterized by apathy, inertia, and irritability, and (d) general slowing of all thought processes. Considerable variability in presentation has been reported (6). Impor-

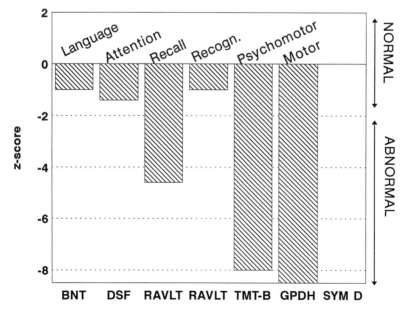

FIG. 1. Typical neuropsychological profile of a 53-year-old homosexual man with moderate HIV dementia. Vertical axis indicates z score of performance (standard deviation units). Note relatively preserved language (LANG), attention (ATTN), and recognition memory (RCOG), but severely impaired recall memory (RCAL) and tests of psychomotor speed (TMT-B, GPDH).

tant considerations in using neuropsychological testing include: premorbid conditions (e.g., head trauma); age and education; and the effects of systemic illness or substance abuse. Figures 1 and 2 shows examples of neuropsychological profiles.

The most useful tests for screening for HIV dementia are those that examine psychomotor speed: Trail-Making, Grooved Pegboard, and Symbol Digit. With advancing dementia, new learning and memory deteriorate, there is a further slowing of mental processing, and language impairment becomes more obvious. The terminal phases of the syndrome are characterized by a global impairment with severe psychomotor retardation and mutism. Price and colleagues have developed a staging scheme (Table 2) that is useful both in clinical practice and for research studies (3). Without treatment, the dementia is rapidly progressive, with a mean survival of about 6 months, less than half the average survival of nondemented AIDS patients (2,8).

Neurological examination is often normal in the early stages of HIV dementia, although there may be demonstrable impairments of rapid eye and limb movements and diffuse hyperreflexia. As HIV dementia progresses, increased tone develops, particularly in the lower extremities, and is usually associated with tremor, clonus, frontal release signs, and hyperactive re-

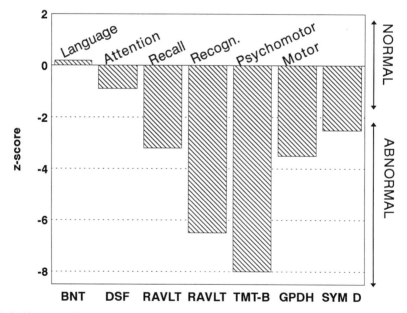

FIG. 2. Neuropsychological profile of a 64-year-old homosexual man with HIV dementia *and* heavy alcohol use. BNT, Boston Naming Test; DSF, Digit Span Forward (WAIS-R); RAVLT, Rey Auditory Verbal Learning Test; TMT-B, Trail-Making Test B; GPDH, Grooved Pegboard Dominant Hand; SYM D, Symbol Digit Test. Note difference in profiles with impaired recognition memory (Recogn) and less impairment on Grooved Pegboard (GPDH).

TABLE 2. *Clinical staging of HIV dementia*[a]

Stage 0 (normal)
Normal mental and motor function
Stage 0.5 (equivocal/subclinical)
Absent, minimal, or equivocal symptoms without impairment of work or capacity to perform aspects of daily life (ADL). Mild signs (snout response, slowed ocular or extremity movements) may be present. Gait and strength are normal.
Stage 1 (mild)
Able to perform all but the more demanding aspects of work or ADL but with unequivocal evidence (signs or symptoms that may include performance on neuropsychological testing) of functional intellectual or motor impairment. Can walk without assistance.
Stage 2 (moderate)
Able to perform basic activities of self-care but cannot work or maintain the more demanding ADL. Ambulatory, but may require a single prop.
Stage 3 (severe)
Major intellectual incapacity (cannot follow news or personal events, cannot sustain complex conversation, considerable slowing of all outputs) or motor disability (cannot walk unassisted, requiring walker or personal support, usually with slowing and clumsiness of arms as well).
Stage 4 (end stage)
Nearly vegetative. Intellectual and social comprehension and output are at a rudimentary level. Nearly or absolutely mute. Paraparetic or paraplegic with urinary and fecal incontinence.

[a] Developed at Memorial Sloan Kettering Center (3).

flexes. Some of these signs may reflect the effects of an accompanying HIV-related myelopathy (9), and a peripheral neuropathy may develop concurrently.

In the early stages of HIV dementia, diagnosis is particularly difficult because the initial symptoms can be confused with depression, anxiety disorders, or the effects of psychoactive substances. Often detailed historical information from friends, family, or co-workers is helpful, and psychiatric consultation may be indicated. Differentiation from infections such as CMV encephalitis, cerebral toxoplasmosis, neurosyphilis, and cryptococcal or tuberculous meningitis is critical. Table 3 lists features that may be helpful in

TABLE 3. *Clinical features useful for diagnosis of HIV-1-related dementia*

- HIV-1 seropositivity (Western blot confirmation)
- History of *progressive* cognitive/behavioral decline with apathy, memory loss, slowed mental processing
- Neurological exam: diffuse CNS signs, including slowed rapid eye/limb movements, hyperreflexia, hypertonia, and release signs
- Neuropsychological assessment: progressive deterioration on serial testing in at least two areas, including frontal lobe, motor speed, and nonverbal memory
- CSF analysis: elevated β_2-microglobulin, nonspecific abnormalities of IgG and protein, exclusion of neurosyphilis and cryptococcal meningitis
- Imaging studies: diffuse cerebral atrophy with ill-defined white matter hyperintensities on MRI in the absence of opportunistic process
- Absence of major psychiatric disorder or intoxication
- Absence of metabolic derangement (e.g., hypoxia, sepsis)
- Absence of active CNS opportunistic processes

TABLE 4. *Common brain diseases complicating AIDS: clinical differentiation[a]*

Disorder	Presentation	Alert	Fever/HA[b]	Focal exam
HIV dementia	weeks/months	NL[c]	0	0
Toxoplasmosis	<2 weeks	↓	+	+ + +
Primary lymphoma	2–8 weeks	↓ or NL	0	+
Progressive multifocal leukoencephalopathy	weeks/months	NL	0	+ +
Cryptococcus	<2 weeks	↓	+ + +	0
CMV encephalitis	<2 weeks	↓ or NL	+	0

[a] Modified from ref. 9a.
[b] HA, headache
[c] NL, normal

establishing the diagnosis of HIV dementia. Table 4 indicates the clinical features that distinguish HIV dementia from other CNS processes. One frequent CNS opportunistic infection that is easily mistaken for HIV dementia is CMV encephalitis. This presents in about 10 percent of all patients with AIDS as a rapidly developing encephalopathy. Distinguishing features from HIV dementia include: coexisting CMV infection (retinitis, colitis, etc.); electrolyte abnormalities reflecting CMV adrenalitis; and periventricular abnormalities on magnetic resonance imaging (MRI) consistent with a periventriculitis (10).

Laboratory Findings

The majority of patients with HIV dementia will have abnormalities of routine CSF studies; however, these are usually nonspecific because similar cerebrospinal fluid (CSF) abnormalities are frequently found in neurologically *normal* HIV carriers. At present, no single CSF test or combination of tests can reliably predict HIV dementia. Lumbar puncture is important, however, to exclude opportunistic infections (OIs) in the patient with suspected HIV dementia. Elevated total protein is found in about 65 percent of cases, and increased total immunoglobulin (IgG) fraction is found in up to 80 percent (2). Oligoclonal bands are found in up to 35 percent, but myelin basic protein is usually not elevated. Intrathecal synthesis (ITS) of anti-HIV-1 IgG is not specific because ITS can be detected in up to 45 percent of neurologically normal HIV carriers (11). The CSF is usually acellular, but may show a mild lymphocytic pleocytosis with proportions of $CD4^+$ and $CD8^+$ lymphocytes that parallel peripheral blood (12). Markers of immune activation in the CSF such as neopterin and β_2-microglobulin have been studied in HIV dementia and are frequently elevated (13,14). β_2-Microglobulin is useful in diagnosis, particularly in mild dementia; in the absence of OIs, it has a positive predictive value of 88 percent (15). Quinolinic acid, a metabolite of tryptophan, is also elevated during HIV dementia and may reflect macrophage activation within the CNS (16). All of these substances are increased in opportunistic processes and are relatively nonspecific markers.

Imaging studies are critical in the evaluation of suspected HIV dementia to exclude opportunistic processes. Radiologic features of HIV dementia include both central and cortical atrophy and white matter rarefaction. In children, calcifications of the basal ganglia are commonly seen on computed tomographic (CT) scan. Diffuse cerebral atrophy can often be observed to progress in parallel with clinical deterioration. MRI demonstrates white matter abnormalities in HIV dementia that appear as ill-defined areas of increased signal intensity on T2-weighted images (17,18). These often evolve from small ill-defined hyperintensities seen in deep white matter in patients with early HIV dementia to more diffuse abnormalities in severely demented individuals. Quantitative MRI studies have shown that selective caudate region atrophy occurs in HIV dementia (19), and that there is loss of gray matter volume overall (20). Table 5 contrasts the different radiological patterns.

Both single positron emission computed tomography (SPECT) and positron emission tomography (PET) have been used in small numbers of individuals with HIV dementia. Using PET, Rottenberg et al. (21) demonstrated subcortical hypermetabolism in the early stages of HIV dementia, with later progression to cortical and subcortical hypometabolism. Normalization of PET abnormalities has also been shown with administration of antivirals (22). With SPECT, abnormalities in cerebral blood flow have been identified in most individuals with HIV dementia and in neurologically normal HIV-1 carriers, suggesting that SPECT might be a useful predictive tool (23). It appears, however, that some of these changes may be mimicked by the effects of cocaine (24), and so the usefulness of SPECT in detection of HIV dementia or in assessing treatment effects remains to be determined.

Minor electroencephalographic abnormalities have been reported by some investigators in asymptomatic HIV seropositives (25), but have not been confirmed by others (26). As with the neuropsychological tests, their clinical significance is uncertain. The electroencephalogram (EEG) has not been systematically studied in either the diagnosis or staging of HIV dementia. In

TABLE 5. *Radiological pattern of HIV-related CNS disease[a]*

Disorder	Number	Pattern	Enhance	Location
HIV dementia	Diffuse	Ill-defined	0	Deep white
Toxoplasmosis	One to many	Ring mass	+ +	Basal ganglia
Primary lymphoma	One to several	Solid mass	+ + +	Periventricular
Progressive multifocal leukoencephalopathy	One to several	No mass	0	Subcortical white
Cryptococcus	One to many	Punctate	0	Basal ganglia
CMV encephalitis	One to several	Confluent	+ +	Periventricular

[a] Modified from ref. 9a.

the late stages of HIV dementia a diffuse slowing is frequently noted (6); however, in less advanced stages of dementia the EEG may be normal in 50 percent of patients (2). The specificity of electroencephalography in differentiating psychiatric disorders from early dementia is uncertain, and in general neither standard electroencephalography nor computerized spectral analysis adds little information.

Pathological Features

HIV infection of the brain causes the distinct neuropathological changes termed *HIV encephalitis* and *HIV leukoencephalopathy* (27). Other abnormalities, including (a) astrocytic and microglial proliferation and (b) cortical neuronal loss, have also been found in patients with AIDS, and are likely to be related to productive HIV infection in the brain (27–35). The relationship of any of these pathological changes to the clinical features of progressive dementia in AIDS remains unclear. There have been only a few studies specifically addressing clinical–neuropathological correlation in AIDS dementia, and none in which the clinical diagnosis of AIDS dementia was based on prospective patient identification. The original description of the "AIDS dementia complex" involved a retrospective chart review, and carefully correlated neuropathological changes with the presence or absence of dementia (36). A correlation was found between the presence of multinucleated giant cells (MNGCs), myelin pallor, and the severity of dementia. However, not all patients with dementia showed these changes (Fig. 3). Schmidbauer et al. (37) found that myelin pallor, vacuolar myelin damage, and angiocentric

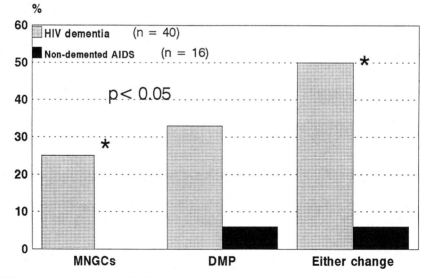

FIG. 3. Neuropathological findings in HIV dementia (MNGCs, multinucleated giant cells; DMP, diffuse myelin pallor).

demyelinating foci correlated with the severity of AIDS dementia. We have recently completed a prospective analysis of AIDS dementia from our AIDS Brain Bank (38). We found that only 25 percent of cases with AIDS dementia had MNGCs, the defining element of HIV encephalitis, and 50 percent showed neither MNGCs nor white matter pallor. These findings suggest that other neuropathological correlations must be sought to explain the clinical syndrome of AIDS dementia. Based on the paucity of prospective clinical–pathological correlations, and our observation of a striking discordance between clinical expression of disease and neuropathological findings, we believe that the pathological substrate of AIDS dementia remains undetermined. Although the structural basis for dementia has yet to be delineated, several pathogenetic mechanisms have been proposed. *In vitro* culture systems of neurons from humans and rodents have identified a collection of putative neurotoxins that may play a role in AIDS dementia. These neurotoxins include quinolinic acid (16), macrophage/microglia-derived neurotoxins (39,40), and viral proteins such as gp120 (41,42). Cytokines have also been implicated in neurological injury in AIDS (43), especially tumor necrosis factor alpha (TNF-α). Genis et al. (44) have recently shown that arachidonic acid metabolites may amplify cytokine-induced neuronotoxicity. Many of these *in vitro* systems rely on a pathological endpoint (e.g., neuronal loss, gliosis, myelin damage), so an improved understanding of the pathological substrate of human disease is essential.

The recent consensus statement has helped to define the neuropathological changes associated with HIV, including the following:

1. HIV encephalitis (5,27,36,45) has been identified in 30–90 percent of patients dying with AIDS (46). The presence of MNGCs correlates both with degree of dementia and the detection of HIV-1 DNA (47). These giant cells are thought to reflect HIV replication, since MNGCs form in HIV-1 macrophage cultures (48). Perivascular infiltrations of lymphocytes and monocytes/macrophages are also frequently seen (36,46,49,50). The inflammatory infiltrates, MNGCs and endothelial cells have been demonstrated to contain viral nucleic acid sequences (50).

2. HIV leukoencephalopathy represents a frequent finding of diffuse myelin pallor, particularly in deep areas of the centrum semiovale. Perivascular macrophages and MNGCs are frequently seen.

3. Diffuse poliodystrophy includes changes in gray matter with a loss of neuronal numbers, particularly in frontal, parietal, and temporal areas (28,29,33). Other neuronal changes include a loss of synapses and dendritic simplification (30).

EPIDEMIOLOGY OF HIV DEMENTIA

Early in the epidemic, numerous studies indicated that nervous system invasion could occur early. The evidence for this included (a) the frequency of CSF abnormalities (51) during the early phase of HIV infection and (b) the descriptions of the development of cognitive impairment before other AIDS-defining illnesses (52). Since then, tremendous efforts have been poured into large-scale natural history studies of HIV-infected cohorts to define the frequency of neurological disease. These studies have been useful from several standpoints. They have given us information about the natural history of HIV neurologic disease as distinct from opportunistic CNS infection. Thus, while CNS infection with HIV may occur early after primary HIV infection, in most patients neurologic disease is delayed and develops only later with the onset of immune deficiency, medical symptoms, and other AIDS-defining illnesses. Natural history studies of neurologic disease have assisted with the development of public health policy and employment policy and allowed for more accurate prognosis and prediction of neurologic disease and have treatment implications, specifically when antiretroviral therapy should be started and how it should be used. In adults, only 3 percent of AIDS cases present with dementia; more typically, dementia develops after constitutional symptoms, immune deficiency, and systemic opportunistic processes (1,2,52).

NEUROPSYCHOLOGICAL STUDIES IN ASYMPTOMATIC HIV INFECTION

Rather than a true state of viral latency during the asymptomatic phase of HIV infection, there seems to be a slow replication with continuous low-level viral transcription, gradually accumulating viral burden, and $CD4^+$ lymphocyte depletion. Early studies described high rates of neuropsychological test abnormalities in healthy HIV-1-infected homosexual men (53,54) and in intravenous drug users (55). The clinical significance of these findings was uncertain because the neuropsychological abnormalities were not severe or progressive and may reflect the effects of low education, age, or alcohol and drug use rather than HIV infection. Nonetheless, these studies were helpful in developing hypothetical models for HIV-associated dementia (see Fig. 4). The original San Diego study suggested a progressive decline beginning soon after initial infection with HIV, with an incremental rise in the frequency of neurocognitive impairment as HIV disease advances. Studies with larger sample sizes in homosexual men, hemophiliacs, and intravenous drug users have not confirmed these observations and show that there is no significant neurocognitive decline during the asymptomatic phase of infection (see Tables 6 and 7).

As one example, among several hundred HIV-seropositive men without AIDS or constitutional symptoms in the Multicenter AIDS Cohort Study (MACS), the prevalence of HIV dementia was less than 1 percent, and overall the frequency of neuropsychological impairment was not significantly

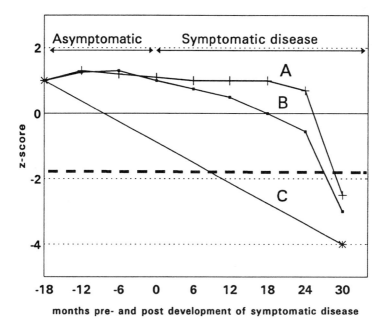

FIG. 4. Hypothetical model of neurocognitive decline with progression to symptomatic disease. Pattern A illustrates relative stable performance until late-stage disease. Pattern B illustrates stable performance until development of symptomatic disease, followed by slow progression. Pattern C illustrates linear decline from time of seroconversion.

TABLE 6. *Cross-sectional neuropsychological studies in asymptomatic HIV infection*

Author	Year	Cases/control
Studies that have suggested an increased frequency of cognitive impairment among asymptomatic HIV-seropositives		
Grant, Atkinson, Hesselink, et al.	1987	44/11
Poutianen, Iivanainen, et al.	1988	13/10
Fitzgibbon, Cella, Humfleet, et al.	1989	25/25
Perry, Belsy-Barr, Barr, et al.	1989	20/20
Krikorian, Wrobel, Meinecke, et al.	1990	38/16
Wilkie, Eisdorfer, Morgan, et al.	1990	46/13
Studies that have not suggested an increased frequency of cognitive impairment among asymptomatic HIV-seropositives		
Helmsteadtler, Riedel, et al.	1988	181/28
Goethe, Mitchell, Marshall, et al.	1989	83/18
Tross, Price, Navia, et al.	1988	100/20
Miller, Selnes, McArthur, et al.	1990	727/769
Arday, Brundage, et al.	1991	1283/6415

TABLE 7. *Longitudinal neuropsychological studies in asymptomatic HIV infection*

Study	Year	Cohort	Follow-up (months)	Cases/controls
Selnes et al.	1990	Homosexuals	18	238/170
Saykin et al.	1991	Homosexuals	18	21/21
Gastaut et al.	1990	Homosexuals	6–18	50/8
Selnes et al.	1992	Intravenous drug users	12	37/69
Helmsteadtler et al.	1992	Hemophiliacs	20	62/—
Whitt et al.	1992	Hemophiliacs	24	25/25
Robertson et al.	1992	Homosexuals	24	118/0
Karlsen et al.	1993	Homosexuals	24	36/—
Selnes et al.	1992	Intravenous drug users	36	19/40

higher than in HIV-1-seronegative controls (56,57). Similar results have been described in intravenous drug users (58).

From longitudinal neuropsychological evaluation in the MACS and among intravenous drug users, as well as among other groups such as hemophiliacs, no evidence for significant cognitive decline has been found during the asymptomatic phase of infection (59,60). These U.S. studies have been confirmed by the World Health Organization (WHO) Multicenter Study, which also showed no significance rise in the frequency of neurocognitive impairment during asymptomatic HIV infection. The 1988 WHO report on neuropsychiatric aspects of HIV-1 infection concluded that "at present, there is no evidence for an increase of clinically significant neuropsychiatric abnormalities in CDC groups II or III HIV-seropositive (i.e., otherwise asymptomatic) individuals as compared to HIV-1-seronegative controls" (61).

PATTERNS OF COGNITIVE DECLINE IN HIV DEMENTIA

HIV dementia develops and progresses in parallel with the later stages of AIDS; typically, the onset is relatively abrupt, rather than developing insidiously (62). In preliminary longitudinal analyses from the MACS, examining the performance of subjects who had progressed to symptomatic disease, we found no evidence of decline in longitudinal neuropsychological testing (Grooved Pegboard) until $CD4^+$ levels dropped below 50 (63). After studying 29 asymptomatic and 19 subjects with AIDS-related complex (ARC) or AIDS with serial CD4 measurements and neuropsychological assessments, Bornstein et al. (64) suggested that rate of decline in $CD4^+$ lymphocytes is related to poor performance in neuropsychological tests. Dunbar et al. (65) studied change in cognition associated with progression from ARC to AIDS. The performance of both progressors (to AIDS) and nonprogressors deteriorated somewhat over time relative to seronegative controls, but there were no specific changes associated with progression to AIDS. Therefore, progression to AIDS in and of itself does not predict specific changes in

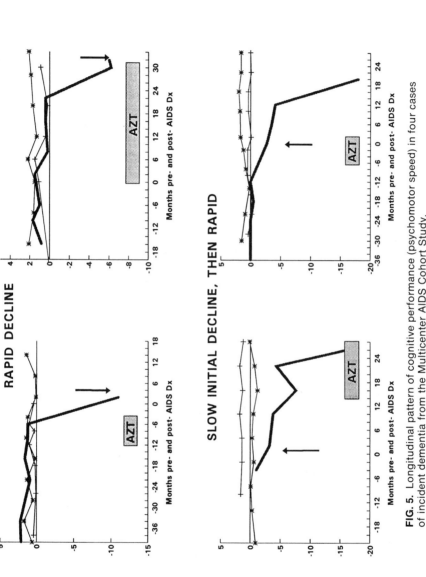

FIG. 5. Longitudinal pattern of cognitive performance (psychomotor speed) in four cases of incident dementia from the Multicenter AIDS Cohort Study.

neuropsychological performance. From observations of individual patients studied within the MACS who had repeated neuropsychological performance testing before onset of dementia, we have noticed different patterns of cognitive decline depending on whether dementia occurred as a primary or secondary AIDS-defining illness. Figure 5 gives examples of these different patterns. Among individuals with HIV dementia as the first AIDS defining illness, a period of cognitive stability during the asymptomatic phase of HIV infection appeared to be followed by a gradual and relatively modest decline in psychomotor performance. Other cognitive domains remained well preserved. A different pattern of cognitive decline was seen among those who developed dementia after other AIDS-defining illnesses. All had had a long period of cognitive stability (or only very gradual decline in psychomotor performance) which was then followed by an abrupt, steep decline in psychomotor performance with the onset of HIV dementia.

FREQUENCY OF HIV DEMENTIA: INCIDENCE, PREVALENCE, AND RISK FACTORS

Estimates of the frequency of HIV dementia in selected neurological referrals series have ranged from 16 percent to 67 percent in patients with symptomatic HIV disease (2,66,67). It has been difficult to interpret the differences in frequency, which may reflect (a) referral biases, (b) differences in diagnostic criteria, or (c) examination of patients at more advanced stages of HIV disease (e.g., in patients with AIDS). Surveillance figures from the Centers for Disease Control showed that HIV dementia is reported in 7.3 percent of persons with AIDS and in 2.8 percent of patients with the initial AIDS-defining illness (1). These estimates only apply to dementia as the initial manifestation of AIDS because the CDC AIDS reporting system does not often capture secondary diagnoses occurring after AIDS. In 1990, in persons 20–59 years old, the incidence of HIV dementia was 1.9 per 100,000 population. Because survival times for AIDS patients have increased with improvements in antiretroviral treatments (68–71) and prophylaxis of opportunistic infections, it has been projected that the incidence of neurological disorders will increase (72). More widespread and earlier use of zidovudine was initially thought to have reduced the incidence of HIV dementia, with an encouraging drop in the incidence of HIV dementia from 53 percent before zidovudine was available to 10 percent after its initiation (73). These initially encouraging statistics do not appear to have held up with prospective studies.

Recent MACS data regarding 492 homosexual men who developed AIDS-defining illnesses during the period 1984 through 1991 have allowed a more accurate estimate of (a) incidence figures for HIV dementia after AIDS and (b) risk factors for its development. A prospective study of the natural history of HIV infection among homosexual men was conducted in the Baltimore and Los Angeles sites of the MACS (71,74,75). In 1986, neurological and neuropsychological instruments were added to the semiannual medical and immunological evaluations. HIV dementia was recognized through prospective neuropsychological evaluation and was confirmed with neurological and neurodiagnostic evaluation, including MRI, CSF analysis, and other exclusionary tests. Sixty-four dementia cases were identified from a total of 492 AIDS cases; and a wide range of demographic, clinical, and laboratory variables were analyzed to identify risk factors. For 3 percent of the AIDS cases, dementia was diagnosed concurrently with the initial AIDS-defining illness. The incidence of HIV dementia during the first two years after AIDS was 7 percent per year, and a total of 15 percent of the cohort developed dementia before death (see Fig. 6). The median survival after dementia was 6.0 months compared to 7.8 months for nondemented subjects with a second AIDS-defining illness. Using a proportional hazards model, risk factors for hazard of dementia were lower hemoglobin and body mass index 1–6 months before AIDS, more constitutional symptoms 7–12 months before AIDS, and older age at AIDS. In a multivariate model, pre-AIDS hemoglobin remained the most significant predictor of dementia, and no significant risk was defined from demographic characteristics, specific AIDS-defining illnesses, zidovudine use before AIDS, or $CD4^+$ lymphocyte count before AIDS (see Table 8 and Fig. 7). The observed association between anemia, low weight, constitutional symptoms, and dementia suggests a role for cytokines inducing both systemic and neurologic disease.

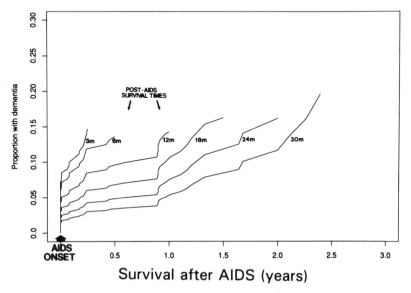

FIG. 6. Cumulative probability (prevalence) of HIV dementia after initial AIDS diagnosis based on length of survival after AIDS.

TABLE 8. *Final multivariate model for hazard of HIV dementia, adjusted for post-AIDS survival time*

Variable	Relative hazard (95% C.I.[a])	p value
Hemoglobin 1–6 months before AIDS (per 2 additional g/dl)	0.60 (0.38–0.96)	0.03
Body mass index 1–6 months before AIDS (per additional 5 kg/m^2)	0.79 (0.45–1.39)	0.41
Age at first AIDS diagnosis (per additional decade)	1.12 (0.64–1.95)	0.70
CD4$^+$ count 1–6 months before AIDS (per additional 100 × 10^6/liter)	1.00 (0.74–1.35)	0.99
Zidovudine use before AIDS	1.54 (0.66–3.63)	0.32
Kaposi's sarcoma as first AIDS diagnosis	1.03 (0.46–2.30)	0.94
Clinical symptoms 1–6 months before AIDS (per additional symptom)	1.00 (0.75–1.27)	0.99

[a] C.I., confidence interval

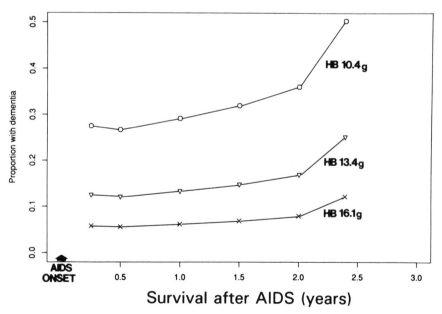

FIG. 7. Probability of developing HIV dementia stratified by hemoglobin 1–6 months prior to AIDS and post-AIDS survival.

ANTIRETROVIRALS AND HIV DEMENTIA

Despite the unresolved questions in the pathogenesis of HIV dementia, antiretroviral agents are currently used for its treatment. Three antiretroviral agents are current licensed in the United States: zidovudine (AZT, Retrovir), didanosine (ddI, Videx), and dideoxycytidine (ddC, Hivid). All are nucleoside analogues that act by inhibiting reverse transcriptase, an enzyme critical in HIV's life cycle. The nucleoside analogues are only active against replicating HIV, not latent provirus, and resistance can develop to all of them within 6–12 months of use. Open-label studies with AZT in demented individuals showed promising improvements in clinical functioning, neuropsychological performance, and, in one case, normalization of PET scans (22). Evidence from the multicenter licensing trial of AZT (76) in patients with AIDS or ARC suggested improvements in neuropsychological functioning, particularly in measures of psychomotor speed (77). Children treated with intravenous AZT showed improvements in neuropsychological performance, although no clear dose response was seen (78). Data from the only placebo-controlled trial of AZT in HIV dementia suggested that the neurocognitive improvement is seen only with very high doses of AZT, around 2000 mg/day (79). The optimal dose of AZT for treatment of HIV dementia has not been determined, and most of the studies discussed above have used doses of 1000–2000 mg/day. However, the current recommended dose of AZT for systemic use has been reduced to 500 mg because this dose has equivalent efficacy in preventing systemic infections (80). Whether significant neurological improvement in HIV dementia can be induced with lower doses of AZT, or with other antiretrovirals, remains to be determined.

While the issue of optimal zidovudine dose for treatment of HIV dementia has not yet been determined, and little information about the therapeutic response to ddI or ddC exist, except for very little open-label studies (81), there are some data which indicate that antiretrovirals may have a neuroprotective effect when started before onset of dementia. In the original placebo-controlled licensing trial of zidovudine, dementia developed in 9 of 32 (28 percent) patients with symptomatic HIV disease, at an annual rate of 14 percent (82). There was no hint of a neuroprotective effect of zidovudine in this study; similarly, in the MACS study, no protective effect was found from zidovudine therapy started before AIDS. It is noteworthy that most of the MACS subjects were taking doses averaging 600 mg or less daily (83). Two studies have suggested that early, high-dose zidovudine may prevent HIV dementia. In the first study, a controlled trial of early versus late treatment with zidovudine in symptomatic HIV infection, Hamilton et al. (84) noted that dementia developed in 6 of 168 (3.6 percent) patients who began zidovudine only after development of an AIDS-defining opportunistic infection, compared to none of the 170 patients who began zidovudine early. In a second study comparing three dosing strata of zidovudine in advanced HIV

TABLE 9. *Nordic MRC HIV therapy group (85)*

	Zidovudine use			
	400 mg (n = 160)	800 mg (n = 158)	1200 mg (n = 156)	p value
Died (%)	23	23	19	0.48
PCP (%)	19	15	13	0.15
CMV (%)	8	4	4	0.24
Dementia (%)	8	6	3	0.06

infection, a dose response was noted with fewer dementia cases in the group receiving the highest doses of zidovudine (see Table 9). These two studies suggest a "neuroprotective" effect of zidovudine on the development of dementia, but only with the initiation of zidovudine before AIDS and only for doses above 1000 mg/day. Thus, both the timing and the dose of zidovudine may be critical with respect to prophylactic efficacy for neurologic disease.

FUTURE PROJECTIONS AND CONCLUSION

Our understanding of the pathogenesis of HIV dementia is only in its early stages, and there is a clear need to better define its neuropathological substrate. Equally critical is the effect of antiretroviral therapy on the development and course of HIV dementia and the severity of neuropathological changes in brain. HIV dementia is uncommon during the early, asymptomatic phases of HIV infection and tends to develop only after profound immunodeficiency and AIDS-defining illnesses. Its annual incidence after AIDS is about 7 percent and will occur in approximately 20 percent of individuals with advanced HIV disease. With an estimated one million individuals already infected with HIV in the United States alone, we can anticipate an annual incidence of 40,000 cases of HIV dementia, approximately five times the annual incidence of multiple sclerosis. HIV dementia will likely become the leading cause of dementia in young Americans.

REFERENCES

1. Janssen RS, Nwanyanwu OC, Selik RM, Stehr-Green JK. Epidemiology of human immunodeficiency virus encephalopathy in the United States. *Neurology* 1992;42:1472–1476.
2. McArthur JC. Neurologic manifestations of AIDS. *Medicine (Baltimore)* 1987;66:407–437.
3. Price RW, Brew BJ. The AIDS dementia complex. *J Infect Dis* 1988;158:1079–1083.
4. Centers for Disease Control. Revision of the CDC surveillance case definition for acquired immunodeficiency syndrome. *MMWR* 1987;36(suppl 1S):3S–15S.
5. Snider WD, Simpson DM, Nielsen S, Gold JW, Metroka CE, Posner JB. Neurological complications of acquired immune deficiency syndrome: analysis of 50 patients. *Ann Neurol* 1983;14:403–418.

6. Navia BA, Jordan BD, Price RW. The AIDS dementia complex. I. Clinical features. *Ann Neurol* 1986;19:517–524.
7. Janssen RS, Cornblath DR, Epstein LG, et al. Nomenclature and research case definitions for neurological manifestations of human immunodeficiency virus type-1 (HIV-1) infection. Report of a Working Group of the American Academy of Neurology AIDS Task Force. *Neurology* 1991;41:778–785.
8. Rothenberg R, Woelfel M, Stoneburner R, Milberg J, Parker R, Truman B. Survival with the acquired immunodeficiency syndrome: experience with 5833 cases in New York City. *N Engl J Med* 1987;317:1297–1302.
9. Petito CK, Navia BA, Cho ES, Jordan BD, George DC, Price RW. Vacuolar myelopathy pathologically resembling subacute combined degeneration in patients with the acquired immunodeficiency syndrome. *N Engl J Med* 1985;312:874–879.
9a. Price R. American Academy of Neurology. April, 1990.
10. Power C, Holland NR, Mathews VP, Glass JD, McArthur JC. CMV encephalitis in AIDS: distinction from HIV dementia. [Abstract]. *Neurology* 1992;42:211.
11. Van Wielink G, McArthur JC, Moench T, Farzadegan H, Johnson RT, Saah A. Intrathecal synthesis of anti-HIV-IgG: correlation with increasing duration of HIV-1 infection. *Neurology* 1990;40:816–819.
12. McArthur JC, Sipos E, Cornblath DR, et al. Identification of mononuclear cells in CSF of patients with HIV infection. *Neurology* 1989;39:66–70.
13. Brew BJ, Bhalla RB, Paul M, et al. Cerebrospinal fluid β2 microglobulin in patients with AIDS dementia complex: an expanded series including response to zidovudine treatment. *AIDS* 1992;6:461–465.
14. Brew BJ, Bhalla RB, Paul M, et al. Cerebrospinal fluid neopterin in human immunodeficiency virus type-I infection. *Ann Neurol* 1990;28:556–560.
15. McArthur JC, Nance-Sproson TE, Griffin DE, et al. The diagnostic utility of elevation in cerebrospinal fluid β2 microglobulin in HIV-1 dementia. *Neurology* 1992;42:1707–1712.
16. Heyes MP, Brew BJ, Martin A, et al. Quinolinic acid in cerebrospinal fluid and serum in HIV-1 infection: relationship to clinical and neurologic status. *Ann Neurol* 1991;29:202–209.
17. Levy RM, Rosenbloom S, Perrett LV. Neuroradiologic findings in AIDS: a review of 200 cases. *AJR* 1986;147:977–983.
18. Price RW, Navia BA. Infections in AIDS and in other immunosuppressed patients. In: Kennedy PGE, Johnson RT, eds. *Infections of the nervous system.* London: Butterworths, 1987.
19. Dal Pan GJ, McArthur JH, Aylward E, et al. Patterns of cerebral atrophy in HIV-1 infected individuals: results of a quantitative MRI analysis. *Neurology* 1992;42:2125–2130.
20. Aylward E, Henderer JD, McArthur JC, Harris GJ, Barta PE, Pearlson GD. Atrophy in gray tissue, but not white tissue, in HIV-1 infected homosexual males. *Neurology* 1992 *(in press).*
21. Rottenberg DA, Moeller JR, Strother SC, et al. The metabolic pathology of the AIDS dementia complex. *Ann Neurol* 1987;22:700–706.
22. Yarchoan R, Berg G, Brouwers P, et al. Response of human-immunodeficiency-virus-associated neurological disease to 3'-azido-3'-deoxythymidine. *Lancet* 1987;1:132–135.
23. LaFrance N, Pearlson GD, Schaerf FW, et al. I-123 IMP-SPECT in HIV-related dementia. *Adv Funct Imaging* 1988;1:9–15.
24. Handelsman L, Aronson M, Maurer G, et al. Neuropsychological and neurological manifestations of HIV-1 dementia in drug users. *J Neuropsychiatr Clin Neurosci* 1992;4:21–28.
25. Koralnik IJ, Beaumanoir A, Hausler R, et al. A controlled study of early neurologic abnormalities in men with asymptomatic human immunodeficiency virus infection. *N Engl J Med* 1990;323:864–870.
26. Nuwer MR, Miller EN, Visscher BR, et al. Asymptomatic HIV infection does not cause EEG abnormalities: results from the Multicenter AIDS Cohort Study (MACS). *Neurology* 1992;42:1214–1219.
27. Budka H, Wiley CA, Kleihues P, et al. HIV-associated disease of the nervous system: review of nomenclature and proposal for neuropathology-based terminology. *Brain Pathol* 1991;1:143–152.
28. Ketzler S, Weis S, Haug H, Budka H. Loss of neurons in the frontal cortex in AIDS brains. *Acta Neuropathol (Berl)* 1990;80:92–94.

29. Wiley CA, Masliah E, Morey M, et al. Neocortical damage during HIV infection. *Ann Neurol* 1991;29:651–657.
30. Masliah E, Ge N, Morey M, Deteresa R, Terry RD, Wiley CA. Cortical dendritic pathology in human immunodeficiency virus encephalitis. *Lab Invest* 1992;66:285–291.
31. Gray F, Gherardi R, Keohane C, Favolini M, Sobel A, Poirier J. Pathology of the central nervous system in 40 cases of acquired immune deficiency syndrome (AIDS). *Neuropathol Appl Neurobiol* 1988;14:365–380.
32. Vazeux R, Lacroix-Ciaudo C, Blanche S, et al. Low levels of human immunodeficiency virus replication in the brain tissue of children with severe acquired immunodeficiency syndrome encephalopathy. *Am J Pathol* 1992;140:137–144.
33. Everall IP, Luthert PJ, Lantos PL. Neuronal loss in the frontal cortex in HIV infection. *Lancet* 1991;337:1119–1121.
34. Ciardi A, Sinclair E, Scaravilli F, Harcourt-Webster NJ, Lucas S. The involvement of the cerebral cortex in human immunodeficiency virus encephalopathy: a morphological and immunohistochemical study. *Acta Neuropathol (Berl)* 1990;81:51–59.
35. Sinclair E, Scaravilli F. Detection of HIV proviral DNA in cortex and white matter of AIDS brains by non-isotopic polymerase chain reaction: correlation with diffuse poliodystrophy. *AIDS* 1992;6:925–932.
36. Navia BA, Cho ES, Petito CK, Price RW. The AIDS dementia complex. II. Neuropathology. *Ann Neurol* 1986;19:525–535.
37. Schmidbauer M, Huemer M, Cristina S, Trabattoni GR, Budka H. Morphological spectrum, distribution and clinical correlation of white matter lesions in AIDS brains. *Neuropathol Appl Neurobiol* 1992;18:489–501.
38. Glass JD, Wesselingh SL, Selnes OA, McArthur JC. Clinical–pathological correlation in HIV-associated dementia. *Neurology (in press)*.
39. Giulian D, Vaca K, Noonan CA. Secretion of neurotoxins in mononuclear phagocytes infected with HIV-1. *Science* 1990;250:1593–1596.
40. Pulliam L, Herndier BG, Tang NM, McGrath MS. Human immunodeficiency virus-infected macrophages produce soluble factors that cause histological and neurochemical alterations in cultured human brains. *J Clin Invest* 1991;87:503–512.
41. Lipton SA. HIV-related neurotoxicity. *Brain Pathol* 1991;1:193–199.
42. Brenneman D, Buzy J, Ruff M. Peptide T sequences prevent neuronal cell death produced by the protein gp120 of the human immunodeficiency virus. *Drug Dev Res* 1988;15:361–369.
43. Tyor WR, Glass JD, Griffin JW, et al. Cytokine expression in the brain during AIDS. *Ann Neurol* 1992;31:349–360.
44. Genis P, Jett M, Bernton EW, et al. Cytokines and arachidonic metabolites produced during human immunodeficiency virus (HIV)-infected macrophage–astroglia interactions: implications for the neuropathogenesis of HIV disease. *J Exp Med* 1992;176:1703–1718.
45. Sharer LR, Kapila R. Neuropathologic observations in acquired immunodeficiency syndrome (AIDS). *Acta Neuropathol (Berl)* 1985;66:188–198.
46. de la Monte SM, Ho DD, Schooley RT, Hirsch MS, Richardson EP Jr. Subacute encephalomyelitis of AIDS and its relation to HTLV-III infection. *Neurology* 1987;37:562–569.
47. Price RW, Sidtis J, Rosenblum M. AIDS dementia complex: some current questions. *Ann Neurol* 1988;23(suppl):S27–S33.
48. Gartner S, Markovits P, Markotivz DM, Kaplan MH, Gallo RC, Popovic M. The role of mononuclear phagocytes in HTLV-III/LAV infection. *Science* 1986;233:215–219.
49. Rhodes RH. Histopathology of the central nervous system in the acquired immunodeficiency syndrome. *Hum Pathol* 1987;18:636–643.
50. Wiley CA, Schrier RD, Nelson JA, Lampert PW, Oldstone MB. Cellular localization of human immunodeficiency virus infection within the brains of acquired immune deficiency syndrome patients. *Proc Natl Acad Sci USA* 1986;83:7089–7093.
51. McArthur JC, Cohen BA, Farzedegan H, et al. Cerebrospinal fluid abnormalities in homosexual men with and without neuropsychiatric findings. *Ann Neurol* 1988;23:S34–S37.
52. Navia BA, Price RW. The acquired immunodeficiency syndrome dementia complex as the presenting or sole manifestation of human immunodeficiency virus infection. *Arch Neurol* 1987;44:65–69.
53. Grant I, Atkinson JH, Hesselink JR, et al. Evidence for early central nervous system involvement in the acquired immunodeficiency syndrome (AIDS) and other human immuno-

deficiency virus (HIV) infections. Studies with neuropsychologic testing and magnetic resonance imaging. *Ann Intern Med* 1987;107:828–836. [Published erratum appears in *Ann Intern Med* 1988;108(3):496].

54. Janssen RS, Saykin AJ, Kaplan JE, et al. Neurological complications of human immunodeficiency virus infection in patients with lymphadenopathy syndrome. *Ann Neurol* 1988;23: 49–55.

55. Silberstein CH, McKegney FP, O'Dowd MA, et al. A prospective longitudinal study of neuropsychological and psychosocial factors in asymptomatic individuals at risk of HTLV-III/LAV infection in a methadone program: preliminary findings. *Int J Neurosci* 1987;32: 669–676.

56. McArthur JC, Cohen BA, Selnes OA, et al. Low prevalence of neurological and neuropsychological abnormalities in otherwise healthy HIV-1-infected individuals: results from the Multicenter AIDS Cohort Study. *Ann Neurol* 1989;26:601–611.

57. Miller EN, Selnes OA, McArthur JC, et al. Neuropsychological performance in HIV-1 infected homosexual men: the Multicenter AIDS Cohort Study (MACS). *Neurology* 1990; 40:197–203.

58. Royal W, Updike M, Selnes OA, et al. HIV-1 infection and nervous system abnormalities among a cohort of intravenous drug users. *Neurology* 1991;41:1905–1910.

59. Selnes OA, Miller E, McArthur JC, et al. HIV-1 infection: no evidence of cognitive decline during the asymptomatic stages. *Neurology* 1990;40:204–208.

60. Selnes OA, McArthur JC, Royal W, et al. HIV-1 infection and intravenous drug use: longitudinal neuropsychological evaluation of asymptomatic subjects. *Neurology* 1992;42: 1924–1930.

61. World Health Organization. *Report on the consultation on the neuropsychiatric aspects of HIV infection.* Geneva: WHO, 1988.

62. Selnes OA, McArthur JC, Gordon B, Miller EN, McArthur JH, Saah A. Patterns of cognitive decline in incident HIV-dementia: longitudinal observations from the Multicenter AIDS Cohort Study [Abstract 497P]. *Neurology* 1991;41(suppl 1):252.

63. Selnes OA, McArthur JC, Concha M, Dal Pan G, Saah A. Neuro-cognitive abnormalities with progression to AIDS: association with low CD4+ levels [Abstract]. In: *VIII International Conference on AIDS/III STD World Congress*, 1992:673.

64. Bornstein RA, Nasrallah HA, Para MF, Fass RJ, Whitacre CC, Rice RR Jr. Rate of CD4 decline and neuropsychological performance in HIV infection. *Arch Neurol* 1991;48: 704–707.

65. Dunbar N, Perdices M, Grunseit A, Cooper DA. Changes in neuropsychological performance of AIDS-related complex patients who progress to AIDS. *AIDS* 1992;6:691–700.

66. Levy RM, Bredesen DE, Rosenblum ML. Neurological manifestations of the acquired immunodeficiency syndrome (AIDS): experience at UCSF and review of the literature. *J Neurosurg* 1985;62:475–495.

67. Price RW, Sidtis JJ, Navia BA, Pumarola-Sune T, Ornitz DB. The AIDS dementia complex. In: Rosenblum ML, Levy RM, Bredesen DE, eds. *AIDS and the nervous system*. New York: Raven Press, 1988:203–219.

68. Piette J, Mor V, Fleishman J. Patterns of survival with AIDS in the United States. *Health Serv Res* 1991;26:75–95.

69. Moore RD, Hidalgo J, Sugland BW, Chaisson RE. Zidovudine and the natural history of the acquired immunodeficiency syndrome. *N Engl J Med* 1991;324:1412–1416.

70. Friedman Y, Franklin C, Freels S, Weil MH. Long-term survival of patients with AIDS, *Pneumocystis carinii* pneumonia, and respiratory failure. *JAMA* 1991;266:89–92.

71. Graham NMH, Zeger SL, Park LP, et al. The effects on survival of early treatment of human immunodeficiency virus infection. *N Engl J Med* 1992;326:1037–1042.

72. Pluda JM, Yarchoan R, Jaffe ES, et al. Develpoment of non-Hodgkin lymphoma in a cohort of patients with severe human immunodeficiency virus (HIV) on long-term antiretroviral therapy. *Ann Intern Med* 1990;113:276–282.

73. Portegies P, de Gans J, Lange JM, et al. Declining incidence of AIDS dementia complex after introduction of zidovudine treatment. *Br Med J* 1989;299:819–821. [Published erratum appears in *Br Med J* 1989;299(6708):1141.]

74. Kaslow RA, Ostrow DG, Detels R, Phair JP, Polk BF, Rinaldo CR. The Multicenter AIDS Cohort Study (MACS): rationale, organization, and selected characteristics of the participants. *Am J Epidemiol* 1987;126:310–318.

75. Polk BF, Fox R, Brookmeyer R, et al. Predictors of the acquired immunodeficiency syndrome developing in a cohort of seropositive homosexual men. *N Engl J Med* 1987;316: 61–66.
76. Fischl MA, Richman DD, Grieco MH, et al. The efficacy of azidothymidine (AZT) in the treatment of patients with AIDS and AIDS-related complex. *N Engl J Med* 1987;317: 185–191.
77. Schmitt FA, Bigley JW, McKinnis R, et al. Neuropsychological outcome of zidovudine (AZT) treatment of patients with AIDS and AIDS-related complex. *N Engl J Med* 1988; 319:1573–1578.
78. Pizzo PA, Eddy J, Falloon J, et al. Effect of continuous intravenous infusion of zidovudine (AZT) in children with symptomatic HIV infection. *N Engl J Med* 1988;319:889–896.
79. Sidtis JJ, Gatsonis C, Price RW, et al. Zidovudine treatment of the AIDS dementia complex: results of a placebo-controlled trial. *Ann Neurol* 1993 **(in press)**.
80. Volberding PA, Lagakos SW, Koch MA, et al. Zidovudine in asymptomatic human immunodeficiency virus infection. A controlled trial in persons with fewer than 500 CD4-positive cells per cubic millimeter. *N Engl J Med* 1990;322:941–949.
81. Yarchoan R, Pluda JM, Thomas RV, et al. Long-term toxicity/activity profile of 2′,3′-dideoxyinosine in AIDS and AIDS-related complex. *Lancet* 1990;336:526–529.
82. Day JJ, Grant I, Atkinson JH, et al. Incidence of AIDS dementia in a two-year follow-up of AIDS and ARC patients on an initial Phase II AZT placebo-controlled study: San Diego cohort. *J Neuropsychiatry* 1992;4:15–20.
83. Graham NMH, Zeger SL, Kuo V, et al. Zidovudine use in AIDS-free HIV-1 seropositive homosexual men in the Multicenter AIDS Cohort Study (MACS) 1987–1989. *J AIDS* 1991; 4:267–276.
84. Hamilton JD, Hartigan PM, Simberkoff MS, et al. A controlled trial of early versus late treatment with zidovudine in symptomatic human immunodeficiency virus infection. *N Engl J Med* 1992;326:437–443.
85. Nordic Medical Research Councils HIV Therapy Group. Double blind dose–response study of zidovudine in AIDS and advanced HIV infection. *Br Med J* 1992;304:13–17.

HIV, AIDS and the Brain, edited by
R. W. Price and S. W. Perry.
Raven Press, Ltd., New York © 1994.

15

Evaluation of the AIDS Dementia Complex in Adults

John J. Sidtis

Department of Neurology, University of Minnesota Medical School, Minneapolis, MN 55455

Infection by human immunodeficiency virus type 1 (HIV-1) is complicated by a number of neurological disorders, but perhaps the most important is the AIDS dementia complex (ADC), a syndrome of "subcortical dementia" (1). During the brief history of this syndrome, its recognition as a clinical entity has reflected two extremes. The incorrect attribution of the symptoms of ADC to depression, a problem early in the history of this disease, has become less common as the syndrome has become better recognized. In contrast, the search for early signs of ADC has led some to equate HIV-1 infection alone with subclinical neurological disease. Between these extremes, progress has been made in characterizing the clinical features of ADC, identifying its place in the broader context of HIV-1 infection, and studying its response to therapy. The development of systematic, standardized approaches to the clinical evaluation of ADC have been central to these efforts. This chapter will describe (a) an approach to evaluation that incorporates neurological and neuropsychological components and (b) a staging scheme that characterizes the severity of ADC. This approach has proven valuable in clinical trials, and should play a key role in eventually understanding the pathophysiology of ADC.

THE DIAGNOSIS OF ADC

The diagnosis of ADC requires the documentation of HIV-1 infection, evidence of an acquired neurological deficit, and exclusion of other neurological or psychiatric problems as its cause. Furthermore, the acquired abnormalities in cognitive, motor, and/or behavioral functions must be characteristic of ADC. In the cognitive area this may include early symptoms of impaired concentration and slowed thinking. Complaints of forgetfulness are common,

TABLE 1. *Frequent early symptoms of ADC in the areas of cognitive, motor, and behavioral function*

Cognitive
  Mental slowing (not as quick, less verbal, loss of spontaneity)
  Poor concentration (losing track of conversations, reading)
  Forgetfulness (names, appointments, historical details)
  Confusion (time, place)
  Reduced initiation
Motor
  Unsteady gait
  Leg weakness
  Loss of coordination, impaired handwriting
  Tremor
Behavior
  Apathy, withdrawal
  Agitated psychosis
  Personality change

---

but formal testing may reveal normal function early in ADC. Cognitive changes may evolve to significant impairments in abstraction, profound slowing, failures in concentration and memory, and, subsequently, global dementia. In the motor area, changes characteristic of ADC include early slowing of rapid movements of the extremities; this may evolve to clumsiness and ataxia of gait, accompanied by impaired hand coordination. Subsequent progression can lead to paraplegia with incontinence in the most severe cases. Behavioral dysfunction has been less useful for diagnosis, but characteristic abnormalities include personality change and apathy without dysphoria, which may progress in parallel with psychomotor retardation. A subgroup of patients may exhibit psychosis, agitation, or even frank mania. Some of the most frequent early symptoms of ADC are listed in Table 1.

THE EVOLUTION OF THE EVALUATION SCHEME

The neurological evaluation for ADC has developed from an extensive clinical experience with this disorder dating to its recognition as a significant complication of AIDS (2). The evolution of this evaluation scheme has been shaped by several forces, with sensitivity and efficiency being major concerns. Throughout its development, however, the process has been concerned with establishing an appropriate diagnosis, assessing functional status, and objectively measuring performance using neuropsychological tests. Initially, a complete neurological examination and broad neuropsychological battery were coupled with functional status measures used in the study of other diseases (3–5). After analyzing this experience, the neurological history and examination began to focus on the cardinal features of ADC, and the neuropsychological battery was modified and shortened. The functional status scales were replaced with clinical impairment ratings of the patient's cognition, motor function, and behavior made by the examining neurologist.

As the need for a practical examination for clinical trials grew, standardization became more important and the relative roles of the neurological and neuropsychological examinations in diagnosis and quantitation, respectively, became apparent (6). With increasing experience, the neurological history and examination were further focused on ADC, impairment ratings were replaced with ADC staging, and a neuropsychological summary measure based on normalized scores was developed. Components of this evaluation system make up the long and short forms of the neurological evaluations widely used in clinical trials.

ADC STAGING

Although an ADC stage is assigned based on the results of the neurological history and examination, staging will be considered first because it provides a context in which the rest of the evaluation can be considered. The development of a staging scheme to provide a functional classification based on neurological disease severity became particularly important with increasing

TABLE 2. *Staging scheme for the AIDS dementia complex (ADC)[a]*

ADC stage	Characteristics
Stage 0 (normal)	Normal mental and motor function.
Stage 0.5 (equivocal/ subclinical)	Either minimal or equivocal *symptoms* of cognitive or motor dysfunction characteristic of ADC, or mild signs (snout resonse, slowed extremity movements), but *without impairment of work or capacity to perform activities of daily living* (ADL). Gait and strength are normal.
Stage 1 (mild)	Unequivocal evidence (symptoms, signs, neuropsychological test performance) of functional intellectual or motor impairment characteristic of ADC, but able to perform *all but the more demanding aspects of work or ADL.* Can walk without assistance.
Stage 2 (moderate)	Cannot work or maintain the more demanding aspects of daily life, but able to perform *basic activities of self care.* Ambulatory, but may require a single prop.
Stage 3 (severe)	*Major intellectual incapacity* (cannot follow news or personal events, cannot sustain complex conversation, considerable slowing of all output), *or motor disability* (cannot walk unassisted, requiring walker or personal support, usually with slowing and clumsiness of arms as well).
Stage 4 (end stage)	*Nearly vegetative.* Intellectual and social comprehension and response are at a rudimentary level. Nearly or absolutely mute. Paraparetic or paraplegic with double incontinence.

[a] ADC Stages 1 through 4 are reserved for unequivocal abnormalities that impair the patient's functional capacity. Stage 0.5 is reserved for patients with minor symptoms or "soft" signs, for whom ADC must be considered subclinical or equivocal. Developed at Memorial Sloan Kettering Center (7).

recognition of ADC earlier in its course (7). ADC staging, like the staging of systemic HIV-1 disease, provides critical reference points for understanding and tracking the onset and progression of disease from its earliest subclinical presentation to its end stage (1,8). The stage, which is applied only after establishing a clinical diagnosis of ADC, is based on the patient's functional status as it is affected by the neurological complications of HIV-1 infection, excluding the effects of neoplasms and opportunistic infections of the central nervous system. The ADC staging system is presented in Table 2. The stages range from 0 (Normal) through 4 (end stage), at which point the patient is nearly vegetative. ADC stages 1 through 4 are reserved for unequivocal abnormalities that impair the patient's functional capacity. Stage 0.5 is included in the staging in order to allow inclusion of patients with minor symptoms or "soft" neurological signs in which there is no clear evidence of functional incapacity related to ADC.

THE LONG AND THE SHORT EVALUATION: THE MACRO AND MICRO EXAMINATIONS

In order to provide standardization to the neurological evaluation for ADC to as broad a group of examiners as possible, the neurological evaluation was divided into two versions whereby the briefer version (the MICRO examination) consisted of a subset of items from the longer version (the MACRO examination). The MACRO neurological examination is briefer than a full examination, but it is focused on characterizing ADC, especially for longitudinal studies or clinical trials. The MICRO neurological examination, which was developed to obtain limited neurological data in clinical trials, consists of a small subset of items from the MACRO examination that have recently been incorporated into a self-report questionnaire. The neuropsychological examination for ADC follows a structure parallel to the MACRO and MICRO neurological examinations, with versions that provide summary measures based on eight, four, or two tests.

THE NEUROLOGICAL HISTORY AND EXAMINATION

The neurological evaluation for ADC has evolved to characterize the most salient and reliable features of cognitive, motor, and behavioral abnormalities in this disorder, with an emphasis on changes in cognition and motor function. As indicated above, the neurological history and examination has two major purposes: to establish an appropriate diagnosis, and to define the functional context for the neurological deficit.

General Considerations

It is important to document any history of significant background neurologic or psychiatric disease, as well as any other confounding factors because they may affect the results of the patient's neurological and neuropsychological examinations independent of his or her ADC status. In addition to preexisting diseases, confounding factors can include a history of head injury, drug or alcohol abuse, and developmental abnormalities. In instances where potential confounding factors exist, their functional significance should be a consideration in making a diagnosis of ADC and subsequent staging. Medication history should also be documented, and it is important to maintain current information regarding the patient's status with respect to systemic disease and immunological function, actual and potential work status, and level of function in activities of daily living.

The Neurological History for ADC

The patient should be carefully questioned about changes in cognitive, motor, and behavioral function, specifically as such changes pertain to ADC.

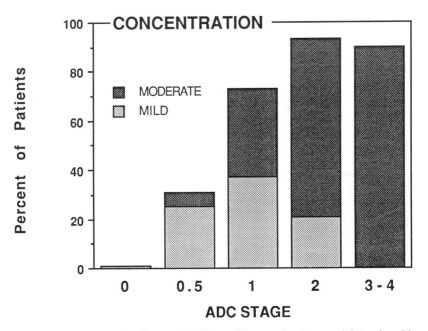

FIG. 1. The percentage of patients with either mild or moderate complaints of problems with concentration as a function of ADC stage. The percentages of patients with mild complaints are indicated by the lighter bars, while the percentages of patients with moderate complaints are indicated by the darker bars. These data were collected using the MACRO neurological history.

In the area of cognition, the history focuses on the patient's concentration, speed of thought, capacity to read or follow a plot on television, recall information, find words, and communicate coherently. With respect to motor function, the history particularly addresses gait and coordination in the upper and lower extremities, the presence of involuntary movements, and bladder incontinence. Changes in the patient's social behavior, mood, and emotional control should also be documented, as should sensory changes and the presence of headache and seizures.

Figure 1 depicts the percentage of patients with either mild or moderate complaints of problems, with concentration as a function of ADC stage. Complaints were elicited while taking the history using the MACRO neurological evaluation. Data on complaints are often missing in the most advanced patients because of obvious limitations in their ability to respond due to their dementia.

The Neurological Examination for ADC

As with the history, the neurological examination is directed toward the cardinal features of ADC. The major sections of the examination evaluate

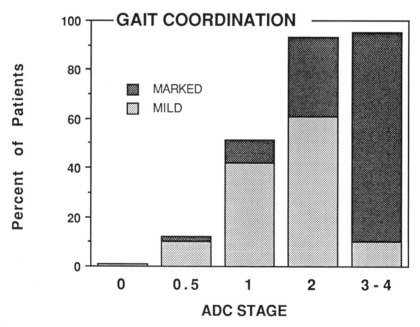

FIG. 2. The percentage of patients with either mild or marked abnormalities in gait coordination as a function of ADC stage. The percentages of patients with mild complaints are indicated by the lighter bars, while the percentages of patients with marked complaints are indicated by the darker bars. These data were collected using the MACRO neurological examination.

mental status, selected cranial nerves, motor strength and coordination, selected reflexes, and sensation. The formal examination begins with a modified mini-mental status examination. The retina is examined, ocular motility is evaluated with respect to smooth pursuits and saccades, and the patient's facial expression is classified with respect to hypomotility. The examination of motor function emphasizes lower-extremity strength, as well as gait and limb coordination. Selected reflexes, including the snout and jaw jerk, are examined, and the patient should be evaluated for neuropathy.

Figure 2 depicts the percentage of patients with either mild or marked abnormalities in gait coordination as a function of ADC Stage. Abnormalities were rated according to the MACRO neurological examination. As with the complaints, not all examination items can be completed in the most advanced patients because of the severity of their disease.

NEUROPSYCHOLOGICAL TESTING

Neuropsychological assessment typically produces a characteristic profile that demonstrates psychomotor slowing and poor performance on tasks of attention and concentration, with relative sparing of language and memory skills early in the course (1,9–13). In the context of this evaluation scheme, neuropsychological tests provide a quantitative neurological examination that can objectively document such changes.

Constraints on the Test Battery

Unlike neurology, neuropsychology has not established a standard examination. Rather, there is a large range of available tests dealing with various mental functions, and there are differing approaches to their use. Traditionally, neuropsychological testing lasted many hours, typically attempting to broadly assess intellectual functions and establish a pattern of deficits consistent with a specific anatomic localization. However, the evolution of the neuropsychological component of this evaluation scheme has been influenced by a number of factors that have kept this test battery relatively brief and efficient. The presence of neurological disease in the context of active systemic disease means that patients are typically undergoing a larger number of examinations, studies, and procedures than is usual for most neurology or psychiatry patients, especially in the later stages of HIV-1 disease. Time, therefore, is an important constraint, as is patient acceptance of the testing procedures. Similarly, the stamina of patients with mid- to later-stage systemic disease in the face of very extensive multidisciplinary clinical and laboratory studies is also a practical concern.

The importance of following patients longitudinally, beginning at earlier stages of their disease, adds another constraint: Tests have to be suited for repeated-measures studies. In our earliest longitudinal studies prior to treatment trials, it became clear that patient acceptance was reduced by long batteries containing tests that, while once challenging, had become rote and tedious in the absence of disease progression. When patients began to recite memory passages before they were presented as material to be remembered, or when they would note that a particular test was the one in which they were supposed to figure this or that out without being told, it became clear that while many multiple versions would be required for some tests, for others the nature of what was being tested would change after the initial administration. With the advent of treatment trials, patient compliance for follow-up evaluations improved, but the repeated-measures issues became more acute, with examinations often occurring weeks rather than months apart.

In addition to brevity and repeatability, it is also desirable that the tests yield quantitative measures derived from simple, objective scoring. The use of objective scores facilitates communication of test results and their significance to nonpsychologists, thereby improving the acceptance of such measures as an important part of the evaluation of HIV-1-infected patients. The use of objectively scored tests also reduces the reliance on experienced neuropsychologists for patient evaluation, thereby making the evaluation more accessible to sites with technical support but limited resources at the professional level. Finally, with the need to compare diverse patient populations, tests suited for (or adaptable to) individuals over a wide range of age, educational attainment, and diverse cultural backgrounds are desirable.

The neuropsychological test battery in this evaluation scheme focuses heavily on psychomotor performance, and it includes self-report measures to assess psychological abnormalities. It has never been intended to be a comprehensive examination, but is tailored to the evaluation of ADC. By itself, the neuropsychological test battery does not yield a diagnosis of ADC, but the measures contained in the battery can contribute significantly to establishing the diagnosis. These measures can play a central role in quantitative, longitudinal studies of the disease course and, more importantly, of therapeutic efficacy.

General Considerations

As with the neurological examination, certain background information is directly relevant to the neuropsychological examination. This includes the patient's handedness, native language, educational level, prior or current neurologic or psychiatric disease, and a history of developmental abnormalities, substance abuse, or head trauma.

The MACRO Neuropsychological Examination

Since its earliest stages, it was hoped that the battery would be widely used at sites dealing with HIV. However, it was also acknowledged that fixed test batteries reduce individual investigator's flexibility and are therefore often not adopted. Furthermore, it was also acknowledged that not every site had the necessary expertise available to conduct extensive neuropsychological testing. To encourage obtaining comparable measures across the widest range of studies and clinical centers, the original test battery was divided into core and supplementary components. The core could serve as a screening examination, as a minimal set of primary data collected by a trained technician at sites with limited resources, or as a set of reference points for studies that also included other neuropsychological, neurological, or psychiatric measures. With some modifications, the original core tests became the components of the neuropsychology summary score, and the supplementary test distinction was dropped in favor of MACRO and MICRO versions of the examination to parallel the neurological evaluation format.

The components of the MACRO neuropsychological examination are listed in Table 3. The vocabulary subtest of the Wechsler Adult Intelligence Scale—Revised (WAIS-R) (14) is only given once, to be used with education level to provide an estimate of premorbid intellectual function. Vocabulary scores remain relatively stable until the later stages of disease (9).

The next eight tests in Table 3 are measures that efficiently assess functions affected in ADC, and can be repeated without adverse practice effects. These tests contribute to the various versions of the neuropsychological summary scores discussed below. The *Timed Gait* test assesses walking speed. A 10-yard distance is clearly marked, and the subject is instructed to walk as

TABLE 3. *Components of the University of Minnesota neuro-AIDS program MACRO neuropsychological examination[a]*

Neuropsychological tests	Summary measures		
	NPZ-8	NPZ-4	NPZ-2
Baseline			
Vocabulary subtest of the WAIS-R			
Repeated measures			
Timed gait	*	*	*
Grooved pegboard (dominant)	*	*	
Grooved pegboard (nondominant)	*		
Trail-making A	*		
Trail-making B	*		
Digit symbol	*	*	*
Finger tapping (dominant)	*		
Finger tapping (nondominant)	*	*	
Auditory verbal learning test			
Profile of mood states			

[a] The vocabulary test is only given once at baseline. All other tests are repeated measures. Three different neuropsychological summary measures based on z-scores (NPZ) are represented on the right side of the table. The NPZ-8 represents the average of the eight tests indicated by an asterisk, the NPZ-4 represents the average of four tests, and the NPZ-2 represents the average of two tests.

quickly as possible (without running) to the 10-yard marker, step over it with one foot, turn around, and return still walking as quickly as possible. The *Grooved Pegboard* test is administered for both the dominant and nondominant hands (15). This test is timed, and it requires fine motor control and rapid eye–hand coordination as well as the use of somatosensory and visual feedback. The *Trail-Making A* and *B* (15) and *Digit Symbol* subtest of the WAIS-R (14) require visual search, performance on sequential tasks, and the ability to switch mental set rapidly. These timed tests add perceptual and cognitive components to the battery. The *Finger Tapping* test is also administered for both the dominant and nondominant hands (15). This test assesses the speed of simple, repetitive movements. It is easy to administer and perform, and it can provide a useful measure of motor speed even relatively late in the disease.

The auditory verbal learning test (15) provides a measure of learning and memory over five repetitions of a 15-item word list. Immediate recall of the word list is challenged using an interference procedure, and recall after a 20-minute delay is also obtained. Recognition testing can also be employed. Finally, the patient's subjective sense of mood is assessed using the Profile of Mood States (16). This self-report questionnaire addresses several psychological states, including depression, anger, vigor, and fatigue.

NEUROPSYCHOLOGICAL SUMMARY MEASURES: THE NPZ SCORES

The psychomotor tests that make up the core of the MACRO examination have several advantages. They are highly sensitive to ADC, can be administered in less than 30 minutes, and require minimal instrumentation. As a group, these tests have been extremely useful in both clinical practice and clinical trials. The results of this group of tests can be summarized by creating an average normalized score referred to as the "neuropsychology z-score" (NPZ score).

To derive the NPZ score, the raw score for an individual's performance on each of the core tests is converted to a z-score by subtracting a reference group mean, and dividing the resulting difference by the reference group's standard deviation. The reference population consists of HIV-1-seropositive individuals classified as ADC Stage 0, with separate reference means and standard deviations determined for patients at different age groups. The NPZ summary measure is simply the average of the individual z-scores.

For the MACRO examination, the NPZ is the average of eight tests (NPZ-8, Table 3). The original MICRO neuropsychological used only two tests (NPZ-2), whereas the current MICRO examination uses four tests (NPZ-4). Figure 3 depicts the NPZ-8 score as a function of ADC stage. There is clearly a significant decline in this performance measure as ADC progresses. Whereas the three versions of the NPZ score reveal nearly identical levels

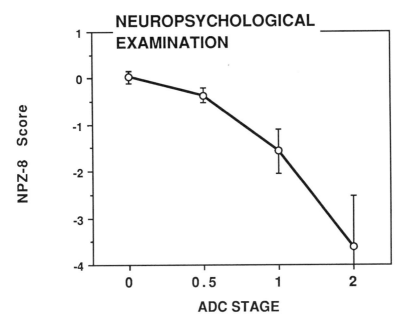

FIG. 3. Changes in the NPZ-8 score derived from the MACRO neuropsychological examination as a function of ADC stage. Error bars represent 95 percent confidence intervals
for each mean.

of decline across ADC stage, the use of eight rather than two tests appears
to provide greater stability across repeated evaluations. Since a larger number of scores are averaged in the NPZ-8 versus the NPZ-2, a single spurious
score will have less of an impact on the former than on the latter. As will
be shown in the next section, this summary measure has also proven advantageous in clinical trials.

AN EXAMPLE FROM A CLINICAL TRIAL

The value of this system of neurological evaluation is perhaps most obvious in clinical trials. A number of observations have suggested that antiretroviral therapy has a beneficial effect on the severity of ADC (17–20). The
AIDS Clinical Trials Group's (ACTG) study of zidovudine [ZDV; 3′-azido-3′-
deoxythymidine (AZT)] for the treatment of ADC in adults used the MACRO
neurological evaluation to study therapeutic efficacy in a randomized, double-blind, placebo-controlled trial (21). The primary assessment of treatment
efficacy was based on (a) an earlier version of the NPZ-8 score, (b) performance on the individual MACRO neuropsychological tests, and (c) improvements in abnormalities noted on the MACRO neurological history and examination.

Forty subjects with a clinical diagnosis of mild to severe ADC based on the presence of characteristic clinical symptoms and signs and exclusion of alternative diagnosis explaining their neurological abnormalities were randomized to one of the three study arms: a "high dose" of 2000 mg/day, a "low dose" of 1000 mg/day, and placebo. The study patients were recruited from nine AIDS Clinical Trials Units sponsored by the National Institute of Allergy and Infectious Disease. Treatment was planned for 16 weeks in the initial stage, after which placebo recipients were re-randomized to one of the two ZDV arms.

For the initial 16 weeks of study, the changes in each of the MACRO neuropsychological tests used in the earlier version of the NPZ score are presented in Fig. 4. While the group comparisons for the individual tests did not reveal significant differences, each test revealed a similar trend in which the treated groups performed better than the placebo group. However, using the NPZ-8 score, the combined mean change of the two treatment arms was significantly different from the mean of the placebo group. In groupwise comparisons of NPZ-8 score changes, only the ZDV 2000 mg/day and the placebo groups differed significantly. After examining selected items from

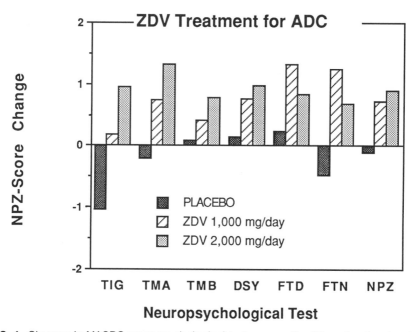

FIG. 4. Changes in MACRO neuropsychological test scores after 16 weeks of a placebo-controlled trial of ZDV for the treatment of ADC (21). Positive z-scores indicate improvement. The tests are as follows: verbal fluency (VF), trail-making A (TMA), trail-making B (TMB), digit symbol substitution (DSY), timed gait (TIG), finger-tapping dominant hand (FTD), and finger-tapping nondominant hand (FTN).

the MACRO neurological history and examination, the two treatment groups showed slightly better improvement compared with the placebo group, but these differences were not statistically significant. In the second stage of the study, patients in the placebo group who were re-randomized to one of the two ZDV arms showed significant improvement on the NPZ-8 score during the subsequent 16 weeks.

Despite the early termination and small number of subjects in this placebo-controlled study, the results extended previous observations indicating a therapeutic benefit of ZDV for the treatment of ADC. Although this study did not resolve the issue of the optimal dose of ZDV for ADC patients, from the standpoint of evaluation, it did demonstrate the effectiveness of complementary roles for the MACRO neurological and neuropsychological evaluations. The MACRO neurological history and examination is best suited for establishing diagnosis and rating functional status as it pertains to ADC. The MACRO neuropsychological examination, and especially the NPZ score summary measure, is best used to quantify treatment effects in the functional context established by the neurological component of the evaluation.

CONCLUDING COMMENTS ON THE EVALUATION OF ADC

The neurological evaluation described in this chapter has been developed to provide a backbone for describing the primary features of ADC. The evaluation has been kept brief enough to encourage both wide clinical use and incorporation into research protocols, and consequently it is extremely well suited for clinical trials.

This type of evaluation scheme may be complemented by the addition of more complicated behavioral tests (22–24), structural or functional brain imaging (25–27), cerebrospinal fluid assays (28,29), or a combination of these (30). Although more sophisticated tests are less widely accessible for clinical trails because they require greater instrumentation and professional support, they may nevertheless play an important role in future studies of pathogenesis and therapeutic response. Whether new means of assessing ADC take the form of behavioral measures, functional images, or assays or cerebrospinal fluid, their significance to ADC will be most usefully interpreted in the context of an evaluation scheme such as the one described in this chapter.

ACKNOWLEDGMENTS

This work was supported by NINDS (NS25701) and by NIAID (AI 276661).

REFERENCES

1. Price RW, Brew B, Sidtis JJ, Rosenblum M, Scheck AC, Cleary P. The brain in AIDS: central nervous system HIV-1 infection and the AIDS dementia complex. *Science* 1988; 239:586–592.
2. Navia BA, Jordan BD, Price RW. The AIDS dementia complex. I. Clinical features. *Ann Neurol* 1986;19:517–524.
3. Blessed G, Tomlinson BE, Roth M. The association between quantitative measures of dementia and of senile change in the cerebral grey matter of elderly subjects. *Br J Psychiatry* 1968;114:797–811.
4. Karnofsky DA, Burchenal JH. The clinical evaluation of chemotherapeutic agents in cancer. In: MacLeod CM, ed. *Evaluation of chemotherapeutic agents*. New York: Columbia University Press, 1949.
5. Kurtzke JF. Rating neurological impairment in multiple sclerosis: an expanded disability status scale (EDSS). *Neurology* 1983;33:1444–1452.
6. Price RW, Sidtis JJ. Evaluation of the AIDS Dementia Complex in clinical trials. *J AIDS* 1990;3(suppl 2):S51–S60.
7. Price RW, Brew BJ. The AIDS dementia complex. *J Infect Dis* 1988;158:1079–1083.
8. Sidtis JJ, Price RW. Early HIV-1 infection and the AIDS dementia complex. *Neurology* 1990;40:323–326.
9. Tross S, Price RW, Navia BA, et al. Neuropsychological characterization of the AIDS dementia complex: a preliminary report. *AIDS* 1988;2:81–88.
10. Janssen RS, Saykin AJ, Cannon L, Campbell J, Pinsky PF, Hessol NA, O'Malley, Lifson AR, Doll LS, Rutherford GW, Kaplan JE. Neurological and neuropsychological manifestations of HIV-1 infection: association with AIDS-related complex but not asymptomatic HIV-1 infection. *Ann Neurol* 1989;26:592–600.
11. Hart RP, Wade JB, Klinger RL, Hamer RM. Slowed information processing as an early change associated with HIV infection. *Neuropsychology* 1990;4:97–104.
12. Perdices M, Cooper DA. Neuropsychological investigation of patients with AIDS and ARC. *J AIDS* 1990;3:555–564.
13. Reinvang I, Froland SS, Skripeland V. Prevalence of neuropsychological deficit in HIV infection. Incipient signs of AIDS dementia complex in patients with AIDS. *Acta Neurol Scand* 1991;83:289–293.
14. Wechsler D. *Wechsler adult intelligence scale—revised*. New York: The Psychological Corporation, 1981.
15. Lezak MD. *Neuropsychological assessment*. New York: Oxford University Press, 1983.
16. McNair D, Lorr M, Droppelman L. *EDITS manual for the profile of mood states*. San Diego: Educational and Industrial Testing Service, 1971.
17. Yarchoan R, Berg G, Brouwers P, et al. Response of human immunodeficiency-virus-associated neurological disease to 3'-azido-3'-deoxythymidine. *Lancet* 1987;8525:132–135.
18. Schmitt FA, Bigley JW, McKinnis R, et al. Neuropsychological outcome of zidovudine (AZT) treatment of patients with AIDS and AIDS-related complex. *N Engl J Med* 1988; 319:1573–1578.
19. Pizzo PA, Eddy J, Falloon J, et al. Effects of continuous intravenous infusion of zidovudine (AZT) in children with symptomatic HIV infection. *N Engl J Med* 1988;319:889–896.
20. Portegies P, de Gans J, Lange JMA, et al. Declining incidence of AIDS dementia complex after introduction of zidovudine treatment. *Br Med J* 1989;299:819–821.
21. Sidtis JJ, Gatsonis C, Price RW, Singer EJ, Collier AC, Richman DD, Hirsch MS, Schaerf FW, Fischl MA, Kieburtz K, Simpson D, Koch MA, Feinberg J, and the AIDS Clinical Trials Group. Zidovudine Treatment of the AIDS Dementia Complex: results of a Placebo-Controlled Trial. *Ann Neurol* 1993;33:343–349.
22. Martin EM, Sorensen DJ, Edelstein HE, Robertson LC. Decision-making speed in HIV-1 infections: a preliminary report. *AIDS* 1992;6:109–113.
23. Miller EN, Satz P, Visscher B. Computerized and conventional neuropsychological assessment of HIV-1 infected homosexual men. *Neurology* 1991;41:1608–1616.
24. Sweeney JA, Brew BJ, Keilp JG, Sidtis JJ, Price RW. Pursuit eye movement dysfunction in HIV-1 seropositive patients. *J Psychiatry Neurosci* 1991;16:247–252.

25. Rottenberg DA, Moeller JR, Strother SC, Sidtis JJ, Navia BA, Dhawan V, Ginos JZ, Price RW. The metabolic pathology of the AIDS dementia complex. *Ann Neurol* 1987;22:700–706.
26. Levin HS, Williams DH, Borucki MJ, Hillman GR, Williams JB, Guinto FC, Amparo EG, Crow WN, Pollard RB. Magnetic resonance imaging and neuropsychological findings in immunodeficiency virus infection. *J AIDS* 1990;3:757–762.
27. Dal Pan GJ, McArthur JH, Aylward E, Selnes OA, Nance-Spronson TE, Kumar AJ, Mellits ED, McArthur JC. Patterns of cerebral atrophy in HIV-1-infected individuals: results of a quantitative MRI analysis. *Neurology* 1992;42:2125–2130.
28. Heyes MP, Brew BJ, Martin A, Price RW, Salazar AM, Yergey JA, Mouradian MM, Sadler AE, Keilp J, Sidtis JJ, Bhalla RB, Rubinow D, Markey SP. Increased cerebrospinal fluid concentrations of the excitotoxin quinolinic acid in HIV infection and AIDS dementia complex. *Ann Neurol* 1991;29:202–209.
29. Brew BJ, Bhalla RB, Paul M, Sidtis JJ, Keilp JG, Sadler AE, Gallardo H, McArthur JC, Schwartz MK, Price RW. Cerebrospinal fluid beta-2-microglobulin in patients with AIDS dementia complex: an expanded series including response to zidovudine treatment. *AIDS* 1992;6:461–465.
30. Sidtis JJ, Rottenberg DA, Worley J, Strother S, Price RW. Continuous performance testing in the AIDS dementia complex: a behavioral contrast agent for functional imaging? *Neurology* 1993;43:A253–A254.

HIV, AIDS and the Brain, edited by
R. W. Price and S. W. Perry.
Raven Press, Ltd., New York © 1994.

16

HIV-1-Associated CNS Disease in Infants and Children

Anita L. Belman

*Department of Neurology, SUNY at Stony Brook School of Medicine,
Stony Brook, NY 11794*

In 1982, four children with unexplained immunodeficiency and opportunistic infections were reported to the Centers for Disease Control and Prevention (CDC). The following year the clinical and immunological features of pediatric acquired immunodeficiency syndrome (AIDS) were described for the first time (1). Shortly after these landmark reports, it became apparent that central nervous system (CNS) involvement was a frequent complication. A "progressive encephalopathy" was described (2,3) as well as more stable neurologic impairment (2,4). Neurologic dysfunction in the majority of these young patients was not due to CNS opportunistic infections (OIs) or neoplasms (5–9). It became clear that by the time human immunodeficiency virus type 1 (HIV-1) infection had advanced to "full-blown" AIDS, cognitive and motor impairments of varying duration, progression, and severity were extremely common (5,6). Clinical, neuropathologic, and virologic investigations indicated that the CNS was infected by HIV-1 (10–20). Morphologic and genetic similarities were documented between HIV-1 and visna virus, an ovine retrovirus with well-known neurotropic properties (21). All these studies suggested that the clinical syndromes of "progressive encephalopathy" in children, and the adult counterpart "AIDS dementia complex" (22), were directly related to HIV-1.

In the past decade, much has been learned about the biology of HIV-1. Much has also been learned about systemic and immunologic aspects of pediatric and adult HIV-1 infection and AIDS. Although it is now well recognized that the CNS is infected by the retrovirus, sometimes at a very early stage (HIV-1 has been identified in fetal brain tissue), many questions remain. The route of CNS invasion and factors relating to latency are not yet established. The neuropathophysiologic processes underlying HIV-1-mediated CNS disease syndromes are still uncertain. The issues are further complicated for infected infants and children because of developmental–maturational considerations. Adult HIV-1 CNS infection and disease occurs in mature, fully developed, and completely myelinated nervous systems. The immune system and the CNS elements of the mononuclear phagocyte system (intrinsic microglia) are also fully developed. Vertically transmitted HIV-1 infection occurs in an immature evolving organism. When exposed to the direct or indirect effects of the virus, the developmental stage of the nervous and immune system is likely to be important. Innumerable dynamic interactions occur between these two systems during development, which will interact in complex ways with HIV-1 variables. Much study will be required, and much remains to be learned.

The focus of this chapter is on HIV-1-associated CNS disease in infants and children. Neurologic, neuroimaging, and neuropathologic features will be summarized.

PEDIATRIC HIV-1 INFECTION: DEFINITION AND CLASSIFICATION

The CDC initially defined AIDS in children in the same restrictive fashion as for adults, requiring opportunistic infection of AIDS-related malignancy. Primary (congenital) or secondary immunodeficiency disorders, as well as congenital infections (e.g., TORCH), had to be excluded. Once HIV-1 was identified and serologic testing established, it was realized that only a minority of infected children fit the case definition. Two subsequent CDC case definition revisions have broadened the criteria. In 1987 a major revision listed a spectrum of clinical manifestations. This current classification is based on (a) laboratory evidence of HIV-1 infection, (b) immunologic function, and (c) clinical manifestations of P-2 classes (see ref. 1 for review). HIV-1-immunoglobulin G specific (IgG) antibodies in infants, unlike those in adults or older children, are uninterpretable. Maternal IgG crosses the placenta and may persist up to 15 months. Therefore a seropositive child less than 15 months of age is classified as P-0, indeterminate infection, unless there is clinical and/or laboratory evidence of HIV-1 infection. For surveillance purposes the CDC currently defines recurrent bacterial infections, OIs, neoplasms, lymphoid interstitial pneumonia, and progressive encephalopathy as AIDS-defining illnesses.

NOMENCLATURE

In this chapter the term "HIV-1-associated CNS disease" will be used to encompass all neurologic syndromes (including progressive encephalopathy) that are currently believed to be related to direct or indirect CNS effects of HIV-1. The term "HIV-1-associated progressive encephalopathy (PE) of childhood" will be used according to the recent recommendation of the

Working Group of the American Academy of Neurology AIDS Task Force on nomenclature (24).

In the future, more precise definitions will evolve as clinical features are further delineated and correlated with underlying neuropathophysiologic processes (1).

HIV-1 ASSOCIATED CNS DISEASE SYNDROMES

Pediatric HIV-1-associated CNS disease(s) refers to a syndrome complex (or syndrome complexes) with a characteristic constellation of cognitive, motor, and behavioral manifestations. The *rate* of neurologic deterioration, *severity* of neurologic deficits, and *domains* of function most affected will vary among patient subsets. Initially, two forms of encephalopathy were described: progressive and static. Continued clinical observations suggested that PE could be subdivided based on progression and severity of neurologic deficits. Several patterns of CNS disease were identified (see Fig. 1).

During the past several years, further observations of children both in research studies and clinical care settings have suggested, at least to this investigator, that the spectrum and diversity of pediatric HIV-1-associated CNS disease syndromes is much wider than previously appreciated. This may be due, in part, to inclusion of children with less advanced systemic disease, since vertically infected infants and children are being identified and followed at earlier and less symptomatic disease stages. It may also be due to inclusion of children in a wider age range, since pediatric patients are living longer because of earlier and more aggressive medical management of AIDS-related conditions and opportunistic infections. It is also possible that the natural history of HIV-1-associated CNS disease may be changing with the introduction of antiretroviral agents. Whatever the explanation, clinical variability is apparent and some patterns of CNS disease are not adequately captured by the Task Force classification.

Clinical Features

Manifestations

The most frequent manifestations of HIV-1-associated CNS disease are developmental delays, cognitive impairment, poor brain growth (acquired microcephaly), and corticospinal tract signs (CST). Movement disorders may develop but are usually superimposed upon spasticity. Cerebellar signs occur but less frequently (Table 1).

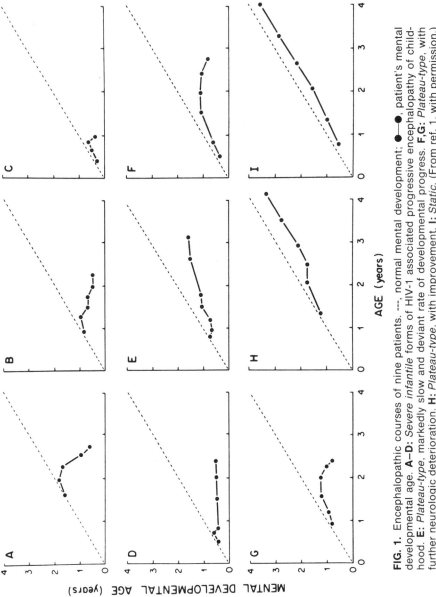

FIG. 1. Encephalopathic courses of nine patients. ---, normal mental development; ●—●, patient's mental developmental age. **A–D:** *Severe infantile* forms of HIV-1 associated progressive encephalopathy of childhood. **E:** *Plateau-type*, markedly slow and deviant rate of developmental progress. **F,G:** *Plateau-type*, with further neurologic deterioration. **H:** *Plateau-type*, with improvement. **I:** *Static.* (From ref. 1, with permission.)

TABLE 1. *Manifestations of HIV-1-related CNS disease*[a]

Cognitive impairment
Developmental delays
Corticospinal tract signs
Acquired microcephaly
Cerebellar signs
  Ataxia
  Tremor
Extrapyramidal tract signs
  Rigidity
  Opisthotonia
  Dystonia
  Tremor

[a] Data from refs. 2 and 6; table taken from ref. 25.

Patterns of Disease

Several patterns of PE are recognized: subacute progressive; plateau, followed by further deterioration or improvement; and static/stable. These terms were introduced to allow further clinical characterization of features and signs. Considerable variability is seen within subdivisions, and this scheme will require modification. Nevertheless, it will be used in the following section because it still remains useful to describe clinical courses. It should be noted, however, that some patients develop severe and progressive CNS dysfunction, with quadriparesis and dementia. Other patients have progressive and disabling motor involvement, with relatively stable cognitive, behavioral, and socially adaptive skills. Other children have greater cognitive impairment than motor deficits (and may not even fit criteria for PE), whereas some patients have relatively minor and stable motor and cognitive impairment.

HIV-1-ASSOCIATED PROGRESSIVE ENCEPHALOPATHY OF CHILDHOOD

Infants and Young Children

Subacute

This is the most severe and devastating syndrome. Characteristic features include (a) progressive CST signs, (b) acquired microcephaly, and (c) loss of previously acquired milestones. Over time, there is deterioration in play and loss of previously acquired language skills and/or adaptive skills (6). Progressive CST signs frequently result in spastic quadriparesis with or without pseudobulbar signs. Movement disorders (rigidity, dystonic posturing, and/or extrapyramidal tremor) may also develop, but are less common and are usually superimposed upon spasticity. Some children develop cerebellar signs. A characteristic facial appearance is an alert and wide-eyed youngster with reduced eye blink and a paucity of spontaneous facial expression and movement ("mask-like" faces). Despite these features, there is little facial weakness evidenced by full movement when crying (1). These youngsters show decreased vocalizations and gestures, and eventually there is progressive apathy and loss of interest in the environment. The end-stage picture is a withdrawn and quadriparetic child with markedly impaired higher cortical functions (6).

Serial head circumference measurements document poor brain growth, and infants and young children develop acquired microcephaly.

Neurologic deterioration in this "subacute PE" is usually insidious. Many patients show a slow decline. Some deteriorate rapidly over weeks, while in others the course is episodic, with periods of deterioration interrupted by variable periods of relative neurologic stability (6) (Fig. 1 and Fig. 1 of ref. 2).

Serial neurodevelopmental evaluations [e.g., Bayley scales of infant development (BSID)] document decline in the mental developmental index (MDI). The mental developmental age (MDA) may initially remain stable, but eventually declines with advancing/end-stage disease (1,2,6).

Plateau

Most children show a more indolent neurologic course (6). Cognitive impairment becomes evident as the rate of mental development declines. Over time, the child may gain further cognitive, language, and socially adaptive skills, but the rate of acquisition of these new skills is slowed. This deviates not only from the norm but in some cases from the child's previous rate of developmental progress (1,6). Serial psychometric evaluations may show a decline in the MDI (or IQ score, depending on the age of the child), even though the mental age remains the same for a period of months or even gradually increases. The MDA mirrors the "raw" scores. There may be an incremental rise over time, but the slope of the curve clearly deviates from the norm (Fig. 2) (1,6,25–29). Some children have more stable, although impaired, cognitive function. Loss of milestones and previously acquired abilities are not observed.

Motor involvement is common, but the progression and severity varies. Some infants and young children develop progressive paraparesis (1,6,25). Early signs are a change of gait. Children begin to toe walk, and show lower-extremity hyperreflexia and increased tone. Some appear to have "a spastic diplegia-type" syndrome (hand use minimally affected), and others have more impairment in fine motor ability; nevertheless, ambulation is maintained for years. In other children, progression is more rapid and some even-

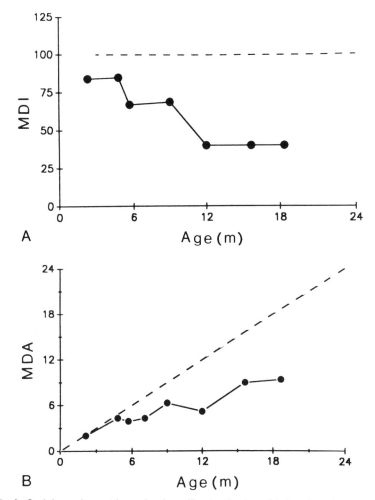

FIG. 2. A: Serial psychometric evaluations [Bayley Scales of Infant Development (BSID)] in this patient show progressive decline in mental developmental index (MDI). Note that scores below 50 are not defined on the BSID. **B:** Serial BSID in the same patient, expressed as equivalent mental developmental age (MDA). Note the plateau between 4 and 8 months of age, decline at 12 months, and a gradual increase in age equivalent thereafter. Note, however, that the slope/curve deviates from the "norm." (From ref. 25.)

tually develop quadriparesis. Motor involvement in some children may be quite mild, manifested only by a mildly spastic gait or hyperreflexia and clumsiness (30). Some children are hypotonic with or without hyperreflexia, with delays in motor milestones (the overlap between this "course" and stable "course" (1,6,25).

Poor brain growth can usually be documented by serial head circumference measurements. Some children will develop acquired microcephaly.

Plateau Followed by Further Deterioration

Some children with a prolonged stable condition ultimately show further neurologic deterioration. The course then becomes similar to that of "subacute PE" (6).

Plateau Followed by Improvement

Some children with "plateau" show "improvement." They steadily acquire additional developmental skills, and their rate of acquisition of new skills accelerates compared to their previous performance. This course then becomes similar to "stable/static" course (6).

School-Age Children

Information on school-age children with congenital HIV-1 infection is limited to clinical observations of small series of patients. Early signs of HIV-1-associated CNS disease and PE are loss of interest in school performance, social withdrawal, increased emotional lability, attention deficits or worsening of attention deficit disorders (ADDs), psychomotor slowing, and worsening of ADD combined with conduct disorders (29,31–33). Over time, motor involvement of varying severity may develop. The most common motor findings are hyperreflexia, with or without increased extensor tone in the lower extremities. Progressive long-tract signs, movement disorders, and cerebellar signs may also occur (1,25,29).

As the disease advances, psychometric tests show a decline in IQ score (6,29,31). In the advanced stages of CNS disease the child has cognitive impairment, and at end stage the child becomes apathetic and abulic (see case 3 in ref. 29).

Adolescents

There is little information currently available on HIV-1-associated CNS disease manifestations in adolescents. It is unknown whether disease differs in early signs and progression from that of adults or children.

"STATIC/STABLE" ENCEPHALOPATHY

In the early years of the AIDS epidemic the term "static" encephalopathy was used to describe a group of youngsters who had (a) histories of developmental abnormalities (delays in acquisition of language and motor milestones), (b) cognitive and/or motor impairment, and (c) no history of "loss of milestones" or progressive neurologic deficits (2,4). Longitudinal studies documented a pattern of continued but impaired development. Developmental and intelligence quotients ranged from low average or borderline to retarded. These scores remained relatively stable during the study period (6,30,39a). The children acquired new skills and abilities at a rate fairly consistent with their level of functioning at initial evaluation, although their rate was slower than expected for age. This was in direct contrast to the deteriorating neurologic pattern described above. Motor dysfunction was also common. The most frequent findings were hyperreflexia, increased tone in the lower extremities, and poor coordination. Some children had a spastic gait (6,30).

It remains unclear what role, if any, HIV-1 plays in this syndrome (1,6,25,39a). It is possible that abnormalities are related to concurrent or previous effects of HIV-1 CNS disease. However, confounding uncontrolled factors (reviewed in ref. 25) have made interpretation and analysis difficult. Preliminary data from one prospective study show that some infants manifest this course in the absence of *in utero* exposure to drugs, prematurity, perinatal complications, or other medical conditions that could explain such findings. These infants and young children have "cognitive impairment" and "delays" in acquisition of motor milestones and mental abilities (26). This suggests that in some cases, HIV-1 compromises the normal developmental process. Further information awaits completion and analysis of large multicenter studies (in progress), as well as better understanding of underlying pathophysiologic mechanisms.

Neuropsychological Profiles of HIV-1-Infected Children

Vertically Acquired HIV-1 Infection

Several domains of cognitive function have been reported to be affected in children with low average/borderline "normal" (IQ > 80) cognitive abilities. These include deficits in perceptual motor function, gait, coordination, attention, and/or expressive language and memory (30–39).

Attentional problems have been reported as an early manifestation of HIV-1-associated dementia in adults. It is not yet clear if attention deficits, with or without hyperactivity, can be attributed to HIV-1 CNS disease in children (see ref. 30 for review). The prevalence of such deficits is relatively high, particularly in children with *in utero* exposure to drugs or who are born prematurely. These confounding conditions occur with significant frequency in this population (see refs. 25 and 31 for review). Whether these behavioral disorders are related to or exacerbated by HIV-1 CNS infection remains to be determined by well-designed studies using suitable controls groups.

Several investigators have noted problems with language, with delayed development of expressive language. Again, well-designed studies of larger cohorts of HIV-1-infected children and appropriate controls will be required to address these issues.

Recently, problems with memory as assessed by the Short-Term Memory subset of the Stanford-Binet 4th edition were noted in a cohort of HIV-1-infected children who had no other evidence of HIV-1-related CNS disease. The HIV-1-infected cohort scored significantly lower than controls. There was no difference between the two groups with regard to language testing or general intelligence (39).

Transfusion-Acquired HIV-1 Infection—Longitudinal Studies in Progress

Prospective neuropsychologic and neurologic studies of children with transfusion-acquired HIV-1 infection are in progress (40–42). Baseline studies in HIV-1-infected hemophiliacs revealed subtle impairments in motor, attentional, memory, and sensory-perceptual functioning, relative to age norms (41,42). However, equally frequent problems were also detected in the age-matched HIV-1-seronegative hemophiliac control patients. Neurological examinations revealed abnormalities in both the HIV-1 infected and non-infected control groups as well, indicating that hemophilia and/or associated treatments may contribute to neurologic dysfunction (41,43).

Cohen et al. (40) studied a cohort of asymptomatic and mildly symptomatic HIV-1-infected children who acquired HIV-1 infection as neonates via blood transfusions. Overall IQ test scores did not differ between the cohort and the HIV-1-seronegative control group. However, the investigators reported small but consistently significant differences in motor speed, visual scanning, and cognitive flexibility. This is in agreement with the studies of Diamond et al. (34) in vertically HIV-1-infected young children (39a).

NEUROIMAGING FINDINGS

Neuroimaging findings are summarized in Table 2. Computed tomographic (CT) examinations of the brain in HIV-1-associated PE usually show variable degrees of cerebral atrophy and white matter (WM) abnormalities (1–7) (see Fig. 3). There may be bilateral symmetrical calcification of the basal ganglia (BG), and less frequently of the frontal WM. Serial studies often show progressive atrophy and WM rarefaction, and in some cases they show progressive calcification of the BG (6,29). It is noteworthy that in some children serial CT studies show no change, even though poor brain growth is demonstrated by serial head circumference and serial clinical examinations show "plateau" or marked delays in mental function (with or without progressive motor findings) (44).

Magnetic resonance imaging (MRI) may reveal atrophy on T1- and T2-weighted images. The T2-weighted images may show abnormal signal inten-

TABLE 2. *Neuroimaging*

Computed tomography
  Cerebral atrophy
    Present in majority of patients
    Serial studies often show progressive atrophy
  Calcification of basal ganglia, ± frontal white matter
    Present in a subset of patients
    Serial studies may show progressive calcification
  White matter
    White matter changes (hypodensity)
    Serial studies often show progressive changes
Magnetic resonance imaging
  Cerebral atrophy
    Present in majority of patients
    Serial studies often show progressive atrophy
  Basal ganglia
    May show abnormal high signal (T2-weighted images) when CT scan is "normal"
    May show abnormal low signal (T2-weighted images) when CT scan shows calcification
  White matter
    May show abnormal high signal (T2 weighted images)

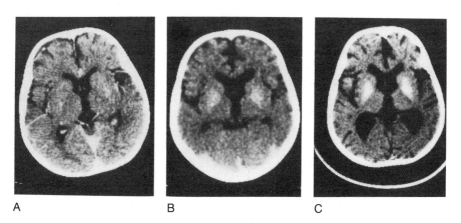

A   B   C

FIG. 3. A: CT scan following intravenous injection of contrast material in a 15-month-old boy with "developmental delays" shows evidence of enhancement in the left basal ganglia regions medial to the enhancing middle cerebral arterial branches in the left sylvian fissure. **B:** Seven months later, punctate and diffuse zones of calcification are present bilaterally in the basal ganglia. There is also evidence of progressive cerebral atrophy. During the 7-month period the child made little developmental progress. **C:** After an additional 8 months, CT scan without contrast shows that both basal ganglia calcification and cerebral atrophy have increased. Neurologic examination showed progressive CST signs and loss of previously acquired mental and motor skills. (Modified from ref. 29.)

sity in the WM and deep gray structures (1,25,29). Tardieu et al. (45) found MRI abnormalities in 40 percent of HIV-1-infected children, in both neurologically normal and symptomatic children. The authors' suggested that this reflected HIV-1 CNS infection. Patients with clinical evidence of HIV-1-associated CNS disease were found to have leukomalacia and cerebral atrophy (45).

MRI is more sensitive to image WM abnormalities and maturational changes in myelination. CT is more sensitive to detect calcification. Cerebral atrophy is well demonstrated by both techniques.

CEREBROSPINAL FLUID STUDIES

Cerebrospinal fluid (CSF) profiles are usually normal, although a mild pleocytosis and elevated protein content have been described. In our experience these findings appear to correlate with neuroimaging abnormalities of marked WM changes and are found more frequently in children during later stages of HIV-1-associated PE or during the development of spastic paraparesis.

HIV-1 has been recovered from the CSF of neurologically normal children, as well as from the CSF of those with HIV-1-related CNS disease. Detectable levels of HIV-1 antigen, intrathecal production of anti-HIV-1 antibodies, oligoclonal bands, and cytokines have been detected in the CSF of some children with PE and static encephalopathy, as well as in the CSF of children with normal neurological exams (5,11,46–51). These findings helped establish that the CNS was infected with HIV-1. They also indicated early CNS invasion. Of interest, interleukin 6 and interleukin 1β have been detected in the CSF of children with PE but not in the CSF of neurologically asymptomatic patients. The prognostic significance of these findings is unclear, and current data are limited to a few cross-sectional studies of small numbers of patients.

NEUROPHYSIOLOGIC STUDIES

Electroencephalographic studies in children with HIV-1-associated PE may show diffuse, mild to moderate slowing of background rhythm (1,2). Abnormal evoked potentials, increased central latencies (prolongation of the 1-V interweave latency), and abnormal response to increased rate of stimulation have also been described in some children with PE (1,2,4).

NEUROPATHOLOGIC FINDINGS

Gross Pathology

Postmortem findings include variable degrees of cerebral atrophy and ventricular enlargement (7,8,52) (see Table 3).

TABLE 3. *Neuropathology*

Brain
  Gross
    Variable degrees of cerebral atrophy
    Ventricular enlargement
    Widening of sulci
    Attenuation of deep cerebral white matter
  Microscopic
    HIV-1 encephalitis
      Foci of inflammatory cells
      Microglia, macrophages, multinucleated giant cells
    HIV-1 leukoencephalopathy
      Myelin loss, reactive astrogliosis, macrophages, multinucleated giant cells
    Calcific vasculopathy
      Basal ganglia, ± white matter
      Mineralization in walls of blood vessels
Spinal cord
  Corticospinal tract "degeneration"
    "Axonopathy type"
    "Myelinopathy type"
  Myelitis
  Vacuolar myelopathy

Microscopic Pathology

HIV Encephalitis

HIV encephalitis characterized by multiple disseminated foci of microglia, macrophages, and multinucleated giant cells have been described similarly in children's brains and in those of adults (53,54). They are most often scattered throughout the deep gray nuclei, white matter, and brainstem. Although this is one of the most striking pathologic findings, it appears to be a more frequent finding in adults than in young children (8,52,55,56).

Calcific Vasculopathy

Calcific BG vasculopathy is probably the most characteristic and consistent neuropathologic finding (8,29) (see Fig. 4). In some cases, mineralization is also noted in vessels of the centrum semiovale (8). Although calcification of the BG is frequently seen with HIV encephalitis, this association is not invariable. Many cases have BG calcification without inflammatory disease and with no sign of acute infection (8). Nevertheless, accompanying WM changes and gliosis are common.

White Matter Pathology

By definition, HIV leukoencephalopathy (53) (diffuse staining pallor or myelin) involves diffuse damage to WM (including myelin loss, reactive

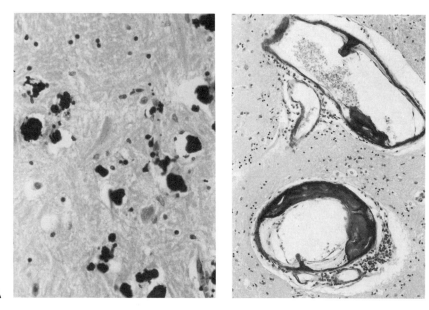

FIG. 4. A: Capillary walls display granular deposits of calcium. Some of the granules have coalesced into larger, irregular calcific nodules; note relative preservation of neurons in between (hematoxylin and eosin, ×100). **B:** Branches of lenticulostriate vessels show massive calcification (hematoxylin and eosin, ×40). (From ref. 29.)

astrogliosis, and presence of macrophages and multinucleated giant cells), but the presence of little or no inflammatory infiltrates is frequently seen in pediatric AIDS (7,8).

Spinal Cord

Unlike adults with HIV-associated myelopathy, the most common and striking pathologic finding in the spinal cord of young children is myelin pallor restricted to the CST (8,57) (see Fig. 5). In some cases there is both axonal and myelin pathology, suggesting that CST findings are due to axonal injury. In others, pathologic findings are predominantly related to myelin. Because the CST are the last tracts to myelinate, it has been hypothesized that HIV-1 in some way (direct or indirect) affects the developmental–maturational process. Injury may occur to myelinating glial cells, newly formed myelin, or even antenatally to proliferating glial precursor cells (57).

Vacuolar myelopathy has been reported infrequently, most often in older children (58).

Myelitis has also been described, but is not a common finding.

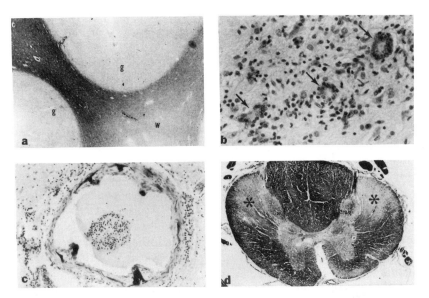

FIG. 5. **(a)** Section of deep cerebral white matter (W) shows staining pallor on myelin stain; g indicates gray matter (luxol fast blue, original magnification ×20). **(b)** Section of basal ganglia shows three multinucleated giant cells *(arrows)* (hematoxylin and eosin, original magnification ×320). **(c)** Large artery in basal ganglia shows multifocal intimal proliferation with dystrophic calcification (hematoxylin and eosin, original magnification ×200). **(d)** Spinal cord cross section with myelin stain shows pallor in both lateral *(asterisks)* and anterior funiculi (luxol fast blue, original magnification ×8). (From ref. 6.)

LOCALIZATION

HIV-1 localizes to monocytes, macrophages, multinucleated cells, and microglia (see refs. 53 and 59 for review). HIV-1 gp-41-positive microglia associated with HIV encephalitis have a characteristic distribution. They are most numerous in deep gray matter [globus pallidus (medial > lateral), corpus striatum, putamen, and thalamus], white matter, ventral midbrain, substantia nigra, and dentate nuclei of the cerebellum. Once again this finding is more common in adults than in children (56).

PATHOPHYSIOLOGY

Although the above syndrome complexes are believed to be due to HIV-1 CNS infection, underlying pathophysiologic mechanisms are not yet elucidated. They remain a focus of ongoing research efforts.

It is unclear whether one or several neuropathophysiologic processes are involved in various syndromes. It is most likely that different pathogenetic mechanisms account, at least in part, for different clinical expressions and patterns of HIV-1-associated CNS disease.

Distinct clinical CNS syndromes may in some subsets of patients reflect a continuum of the disease process, with different stages of disease progression. In others, clinical findings may reflect separate and distinct pathologic processes. In still other subsets of patients, these processes may be interlinked and manifest clinically by overlapping signs and symptoms.

The time and route of HIV-1 CNS invasion remain uncertain. In some patients the CNS is probably infected quite early. The timing of maternal–fetal transmission (i.e., perinatal versus during gestation, and which trimester) appears to vary with subsets of patients. Therefore, the maturational stage of CNS development exposed to direct or indirect local effects will also vary, and this is likely to influence different patterns of HIV-1 CNS disease.

It is unknown whether CNS invasion occurs by entry of infected macrophages, entry of cell-free virus, infection of endothelial cells, or invasion of choroid plexus. The frequent finding of calcific vasopathy suggests a hematogenous route consistent with early CNS infection (6). It also points to the vulnerability of this immature vasculature, and perhaps to selective tropism for BG and its resident microglia (56) (see above).

Cerebral atrophy is a common finding in both adults and children. Recent quantitative and morphometric studies in adults have identified (a) loss of neurons with a frontal and temporal predominance and (b) loss of dendritic arborizations (60–63). Similar studies have not been performed in pediatric AIDS. However, it is tempting to speculate that similar abnormalities result in poor brain growth and acquired microcephaly. Interference with synaptogenesis would explain (in part) developmental delays and cognitive impairment.

THERAPY

Antiretroviral agents offer promising therapeutic interventions. Improvements in cognitive and behavioral function were documented in the initial clinical trials of 3′-azido-2′,3′-dideoxythymidine (AZT), administered via continuous parenteral infusion and in some children treated with orally administered agents (64–70). Not all children show neurologic "improvement" with intermittent orally administered antiretroviral agents, although stabilization has been noted (67,70,71). Unfortunately, some children who initially seem to have a favorable response to oral antiretroviral therapy subsequently "relapse" with clinical and neuroimaging signs of HIV-1-associated CNS disease(s) (72). Clinical trials in progress are investigating newer antiretroviral agents, various dosages, combination drug therapies, immunomodulating therapies, and other therapeutic approaches. New protocols are also in development. Rehabilitation programs, early infant intervention programs, therapeutic nursery schools, and special educational classes are being examined in parallel with these pharmacologic studies.

DIAGNOSIS

The diagnosis of HIV-1-associated CNS disease, including differential diagnosis, involves a careful medical and developmental history, HIV-1 systemic disease history, current immunologic status, neurological examination, psychological assessment, and neuroimaging studies (25).

The diagnosis of HIV-1-associated PE is relatively straightforward if the patient has been followed prospectively. Examination reveals progressive motor dysfunction and/or cognitive impairment (when other causes have been ruled out by appropriate studies). The diagnosis is also fairly straightforward if the child presents with motor deficits and if progression of motor impairment can be documented. Documentation is obtained from a careful review of medical records or photographs (again, other causes for progressive motor impairment must be excluded). However, diagnostic difficulties often arise because most HIV-1-infected youngsters are not followed from birth or infancy with formal neurologic and neuropsychologic evaluations. Often there is no description of a neurologic or developmental examination in medical records. The clinician may note "delays" in mental or motor development or both, with or without other reflex and tonal abnormalities, at initial evaluation. Because the rate of neurologic and developmental impairment in this population is high, it is often impossible for the clinician to ascribe the findings to HIV-1 CNS disease and early signs of PE rather than to other factors. The child should then have a formal psychological assessment with reevaluation by the neurologist and psychologist in 2–4 months (25).

Neuroimaging studies are critical. If BG calcification or cerebral atrophy (in the absence of documented perinatal complications, steroid use, or other known causes for atrophy) is present, it is probable that the child has HIV-1 CNS disease. Follow-up neuroimaging studies should be obtained, in addition to the above-mentioned serial neurological and psychological evaluations.

Head circumference measurements are another very useful tool. It is our experience that a careful review of medical records will document at least one or two head circumference measurements. This allows the examiner to plot serial measurements. The pattern of downward deviation with crossing of percentile curves makes the diagnosis more probable. This is especially true if acquired microcephaly (at or less than the second percentile) is documented. Neuroimaging evidence of atrophy, accompanied by acquired microcephaly, strongly supports diagnosis.

NEUROEPIDEMIOLOGY

The true incidence of HIV-1-related CNS disease is not known. Recently Tovo et al. estimated a 23.8 percent rate in their study of a large cohort of 433 HIV-1 perinatally infected P-2 children (73). Information also comes from retrospective studies, longitudinal clinical studies, and preliminary data from prospective studies that are still in progress (5–7,50,74,75).

Investigations early in the AIDS epidemic that give à 55–62 percent prevalence rate were conducted in cohorts of children with advanced HIV-1 infection (most of the children had OIs). In the past few years, cohorts have also included children with less symptomatic and asymptomatic HIV-1 infection, with an 8–19.6 percent estimated rate. Although cohorts have been dissimilar, review of the literature suggests that HIV-1-associated CNS disease and PE parallels progression and severity of immunodeficiency and systemic disease. However, it is also very clear that some patients do develop HIV-1-associated CNS disease syndromes in the absence of other major AIDS-defining diseases, severe immunodeficiency, or severely depressed CD4 cell counts (26,27,74,76).

FUTURE RESEARCH

HIV-1-associated CNS disease frequently complicates the course of HIV-1 infection in infants and children. Neurologic dysfunction in these young patients adds significantly to the morbidity of the disease and is often

TABLE 4. *Research issues*[a]

Prevention of maternal HIV-1 infection
Prevention of maternal–fetal transmission
Timing of congenital HIV-1 infection
Timing and route of HIV-1 CNS invasion
Pathophysiologic mechanisms of HIV-1 associated CNS diseases
Direct
Indirect
Developing nervous system
Further delineation of HIV-1-associated CNS disease syndromes
Neurological
Neuropsychological
Behavioral
Correlation with neuroimaging
Correlation with neurophysiology
Surrogate markers
Uniform measures of mental and motor function
Therapy
Antiretroviral
Immunomodulation
Rehabilitation

[a] List not complete.

a devastating complication (1). Continuing research efforts focus on many aspects of HIV-1-associated CNS disease (Table 4).

In order to care for these children and to design rational approaches for treatment and prevention, it is now critical to develop a better understanding of how HIV-1 affects the developing nervous system (25). Much study will be required, and much remains to be learned.

REFERENCES

1. Belman AL. AIDS and pediatric neurology. *Neurol Clin North Am* 1990;8:571–603.
2. Belman AL, Ultmann MH, Horoupian D, et al. Neurologic complications in infants and children with acquired immune deficiency syndrome. *Ann Neurol* 1985;18:560–566.
3. Epstein LG, Sharer LR, Joshi VV, et al. Progressive encephalopathy in children with acquired immune deficiency syndrome. *Ann Neurol* 1985;17:488–496.
4. Ultmann MH, Belman AL, Ruff HA, Novick BE, Cone-Wesson B, Cohen HJ, Rubinstein A. Develomental abnormalities in infants and children with acquired immune deficiency syndrome (AIDS) and AIDS-related complex. *Dev Med Child Neurol* 1985;27:563–571.
5. Epstein LG, Sharer LR, Oleske JM, et al. Neurologic manifestations of human immunodeficiency virus infection in children. *Pediatrics* 1986;78:678–687.
6. Belman AL, Diamond G, Dickson D, et al. Pediatric AIDS: neurologic syndromes. *Am J Dis Child* 1988;142:29–35.
7. Epstein LG, Sharer LR, Goudsmit J. Neurological and neuropathological features of HIV in children. *Ann Neurol* 1988;23(suppl):S19–S23.
8. Dickson DW, Belman AL, Park YD, et al. Central nervous system pathology in pediatric AIDS: an autopsy study. *APMIS* 1989;8(suppl):40–57.
9. Sharer LR, Epstein LG, Cho ES, et al. Pathologic features of AIDS encephalopathy in children: evidence for LAV/HTLV-III infection of the brain. *Hum Pathol* 1986;17:271–284.
10. Ho DD, Rota TR, Schooley RT, et al. Isolation of HTLV-III from CSF and neural tissues of patients with AIDS related neurologic syndromes. *N Engl J Med* 1985;313:1493–1497.
11. Hutto C, Scott G, Parks E, Fischel M, Parks W. Cerebrospinal fluid (CSF) studies in adults and pediatric HIV infections. In: III International Conference on AIDS, Washington, DC, June 1–5, 1989, p. 38.
12. Levy JA, Shimabukuro J, Hollander H, et al. Isolation of AIDS associated retrovirus from cerebrospinal fluid and brain of patients with neurological symptoms. *Lancet* 1985;2:586–588.
13. Goudsmit J, Wolters EC, Bakker M, et al. Intrathecal synthesis of antibodies to HTLV-III in patients without AIDS or AIDS related complex. *Br Med J* 1986;292:1231–1234.
14. Resnick L, DiMarzo-Veronese F, Schupbach J, et al. Intra-blood-brain barrier synthesis of HTLV-III specific IgG in patients with neurologic symptoms associated with AIDS or AIDS-related complex. *N Engl J Med* 1985;313:1498–1504.
15. Epstein LG, Sharer LR, Cho S-E, et al. HTLV-III/LAV-like retrovirus particles in the brains of patients with AIDS encephalopathy. *AIDS Res* 1985;1:477–454.
16. Wiley CA, Schrier RD, Nelson AS, et al. Cellular localization of human immunodeficiency virus infection within the brains of acquired immune deficiency syndrome patients. *Proc Natl Acad Sci USA* 1986;83:7089–7093.
17. Gabuzda DH, Ho DD, de la Monte, et al. Immunohistochemical identification of HTLV-III antigen in brain of patients with AIDS. *Ann Neurol* 1986;20:289–295.
18. Koenig S, Gendelman HE, Orenstein JM, et al. Detection of AIDS virus in macrophage in brain tissue from AIDS patients with encephalopathy. *Science* 1986;233:109.
19. Pumarola-Sune T, Navia BA, Cordon-Cardo D, et al. HIV antigen in the brains of patients with the AIDS dementia complex. *Ann Neurol* 1987;21:490–496.
20. Shaw GM, Harper ME, Hahn BH, et al. HTLV-III infection in brains of children and adults with AIDS encephalopathy. *Science* 1985;227:177–181.
21. Gonda MA, Wong-Stall F, Gallo RC, et al. Sequence homology and morphologic similarity of HTLV-III and visna virus, a pathogenic lentivirus. *Science* 1985;227:173–177.

22. Navia BA, Jordon BD, Price RW. The AIDS dementia complex. I. Clinical features. *Ann Neurol* 1986;19:517–524.
23. Belman AL, Dickson DW. In: Stuber ML, ed. *Neurologic aspects in children with AIDS.* Washington, DC: American Psychiatric Press, 1992:89–106.
24. American Academy of Neurology AIDS Task Force. Nomenclature and research case definitions for neurologic manifestations of human immunodeficiency virus type I. *Neurology* 1991;41:778–785.
25. Belman AL. AIDS and the child's central nervous system. *Pediatr Clin North Am* 1992; 39:691–714.
26. Belman AL, Marcus J, Muenz L, et al. Neurologic status of infants born to HIV-1 infected mothers and their controls: a prospective study from birth to 24 months of age [Abstract]. *Neurology* 1993;43:A347.
27. Belman AL, Calvelli T, Nozyce M, et al. Neurologic and immunologic correlates in infants with vertically transmitted HIV infection. *Neurology* 1990;1(suppl):40:409.
28. Belman AL, Diamond G, Park Y, et al. Perinatal HIV infection: a prospective longitudinal study of the initial CNS signs. *Neurology* 1989;39(suppl):278–279.
29. Belman AL, Lantos G, Horoupian D, et al. AIDS: calcification of the basal ganglia in infants and children. *Neurology* 1986;36:1192–1199.
30. Ultmann MH, Diamond G, Ruff HA, Belman AL, et al. Developmental abnormalities in infants and children with acquired immune deficiency syndrome (AIDS): a follow up study. *Int J Neurosci* 1987;32:661–667.
31. Brouwers E, Belman AL, Epstein L. Central nervous system involvement: manifestations and evaluation. In: Pizzo PA, Wilfert CM, eds. *Pediatric AIDS: the challenge of HIV infection in infants, children and adolescents.* Baltimore: Williams & Wilkins, 1990; 318–335.
32. Lifschitz M, Hanson C, Wilson G, Shearer WT. Behavioral changes in children with human immunodeficiency virus (HIV) infection. T.B.P. 175. In: V International Conference on AIDS, Montreal, June 4–9, 1989.
33. Moss H, Wolters P, Eddy J, Wiener L, Pizzo P, Brouwers P. The effects of encephalopathy and AZT treatment on the social and emotional behavior of pediatric AIDS patients. In: V International Conference on AIDS, Montreal, June 4–9, 1989.
34. Diamond GW, Kaufman J, Belman AL, et al. Characterization of cognitive functioning in a subgroup of children with congenital HIV infection. *Arch Clin Neuropsychol* 1987;2:1–16.
35. Condini A, Axia G, Viero A, Laverda AM, et al. Study of language in HIV infected Italian children [Abstract]. In: *Neuroscience of HIV-1 infection.* Satellite Conference, VII International Conference on AIDS, Padova, Italy, 1991;25.
36. Wolters P, et al. In: VIII International Conference on AIDS, Florence, Italy, June 1991.
37. Nozyce M, Diamond G, Belman A, et al. The course of neurodevelopmental functioning in the infants of IVDA and HIV-seropositive parents. M.B.O.41. In: V International Conference on AIDS, Montreal, June 4–9, 1989.
38. Hittelman J, Fikrig S, Mendez H, et al. Neurodevelopmental assessment of children with symptomatic HIV infection. T.B.P.180. In: V International Conference on AIDS, Montreal, June 4–9, 1989.
39. Havens J, Whitaker JA, Feldman J, Alverada MA. A controlled study of cognitive and language function in school age HIV-infected children [Abstract]. New York Acad of Science, Washington, DC, 1992.
39a. Diamond GW, Gurdin P, Wiznia AA, Belman AL, et al. Effects of congenital HIV infection on neurodevelopmental status of babies in foster care. *Dev Med Child Neurol* 1990;32: 399–1005.
40. Cohen SL, Mundy T, Kaarassik B, et al. Neuropsychological functioning in children with HIV-1 infected through neonatal blood transfusion. *Pediatrics* 1991;88:58–68.
41. Papavasiliou A, Aronis S, Stamboulis E, et al. Involvement of central and peripheral nervous system of HIV-infected hemophilic children [Abstract]. In: *Neuroscience of HIV-1 infection.* Satellite Conference, VII International Conference on AIDS, Padova, Italy, 1991; 49.
42. Whitt JK, Hooper SR, Tennison MB, et al. Longitudinal patterns of neuropsychologic functioning in HIV-infected children with hemophilia [Abstract]. In: *Neuroscience of HIV-1 Infection.* Satellite Conference, VII International Conference on AIDS, Padova, Italy, 1991;6611.

43. Bale J, Garg B, Tilton A, et al. Neurologic examination in hemophilic subjects. Relationship to human immunodeficiency virus serostatus. *Ann Neurol* 1991;30:508.
44. Wiley CA, Belman AL, Dickson D, Rubinstein A, Nelson JA. Human immunodeficiency virus within the brains of children with AIDS. *Clin Neuropathol* 1990;1:1–6.
45. Tardieu M, Blanche W, Bruneke F, et al. Cerebral MRI studies in HIV-1 infected children born to seropositive mothers. In: *Neuroscience of HIV-1 infection*. Satellite Conference, VII International Conference on AIDS, Padova, Italy, 1991;27.
46. Epstein LG, Goudsmit J, Paul DA, et al. Expression of human immunodeficiency virus in cerebrospinal fluid of children with progressive encephalopathy. *Ann Neurol* 1987;21: 397–401.
47. Gallo P, Laverda AM, DeRossi A, et al. Immunological markers in the cerebrospinal fluid of HIV-1 infected children. *Acta Pediatr Scand* 1991;80:659–666.
48. Laverda AM, Gallo P, Tavolato B, et al. Cerebrospinal fluid findings in neurologically symptomatic and asymptomatic HIV-1 infected children [Abstract]. In: *Neuroscience of HIV-1 infection*. Satellite Conference VII International Conference on AIDS, Padova, Italy, 1991;120.
49. Mintz M, Rapaport R, Oleske M, et al. Elevated serum levels of tumor necrosis factor are associated with progressive encephalopathy in children with acquired immunodeficiency syndrome. *ACJC* 1989;143:771–774.
50. Blanche S, Tardieu M, Duliege AM, et al. Longitudinal study of 94 symptomatic infants with materno fetal HIV infection: evidence for a bimodal expression of clinical and biological symptoms. *Am J Dis Child* 1990;144:1210–1215.
51. Epstein LG, Sharer LR, Oleske JM, et al. Neurologic manifestations of human immunodeficiency virus infection in children. *Pediatrics* 1986;78:678–687.
52. Kozlowski PB, Sher JH, Rao C, et al. Central nervous system in Pediatric AIDS Registry [Abstract]. In: *Pediatric AIDS: clinical, pathologic and basic science perspectives*. New York Academy of Sciences, 1991;11-3.
53. Budka H. Neuropathology of human immunodeficiency virus infection. *Brain Pathol* 1991; 1:163–175.
54. Budka H, Wiley CA, Kleihues P, et al. A HIV-associated disease of the nervous system: review of nomenclature and proposal for neuropathology-based terminology. *Brain Pathology* 1991;1:143–152.
55. Vazeux R, Lacrois-Ciaudo C, Blanche S, et al. Low levels of human immunodeficiency virus replication in the brain tissue of children with severe acquired immunodeficiency syndrome encephalopathy. *Am J Pathol* 1992;140:137–144.
56. Kure K, Weidenheim KM, Lyman WD, Dickson DW. Morphology and distribution of HIV-1 qp 41 positive microglia in subacute AIDS encephalitis. *Acta Neuropathol (Berl)* 1990; 80:393–400.
57. Dickson DW, Belman AL, Kim TS, Horoupian D, Rubinstein A. Spinal cord pathology in pediatric acquired immunodeficiency syndrome. *Neurology* 1989;39:227–235.
58. Sharer LR, Dowling PC, Michaels J, et al. Spinal cord disease in children with HIV-1 infection: a combined molecular and neuropathological study. *Neuropathol Appl Neurobiol* 1990;16:317–331.
59. Johnson RT, McArthur JC, Narayan O. The neurobiology of human immunodeficiency virus infections. *FASEB J* 1988;2:2970–2981.
60. Wiley CA, Masliah JE, et al. Neocortical damage during HIV infection. *Ann Neurol* 1991; 29:651–657.
61. Everal IP, Luthert PJ, Lantos PL. Neuronal loss in the frontal cortex in HIV infection. *Lancet* 1991;337:1119–1121.
62. Ketzier JS, Weis JS, Haug H, Budka H. Loss of neurons in the frontal cortex in AIDS brains. *Acta Neuropathol (Berl)* 1990;80:92–94.
63. Mesliah E, Ge N, Morey M, Deterese R, Terry RD, Wiley C. Cortical dendritic pathology in human immunodeficiency virus encephalitis. *Lab Invest* 1992;66:285–291.
64. Pizzo PA, Eddy J, Balis FM, et al. Effect of continuous intravenous infusion of Zidovudine (AZT) in children with symptomatic HIV infection. *N Engl J Med* 1988;319:889–896.
65. Decarli C, Fugate L, Falloon J, et al. Brain growth and cognitive improvement in children with HIV induced encephalopathy after 6 months of continuous infusion therapy. *SAIDS* 1991;4:585–592.

66. Brouwers P, Moss H, Wolters P, et al. Effect of continuous-infusion zidovudine therapy on neuropsychologic functioning in children with symptomatic human immunodeficiency virus infection. *J Pediatr* 1990;117:980–985.
67. McKinney RE, Maha MA, Conners EM, et al. A multicenter trial of oral zidovudine in children with advanced HIV disease. *N Engl J Med* 1991;324:1018–1025.
68. Butler KM, Husson RN, Balis RM, et al. Dideoxyinosin in children with symptomic human immunodeficiency virus infection. *N Engl J Med* 1990;324:137–144.
69. Pizzo PA, Butler K, Balis F, et al. Dideoxycytidine alone and in an alternating schedule with zidovudine in children with symptomatic human immunodeficiency virus infection. *J Pediatr* 1990;117:799–808.
70. Schmitt B, Seeger J, Kreuz W, Enenkel S, Iacobi G. Central nervous system involvement in children with HIV infection. *Dev Med Child Neurol* 1991;33:535–540.
71. Nozyce M, Hoberman M, Arpade S, et al. The effects of oral AZT on neurodevelopmental, immunological and clinical outcomes in vertically HIV infected children [Abstract]. In: New York Academy of Sciences, 1992. Pediatric AIDS: Clinical and Basic Science Perspectives Nov. 18–21, 1992, Washington.
72. Mintz M, Epstein LG. Neurologic manifestations, clinical features and therapeutic approaches. *Semin Neurol* 1992;12:51–56.
73. Tovo PA, de Martino M, Gabiano C, et al. Prognostic factors in survival in children with perinatal HIV-1 infection. Italian Register for HIV Infection in Children. *Lancet* 1992;339:1249.
74. Scott G. Survival in children with perinatally acquired human immunodeficiency virus type infection. *N Engl J Med* 1989;3211:1791–1796.
75. European Collaborative Study. Cogo P, Laverda AM, Ades ARE, et al. Neurologic signs in young children with human immunodeficiency virus infection. *Pediatr Infect Dis J* 1990;9:402–406.
76. Calvelli TA, Belman AL, Bueti C, Golodner M, Rubinstein A. Divergence of onset of neurologic and immunologic impairment in infants born to HIV seropositive mothers. T.B.P.184. In: V International Conference on AIDS, Montreal, June 4–9, 1989.

HIV, AIDS and the Brain, edited by
R. W. Price and S. W. Perry.
Raven Press, Ltd., New York © 1994.

17

Questions and Prospects Related to HIV-1 and the Brain

Richard T. Johnson

Department of Neurology, Johns Hopkins University School of Medicine, Johns Hopkins Hospital, Baltimore, MD 21287

In the summer of 1981, there was a lull in the area of clinical and laboratory investigation that has become known as *neurovirology*. During the 1950s, the availability of tissue culture in diagnostic laboratories led to an extraordinary increase in the number of viruses associated with acute neurological diseases; the number of different viruses causing meningitis and encephalitis grew from a handful to over a hundred (1). During the 1960s, interest turned to slow infections; over a brief period of 5 years, four chronic neurologic diseases proved to be associated with transmissible agents. The first, the association of a papovavirus with progressive multifocal leukoencephalopathy, was presented at the 1964 meeting of the ARNMD at the Roosevelt Hotel (2). In 1965, measles-like particles were found in subacute sclerosing panencephalitis (3). In 1967 and 1968, kuru and Creutzfeldt–Jakob disease were transmitted to chimpanzees (4,5). At the 1964 meeting of this association, some predicted that many neurological diseases might prove to be of a viral etiology, including amyotropic lateral sclerosis, multiple sclerosis, Parkinson's disease, and others (6).

Then came the lull. A few new agents appeared; for example, in 1969 a new enterovirus appeared causing acute hemorrhagic conjunctivitis and a poliomyelitis syndrome (7), but this agent appeared and faded over a single decade. In 1975, another slow infection, chronic panencephalitis associated with rubella virus, was reported (8,9), but that disease has proved to be extraordinarily rare. Interest in neurovirology waned.

In the summer of 1981, the strange occurrences of Kaposi's sarcoma and pneumocystis pneumonia were noted in otherwise healthy, young gay men (10,11). No one could have predicted that these observations portended an epidemic of nervous system disease that would eclipse all prior viral infections of the nervous system in numbers of cases or in the diversity of syndromes. During the early years of the acquired immunodeficiency disease

(AIDS) epidemic, interest focused on the search for and recovery of the causative agent and study of the hematological, infectious disease and oncological manifestations of the infection. Neurological interest was limited to the opportunistic infections such as unusual manifestations of toxoplasmosis and cryptococcosis and to the high rates of cerebral lymphoma (12).

In 1985 this focus changed. Human immunodeficiency virus (HIV) was isolated from the brain, cerebrospinal fluid (CSF), and peripheral nerve of AIDS patients with neurological diseases (13,14). HIV RNA was demonstrated in microglial nodules of the brains of HIV-infected individuals, and Southern blot analysis showed HIV DNA in the brain at higher levels than found in lymph node, spleen, or lung (15). Finally, increased levels of HIV antibodies were found in the CSF indicating intrathecal antibody synthesis (16). In the same year the virus of AIDS [until then often called human T-lymphotropic virus type III (HTLV III)] was shown to be a lentivirus, a subfamily of retroviruses all of which cause subacute encephalitis (17).

EARLY ISSUES

A variety of diseases are not associated with obvious opportunistic infections and may be the direct result of HIV infection. These diseases involve both the central and peripheral nervous systems. Some—such as acute encephalopathy (18) or acute Guillain–Barré syndrome (19)—occur early in the disease, even at the time of seroconversion. Some occur during the asymptomatic incubation period, such as episodes of aseptic meningitis with chronic headache, episodes of acute or chronic demyelinating polyneuritis, or mononeuritis multiplex (20). The most devastating diseases are seen in patients with AIDS. Dementia is seen in 15–20 percent of patients with AIDS in cross-sectional studies (20) and in up to nearly 70 percent in some autopsy series (21). Signs of myelopathy are found in 10–20 percent of AIDS patients, but vacuolar myelopathy is seen in nearly half of patients by pathological examination (JD Glass, *unpublished observations*). The predominantly sensory neuropathy causes pain in about half of the patients, but pathological evidence of axonal degeneration is found in all patients (22).

This number of diverse neurological syndromes due to a single viral agent is unique. In the past, the concept that measles virus could produce three clinically, pathologically, and virologically distinctive neurological diseases

TABLE 1. *Questions—mid-1980s*

- What is the spectrum of HIV-associated neurological disease?
- How often and how early is the nervous system infected?
- Does infection of CNS initiate progressive cognitive decline?

was regarded with skepticism. Yet an acute demyelinating autoimmune encephalitis develops within a few days after the rash in 1 in 1000 children, a late chronic defective infection of brain (subacute sclerosing panencephalitis) slowly evolves in 1 in 1,000,000 children many years after the acute infection, and an occasional subacute disease with replication of virus in the brain is found in patients with severe immunodeficiency (23). During HIV infection, six to eight varied neurological diseases occur at different times showing very diverse pathologies and suggesting, as in measles, the possibility of different pathogenetic mechanisms (24).

With the recovery of HIV from neural tissues of patients with neurologic disease, the question arose as to whether infection of the nervous system was a late event possibly resulting from virus being carried in by inflammatory cells responding to opportunistic infections. Studies of asymptomatic patients, particularly those of the Multicenter AIDS Cohort Study, showed that infection of the nervous system occurred early during the asymptomatic phase, if not at the time of seroconversion, and that abnormalities in the spinal fluid indicating infection were found in the majority of asymptomatic, gay men (25).

Demonstration of early and frequent nervous system infection in turn led to public concern that a slow deterioration of cognitive function might evolve from the time of the initial infection and ultimately progress to severe dementia in patients with AIDS. Questions were raised by a number of governments to the World Health Organization. The British queried mandatory testing of physicians in fear of their loss of judgment, and the French suggested the testing of all pilots. Over the next several years, most cross-sectional studies showed that seropositive asymptomatic persons were not different on neuropsychological tests from carefully matched seronegative controls (26,27), and most longitudinal studies showed stable function on tests until severe immunodeficiency had developed (28). In 1988 the World Health Organization (29) concluded that, "At present there is no evidence for an increase in clinically significant, neuropsychiatric abnormalities in CDC groups 2 and 3, HIV-1-positive (otherwise asymptomatic individuals) as compared to HIV-1-seronegative controls. Therefore, there is no justification for HIV serological screening as a strategy for detecting such functional impairment in asymptomatic persons."

CLINICAL NEUROLOGICAL DISEASES

A number of aspects of the clinical diseases and their pathological substrate have yet to be clarified. One is why individual patients develop one disease and not another. Are these factors environmental, or are they dependent on the host or the virus? Certain opportunistic infections are more frequent in particular geographic areas, depending on exposure. Kaposi's

TABLE 2. *Clinical questions*

- What are the determinants of different clinical diseases?
- Are dementia, myelopathy, and peripheral neuropathy linked?
- What is the correlation of clinical findings to pathological changes?
- When and how do antiviral agents modify the course of these diseases?

sarcoma is seen primarily in the HIV-infected gay population and is much less frequent among infected intravenous drug users, but the reason for this difference is unknown.

The neurological diseases do not seem to be different between infected gay men and intravenous drug users (30). However, there are striking differences in children infected transplacentally or perinatally. HIV encephalitis has a shorter incubation period and a more destructive pathology (31,32), presumably because of the immaturity of the central nervous system or immaturity of host immune responses. Conversely, infected children only rarely develop vacuolar myelopathy and probably have less peripheral neuropathy, indicating that these complications may be dependent on environmental or host factors (33).

A prospective clinical and pathological study has shown a rather poor correlation between clinical findings and pathological changes (JD Glass, *unpublished observations*). Those patients with all of the pathological findings of HIV encephalitis were uniformly demented. Conversely, many patients with dementia, even severe dementia, failed to show the diffuse myelin pallor and multinucleated giant cells included in the definition of HIV encephalitis. Only mild gliosis or microglia nodules were found, and these findings are common in asymptomatic HIV-infected patients. Clearly, physiological changes occur that are as yet undefined and may be undefinable at a light microscopic level.

Occurrence of neuropsychiatric changes without pathological changes is not surprising in view of the finding that these cognitive deficits are, in part, reversible with antiviral drugs. Intelligence quotients have been shown to rise in children (34), and abnormalities on neuropsychological tests have disappeared in adults after treatment with zidovudine (AZT) (35). It has also been suggested that patients treated with antiviral agents may show less intense pathological changes at autopsy (36). It remains uncertain whether or not any improvement in the clinical or pathological features of the myelopathies and neuropathies results from AZT or other antiviral therapy.

VIROLOGICAL ISSUES

Most studies in adults suggest that infection with HIV virus in the brain is limited to cells of the macrophage lineage: macrophages, perivascular macrophages, and microglia. Nevertheless, the question persists whether

TABLE 3. *Virological questions*

- Are only cells of macrophage lineage infected in the human nervous system?
- Is "viral burden" related to neurological disease and its progression?
- Are there neurotropic and/or neurovirulent strains of HIV?

other cells may be infected at levels undetected by present-day techniques. First, several studies of children with HIV encephalitis have found possible infection of astrocytes (37,38). Second, in early studies, a variety of cells were identified on the basis of anatomical position or because their processes were thought to resemble vascular endothelial cells, neurons, astrocytes, or oligodendrocytes; with the use of double staining for viral antigen and specific cell markers, even cells showing remarkable resemblance (on a morphological basis) to endothelial cells and neural cells have stained for macrophages and microglia (39–41). It is difficult to explain both clinical symptomatology and histological changes found in neurons, astrocytes, and the myelin membranes of oligodendrocytes on the basis of infection confined to macrophages and microglia.

"Viral burden" may represent either numbers of infected cells or quantity of viral protein or infectious virus produced. It is uncertain whether virus burden bears a direct relation to development of neurological disease or to the rate of its progression. Patients with HIV encephalitis, defined pathologically, have larger numbers of macrophage and microglia in which viral antigen can be stained (42), but a similar correlation is lacking between clinical symptomatology and numbers of antigen containing cells. In the systemic infection, the expression ratio of genomic RNA to viral DNA sequences correlates directly with HIV disease state (43). Thus, late in disease there is more active transcription and translation of viral products. The improvement of cognitive deficits following treatment with AZT suggests that the amount of virus replicated may be related to the cognitive deficit. The correlation between amount of virus and disease is much weaker in the vacuolar myelopathy or peripheral neuropathies (44); in support of that lack of correlation, improvement in clinical signs or symptoms have not been documented following AZT treatment.

Are there specific neurotropic and neurovirulent HIV strains? Virus recovered from the brain grows more readily in macrophage, whereas virus grown from blood and CSF grows more readily in activated T lymphocytes (45). Several groups have demonstrated the importance of the V3 envelope region as a determinant of macrophage tropism of HIV *in vitro* (46–48), and from molecularly cloned virus with differing tropism a sequence from the V3 region can be exchanged to alter the tropism for lymphocytes and macrophages. Some preliminary data suggest "brain-specific sequences" in clones derived directly from brain by polymerase chain reaction, and it is assumed that these would be macrophage-tropic (49). It is yet to be determined whether there is a subset of macrophage-tropic changes with even greater consensus found in the brain.

It is important to differentiate ability to enter and replicate in brain (i.e., neuroinvasiveness and neurotropism) from ability to cause disease (i.e., virulence). In other viral infections of the nervous system, these properties may be strikingly discordant. For example, mumps virus is the virus that causes the most frequent infection of the brain. Spinal fluid examinations in patients with otherwise uncomplicated parotitis have shown asymptomatic meningitis in over half the patients. When the symptoms develop in these patients they are usually mild; thus neurotropism or neuroinvasiveness are extremely high, whereas neurovirulence is very low. In contrast, herpes simplex type 1, which causes almost universal infection during life and is latent in sensory ganglia, seldom infects the brain as infectious virus. On those occasions when there is clinical encephalitis, mortality exceeds 50 percent in patients not given antiherpetic drugs. In this case neuroinvasiveness is quite low, whereas neurovirulence is very high (50). During the prolonged incubation period of AIDS, nervous system infection is frequent but unattended by serious disease; but a large percentage of the patients have severe neurological disease after the onset of AIDS. Does this change from low neurovirulence to high neurovirulence result from mutational changes in the virus, from infection of greater numbers of cells or different cells, from an increase in the amount of active replication, or from other factors?

ANIMAL MODELS (TABLE 4)

There is no optimal animal model for HIV infections, since only humans, when infected by HIV, develop an immunodeficiency syndrome and neurological diseases. HIV inoculated into chimpanzees causes infection and a persistent viremia (51). This provides a valuable model in which to study vaccine efficacy and immune responses, but it is of no value in answering questions regarding the pathogenesis of nervous system infections (52). Preliminary studies in the pigtail macaques and possibly in rabbits have also raised the question of infection, but here again there has been no evidence of disease.

An alternative is to establish another animal in which HIV-infected human

---

TABLE 4. *Questions regarding animal models*

- Can HIV infections in animals cause neuropsychiatric disease?
- Can human cells transplanted into rodents and infected with HIV clarify mechanisms of pathogenesis?
- Can *in vitro* studies mimic the infection *in vivo*?
- What can be extrapolated from the studies of other lentiviruses in their natural or unnatural hosts?

cells can be studied. Two intriguing examples in rodents have recently been presented. One is the use of human fetal brain tissue transplanted to the anterior chamber of immunosuppressed adult rats. These xenographs vascularize, form a blood–brain barrier, and differentiate, forming neurons and glia. Xenographs can be infected by HIV or by HIV-infected human monocytes, and pathological damage is noted. Therefore, this provides a model to study the effects of HIV-1 infection on developing human neural tissue and may prove useful for evaluating antiviral therapies (53). An alternative model has been the intracerebral inoculation of human mononuclear cells into the brains of severe combined immunodeficient (SCID) mice. Subsequent intracerebral inoculation of HIV has led to the infection of human macrophages that persist in the brains of the mice; this, in turn, has been accompanied by a widespread gliosis similar to that seen in HIV infections in humans, and this gliosis is found even at sites distant from the infected cells. Furthermore, the infected macrophages appear to persist in the brain—unlike uninfected macrophages, which do not. This provides an interesting model for the study of the pathogenesis of glial and possibly neuronal responses to cytokines and may give insights into trafficking of infected and noninfected mononuclear cells (54).

Another murine model does not involve human cells, but rather the construction of transgenic mice. Initially, transgenic mice containing the entire genome of HIV had no documented infection of the brain reported or any neurological disease (55). Recently, however, transgenic mice have been produced that contain the long terminal repeat of the genome of a number of HIV strains; this segment regulates virus transcription. This transgene has been found to express in neurons and at a variable rate and anatomical location depending on the HIV strain (56). This may provide a model in which to study the neurotropism and neurovirulence of different HIV strains.

In vitro models are readily available. HIV replicates in a variety of human neural cell lines and primary neural cells (57–60). In some cases, these cells have been shown to be infected without expression of the CD4 receptor (61). However, if the neurons or astrocytes are not infected *in vivo,* then studies of their infection *in vitro* may not be relevant. *In vitro* systems have also been used to examine the possible indirect mechanisms of neural damage by mixing infected microglia or macrophages with astrocytes and/or neurons (62). These systems have proved valuable in looking at the toxic effects of cytokines and viral proteins.

A variety of animals have been proposed as possible models. Visna virus infection of sheep has been studied in greatest depth. Visna, the prototype lentivirus, causes a chronic and recurrent leukoencephalitis, but this virus fails to infect CD4 cells and, therefore, does not cause immunodeficiency disease (63). The pathological changes of recurrent demyelinating lesions are localized largely to the white matter and are quite different from those seen in HIV infections in humans. However, the demonstration that visna lesions were mediated by cytokines has been important in directing analogous research in HIV (64). Both feline immunodeficiency virus and simian immune deficiency virus provide better models for HIV, since these viruses also replicate in CD4 cells and cause an immunodeficiency disease as well as a chronic encephalitis. With simian immunodeficiency virus infections, inflammatory cells, multinucleated giant cells, and multiple microglial nodules are seen in the brain, resembling HIV encephalopathy in humans (65). Myelopathy and peripheral neuropathies have not been described, and there is a lack of the diffuse myelin pallor so characteristic of the human disease (33).

PATHOGENESIS

We do not know how HIV invades the nervous system. Because of the prolonged viremia, it is assumed that the virus invades by a hematogenous route. It is not known, however, whether HIV invades the nervous system across cerebrovascular endothelial cells or across the choroid plexus and whether invasion is dependent on free virus in plasma or cell-associated virus. This information may prove important in designing strategies to prevent infection; if free plasma virus is involved, then antibody neutralization of cell-free virus in blood would prevent nervous system invasion; if virus is within cells, then adhesion molecules that may control cell movement across the different vascular endothelium of the brain or choroid plexus would need to be addressed.

The early infection, seen in asymptomatic seropositive persons, might represent only an increase in the T-cell traffic in the spinal fluid, and disease that evolves late may be a manifestation of the infection of the microglia. However, the recent report of a patient inadvertently inoculated with HIV, who died 15 days later and showed antigen-containing cells in perivascular cuffs and a few in the parenchyma (66), testifies for early macrophage and microglial involvement. The percentage of macrophages infected in the brain can be far greater than that found in studies of peripheral blood. This may represent (a) infection of macrophages after they have arrived in the brain, (b) rapid division of infected monocytes after entering the brain, or (c) alterations of the cell surfaces of infected macrophages that cause preferentially traffic into the nervous system.

TABLE 5. *Pathogenesis questions*

- How does virus invade the CNS?
- Does early infection represent T-cell traffic into the CSF, or are microglia infected early?
- What mediates disease?
    - Viral proteins?
    - Excitotoxins?
    - Cytokines?
- What is the role of opportunistic infections?

The question that has received the most discussion and laboratory inquiry is, What mediates disease? Since HIV appears to infect predominantly macrophages and microglial cells of the central nervous system, what causes the clinical signs and symptoms and what causes the proliferation of microglia, the attenuation of neuronal processes and loss of neurons (67), and the diffuse pallor of myelin? These clinical and pathological changes may represent indirect damage mediated by viral proteins (68–70), excitotoxins (71), or cytokines (72,73). Changes could result from a direct effect of proteins or cytokines released by infected macrophages on the target cells or, quite possibly, via a more indirect mechanism whereby cytokines released from macrophages affect glial cells and endothelial cells while their functional changes adversely affect neuronal function (62).

Finally, we must not overlook an early hypothesis. Prior to recognition that HIV infected the nervous system, attempts were made to explain all pathological changes on the basis of opportunistic infections. The role of opportunistic infections as either cofactors or primary factors in some of the HIV-associated neurological syndromes must be kept in consideration. Possibilities range from opportunistic infection with relatively ubiquitous agents such as cytomegalovirus, to the possible pathogenetic role of Mycobacterium avium intracellulare, to the more exotic possibilities of a new mycoplasma (74), to the odd agent associated with cat scratch fever, *Rochalimaea henselae* (75).

CLOSING NOTE

We must not assume that there is one final pathway of injury. Since neurological complications occur at different times during the prolonged infection and since different pathological responses develop, the mechanism of pathogenesis of different syndromes may be different. For example, what we learn in studies of HIV dementia or of HIV encephalitis should not be extrapolated to the spectrum of HIV-associated diseases.

This chapter has presented a summary of the 72nd meeting of the ARNMD. The first meeting held in 1920 was the only prior meeting devoted to a single infectious disease, namely, acute epidemic encephalitis (encephalitis lethargica) (76). Encephalitis lethargica or von Economo's disease was a new "viral" infection of the nervous system that had appeared in Eastern Europe about 5 years before; it had spread across Europe and to the United States in 1918–1919 and was of great concern to the American public in 1920. Yet, the agent of encephalitis lethargica was never recovered, and its mode of transmission and reservoirs were never defined. Cases decreased by the mid-1920s and disappeared in the 1930s before the advent of modern virology. Why the disease simply went away we may never know (50); I do not believe HIV will simply inexplicably vanish, but as we see the number of HIV infections mount to 20 million and as we predict nervous system infections of nearly 20 million people by 2000, I do wish, wistfully, that history could repeat itself.

ACKNOWLEDGMENT

This work was supported by PO-1-NS 2643 from the National Institute of Neurological Diseases and Stroke, The National Institutes of Health.

REFERENCES

1. Meyer HM Jr, Johnson RT, Crawford IP, Dascomb HE, Rogers NG. Central nervous system syndromes of "viral" etiology: a study of 713 cases. *Am J Med* 1960;29:334–347.
2. Zu Rhein GM, Chou S-M. Papova virus in progressive multifocal leukoencephalopathy. *Res Publ Assoc Nerv Ment Dis* 1968;44:307–358.
3. Bouteille M, Fontaine C, Vedrenne CL, Delarue J. Sur un cas de encéphalite subaiguë à inclusions. Étude anatomoclinique et ultrastructurale. *Rev Neurol* 1965;118:454–458.
4. Gajdusek DC, Gibbs CJ Jr, Alpers MP. Transmission and passage of experimental "kuru" to chimpanzees. *Science* 1967;155:212–214.
5. Gibbs CJ Jr, Gajdusek DC, Asher DM, Alpers MP, Beck E, Daniel PM, Matthews WB. Creutzfeldt–Jakob disease (spongiform encephalopathy): transmission to the chimpanzee. *Science* 1968;161:388–389.
6. Gajdusek DC, Gibbs CJ Jr. Slow, latent and termperate virus infections of the central nervous system. *Res Publ Assoc Nerv Ment Dis* 1968;44:254–280.
7. Bharucha EP, Mondkar VP. Neurological complications of a new conjunctivitis. *Lancet* 1972;2:970–971.
8. Weil ML, Itabashi HH, Cremer NE, Oshiro LS, Lennette EH, Carnay L. Chronic progressive panencephalitis due to rubella virus simulating subacute sclerosing panencephalitis. *N Engl J Med* 1975;292:994–998.
9. Townsend JJ, Baringer JR, Wolinsky JS, Malamud N, Mednick JP, Panitch HS, Scott RAT, et al. Progressive rubella encephalitis: late onset after congenital rubella. *N Engl J Med* 1975;292:990–993.
10. Centers for Disease Control. Kaposi's sarcoma and pneumocystis pneumonia among homosexual men—New York City and California. *MMWR* 1981;30:305–308.
11. Centers for Disease Control. Pneumocystis pneumonia—Los Angeles. *MMWR* 1981;30:250–252.
12. Snider WD, Simpson DM, Nielsen S, Gold WM, Metroka CE, Posner JB. Neurological complications of acquired immune deficiency syndrome: analysis of 50 patients. *Ann Neurol* 1983;14:403–418.
13. Levy JA, Shimabukuro J, Hollander H, Mills J, Kaminsky L. Isolation of AIDS-associated retroviruses from cerebrospinal fluid and brain of patients with neurological symptoms. *Lancet* 1985;2:586–588.
14. Ho DD, Rota TR, Schooley RT, Kaplan JC, Allan JD, Groopman JE, Resnick L, et al. Isolation of HTLV-III from cerebrospinal fluid and neural tissues of patients with neurologic syndromes related to the acquired immunodeficiency syndrome. *N Engl J Med* 1985;313:1493–1497.
15. Shaw GM, Harper ME, Hahn BH, Epstein LG, Gajdusek DC, Price RW, Navia BA, et al. HTLV-III infection in brains of children and adults with AIDS encephalopathy. *Science* 1985;227:177–182.
16. Resnick L, DiMarzo-Veronese F, Schüpbach J, Tourtellotte WW, Ho DD, Müller F, Shapshak P, et al. Intra-blood-brain-barrier synthesis of HTLV-III-specific IgG in patients with neurologic symptoms associated with AIDS or AIDS-related complex. *N Engl J Med* 1985;313:1498–1504.

17. Gonda MA, Wong-Staal F, Gallo RC, Clements JE, Narayan O, Gilden RV. Sequence homology and morphologic similarity of HTLV-III and visna virus, a pathogenic lentivirus. *Science* 1985;227:173–177.
18. Carne CA, Tedder RS, Smith A, Sutherland S, Elkington SG, Daly HM, Preston FE, et al. Acute encephalopathy coincident with seroconversion for anti-HTLV III. *Lancet* 1985; 2:1206–1208.
19. Cornblath DR, McArthur JC, Kennedy PGE, Witte AS, Griffin JW. Inflammatory demyelinating peripheral neuropathies associated with human T-cell lymphotropic virus type III infection. *Ann Neurol* 1987;21:32–40.
20. McArthur JC. Neurologic manifestations of AIDS. *Medicine* 1987;66:407–437.
21. Navia BA, Cho E-S, Petito CK, Price RW. The AIDS dementia complex. II. Neuropathology. *Ann Neurol* 1986;19:525–535.
22. Griffin JW, Crawford TO, Tyor WR, Glass JD, Price DL, Cornblath DR, McArthur JC. Sensory neuropathy in AIDS. I. Neuropathology. *Brain* 1993 *(in press).*
23. Johnson RT, Griffin DE, Moench TR. Pathogenesis of measles immunodeficiency and encephalomyelitis: parallels to AIDS. *Microb Pathog* 1988;4:169–174.
24. Johnson RT, McArthur JC, Narayan O. The neurobiology of human immunodeficiency virus infections. *FASEB J* 1988;2:2970–2981.
25. McArthur JC, Cohen BA, Farzedegan H, Cornblath DR, Seines OA, Ostrow D, Johnson RT, et al. Cerebrospinal fluid abnormalities in homosexual men with and without neuropsychiatric findings. *Ann Neurol* 1988;23(suppl):S34–S37.
26. McArthur JC, Cohen BA, Seines OA, Kumar AJ, Cooper K, McArthur JH, Soucy G, et al. Low prevalence of neurological and neuropsychological abnormalities in otherwise healthy HIV-1-infected individuals: results from the multicenter AIDS cohort study. *Ann Neurol* 1989;26:601–611.
27. Goethe KE, Mitchell JE, Marshall DW, Brey RL, Cahill WT, Leger GD, Hoy LJ, et al. Neuropsychological and neurological function of human immunodeficiency virus seropositive asymptomatic individuals. *Arch Neurol* 1989;46:129–133.
28. Selnes OA, Miller E, McArthur JC, Gordon B, Munoz A, Sheridan K, Fox R, et al. HIV-1 infection: no evidence of cognitive decline during the asymptomatic stages. *Neurology* 1990;40:204–208.
29. *Consultation on the neuropsychiatric aspects of HIV infection.* World Health Organization, 1988, Geneva.
30. Royal W III, Updike M, Selnes OA, Proctor TV, Nance-Sproson L, Solomon L, Vlahov D, et al. HIV-1 infection and nervous system abnormalities among a cohort of intravenous drug users. *Neurology* 1991;41:1905–1910.
31. Epstein LG, Sharer LR, Joshi VV, Fojas MM, Koenigsberger MR, Oleske JM. Progressive encephalopathy in children with acquired immunodeficiency syndrome. *Ann Neurol* 1985; 17:488–496.
32. Belman AL, Diamond G, Dickson D, Horoupian D, Llena J, Lantos G, Rubinstein A. Pediatric acquired immunodeficiency syndrome: neurologic syndromes. *Am J Dis Child* 1988;142:29–35.
33. Sharer LR. Pathology of HIV-1 infection of the central nervous system. A review. *J Neuropathol Exp Neurol* 1992;51:3–11.
34. Dewhurst S, Sakai K, Bressler J, Stevenson M, Evinger-Hodges MJ, Volsky DJ. Persistent productive infection of human glial cells by human immunodeficiency virus (HIV) and by infection molecular clones of HIV. *J Virol* 1987;61:3774–3782.
35. Schmitt FA, Bigley JW, McKinnis R, Logue PE, Evans RW, Drucker JL, AZT Collaborative Working Group. Neuropsychological outcome of zidovudine (AZT) treatment of patients with AIDS and AIDS-related complex. *N Engl J Med* 1988;319:1573–1578.
36. Vago L, Castagna A, Lazzarin A, Trabattoni G, Cinque P, Costanzi G. Reduced frequency of HIV-induced brain lesions in AIDS patients treated with Zidovudine. *J AIDS* 1993;6: 42–45.
37. Blumberg BM, Epstein LG, Saito Y, Chen D, Sharer LR, Anand R. Human immunodeficiency virus type 1 nef quasispecies in pathological tissue. *J Virol* 1992;66:5256–5264.
38. Ranki O, Ovod V, Haltia M, Nyberg M, Aavik E, Krohn K. High expression of Nef protein in HIV-infected brain astrocytes associated with rapidly progressing CNS disease. [Abstract]. In: *VII International conference on AIDS,* 1991;TuA10.

39. Pumarola-Sune T, Navia BA, Cordon-Cardo C, Cho E-S, Price RW. HIV antigen in the brains of patients with the AIDS dementia complex. *Ann Neurol* 1987;21:490–496.
40. Stoler MH, Eskin TA, Benn S, Angerer RC, Angerer LM. Human T-cell lymphotropic virus type III infection of the central nervous system. *JAMA* 1986;256:2360–2364.
41. Wiley CA, Schrier RD, Nelson JA, Lampert PW, Oldstone MBA. Cellular localization of human immunodeficiency virus infection with the brains of acquired immunodeficiency syndrome patients. *Proc Natl Acad Sci USA* 1986;83:7089–7093.
42. Budka H. Neuropathology of human immunodeficiency virus infection. *Brain Pathol* 1991; 1:163–175.
43. Michael NL, Vahey M, Burke DS, Redfield RR. Viral DNA and mRNA expression correlate with the stage of human immunodeficiency virus (HIV) type 1 infection in humans evidence for viral replication in all stages of HIV disease. *J Virol* 1992;66:310–316.
44. Rosenblum M, Scheck AC, Cronin K, Brew BJ, Khan A, Paul M, Price RW. Dissociation of AIDS-related vacuolar myelopathy and productive HIV-1 infection of the spinal cord. *Neurology* 1989;39:892–896.
45. Koyanagi Y, Miles S, Mitsuyasu RT, Merrill JE, Vinters HV, Chen ISY. Dual infection of the central nervous system by AIDS viruses with distinct cellular tropisms. *Science* 1987; 236:819–822.
46. Cheng-Mayer C, Shioda T, Levy JA. Host range, replicative, and cytopathic properties of human immunodeficiency virus type 1 are determined by very few amino acid changes in tat and gp120. *J Virol* 1991;65:6931–6941.
47. Shioda T, Levy JA, Cheng-Mayer C. Macrophage and T cell-line tropisms of HIV-1 are determined by specific regions of the envelope gp120 gene. *Nature* 1991;349:167–169.
48. Pang S, Vinters HV, Akashi T, O'Brien WA, Chen ISY. HIV-1 env sequence variation in brain tissue of patients with AIDS-related neurologic disease. *J AIDS* 1991;4:1082–1092.
49. Epstein LG, Kuiken C, Blumberg BM, Hartman S, Sharer LR, Clement M, Goudsmit J. HIV-1 V3 domain variation in brain and spleen of children with AIDS: tissue-specific evolution within host-determined quasispecies. *Virology* 1991;180:583–590.
50. Johnson RT. *Viral infections of the nervous system.* New York: Raven Press, 1982.
51. Alter HJ, Eichberg JW, Masur H, Saxinger WC, Gallo R, Macher AM, Lane HC, et al. Transmission of HTLV-III infection from human plasma to chimpanzees: an animal model for AIDS. *Science* 1984;226:549–552.
52. Gajdusek DC, Gibbs CJ Jr, Rodgers-Johnson P, Amyx HL, Asher DM, Epstein LG, Sarin PS, et al. Infection of chimpanzees by human T-lymphotropic retroviruses in brain and other tissues from AIDS patients. *Lancet* 1985;1:55–56.
53. Cvetkovich TA, Lazar E, Blumberg BM, Saito Y, Eskin TA, Reichman R, Baram DA, et al. Human immunodeficiency virus type 1 infection of neural xenografts. *Proc Natl Acad Sci USA* 1992;89:5162–5166.
54. Tyor WR, Power C, Gendelman HE, Markham R. A model of HIV encephalitis in SCID mice. *Proc Natl Acad Sci USA* 1993 *(in press).*
55. Leonard JM, Abramczuk JW, Pezen DS, Rutledge R, Belcher JH, Hakim F, Shearer G, et al. Development of disease and virus recovery in transgenic mice containing HIV proviral DNA. *Science* 1988;242:1665–1670.
56. Corboy JR, Buzy JM, Zink MC, Clements JE. Expression directed from HIV long terminal repeats in central nervous system of transgenic mice. *Science* 1992;258:1804–1808.
57. Dewhurst S, Sakai K, Zhang XH, Wasiak A, Volsky DJ. Establishment of human glial cell lines chronically infected with the human immunodeficiency virus. *Virology* 1988;162: 151–159.
58. Harouse JM, Bhat S, Spitalnik SL, Laughlin M, Stefano K, Silberberg DH, Gonzalez-Scarano F. Inhibition of entry of HIV-1 in neural cell lines by antibodies against galactosyl ceramide. *Science* 1991;253:320–322.
59. Shapshak P, Sun NCJ, Resnick L, Thornthwaite JT, Schiller P, Yoshioka M, Svenningsson A, et al. HIV-1 propagates in human neuroblastoma cells. *J AIDS* 1991;4:228–237.
60. Yamada M, Watabe K, Saida T, Kim SU. Increased susceptibility of human fetal astrocytes to human T-lymphotropic virus type I in culture. *J Neuropathol Exp Neurol* 1991;50:97–107.
61. Weber J, Clapham P, McKeating J, Stratton M, Robey E, Weiss R. Infection of brain cells by diverse human immunodeficiency virus isolates: role of CD4 as receptor. *J Gen Virol* 1989;70:2653–2660.

62. Genis P, Jett M, Bernton EW, Boyle T, Gelbard HA, Dzenko K, Keane RW, et al. Cytokines and arachidonic metabolites produced during human immunodeficiency virus (HIV)-infected macrophage–astroglia interactions: implications for the neuropathogenesis of HIV disease. *J Exp Med* 1992;176:1703–1718.
63. Narayan O, Clements JE. Biology and pathogenesis of lentiviruses. *J Gen Virol* 1989;70: 1617–1639.
64. Kennedy PGE, Narayan O, Ghotbi Z, Hopkins J, Gendelman HE, Clements JE. Persistent expression of Ia antigen and viral genome in visna-maedi virus-induced inflammatory cells. *J Exp Med* 1985;162:1970–1982.
65. Lackner AA, Dandekar S, Gardner MB. Neurobiology of simian and feline immunodeficiency virus infections. *Brain Pathol* 1991;1:201–212.
66. Davis LE, Hjelle BL, Miller VE, Palmer DL, Llewellyn AL, Merlin TL, Young SA, et al. Early viral brain invasion in iatrogenic human immunodeficiency virus infection. *Neurology* 1992;42:1736–1739.
67. Masliah E, Ge N, Morey M, Deteresa R, Terry RD, Wiley CA. Cortical dendritic pathology in human immunodeficiency virus encephalitis. *Lab Inv* 1992;66:285–291.
68. Brenneman DE, Weatbrook GL, Fitzgerald SP, Ennist DL, Elkins KL, Ruff MR, Pert DB. Neuronal cell killing by the envelope protein of HIV and its prevention by vasoactive intestinal peptide. *Nature* 1988;335:639–642.
69. Lipton SA. HIV-related neurotoxicity. *Brain Pathol* 1991;1:193–199.
70. Sabatier J-M, Vives E, Mabrouk K, Benjouad A, Rochat H, Duval A, Hue B, et al. Evidence of neurotoxic activity of tat from human immunodeficiency virus type I. *J Virol* 1991;65: 961–967.
71. Heyes MP, Brew BJ, Martin A, Price RW, Salazar AM, Sidtis JJ, Yergey JA, et al. Quinolinic acid in cerebrospinal fluid and serum in HIV-1 infection: relationship to clinical and neurologic status. *Ann Neurol* 1991;29:202–209.
72. Tyor WR, Glass JD, Griffin JW, Becker PS, McArthur JC, Bezman L, Griffin DE. Cytokine expression in the brain during the acquired immunodeficiency syndrome. *Ann Neurol* 1992; 31:349–360.
73. Wesselingh SL, Power C, Glass JD, Tyor WR, McArthur JC, Farber JM, Griffin JW, et al. Intracerebral cytokine mRNA expression in AIDS dementia. *Ann Neurol* 1993;33: 576–582.
74. Lo SC, Dawson MS, Wong DM, Newton PB III, Sonoda MA, Engler WF, Wang RYH, et al. Identification of *Mycoplasma incognitus* infection in patients with AIDS: an immuno-histochemical, *in situ* hybridization and ultrastructural study. *Am J Trop Med Hyg* 1989; 41:601–616.
75. Patnaik M, Schwartzman WA, Barka NE, Peter JB. Possible role of *Rochalimaea henselae* in pathogenesis of AIDS encephalopathy. *Lancet* 1992;340:971.
76. Association for Research in Nervous and Mental Diseases. *Acute epidemic encephalitis. Report of the papers and discussions at the meetings of the association, New York City, December 28th and 29th, 1920.* New York: Paul B Hoeber, 1921.

Index

Human immunodeficiency virus-
related neuronal injury
astrocyte, 189–190
human immunodeficiency virus type
1 protein, 189–190
laboratory basis of novel
therapeutic strategies to
prevent, 183–197
N-methyl-D-aspartate antagonist
action sites, 192–193
development, 191–195
N-methyl-D-aspartate redox
modulatory site, 194–195
open-channel blocker, 193–194
oligodendrocyte, 189–190
Human immunodeficiency virus type
1
brain
animal models, 316–318
clinical neurological diseases,
313–314
pathogenesis, 318–319
research issues, 311–320
virological issues, 314–316
central nervous system expression,
72
genetic variability, 5, 55–56
life cycle, 49–51
proviral genomic organization, 53
provirus formation, 49–51
Human immunodeficiency virus type
1-associated cognitive/motor
complex, 8
Human immunodeficiency virus type
1-associated dementia, 8, 9
Human immunodeficiency virus type
1-associated minor cognitive/
motor disorder, 8
Human immunodeficiency virus type
1-associated myelopathy, 8, 9
Human immunodeficiency virus type
1-associated progressive
encephalopathy of childhood,
293–296
Human immunodeficiency virus type
1 encephalitis, 101–102
simian immunodeficiency virus
encephalitis

differences, 140
similarities, 140
Human immunodeficiency virus type
1 env, CD4
antibody neutralization, 62
gp120 shedding, 62
interactions, 59–63
soluble CD4 neutralization, 61
Human immunodeficiency virus type
1 genome, expression, 51
Human immunodeficiency virus type
1 infection, 4–7
central nervous system, 99–100
detection methods, 101
central nervous system pathology
mechanisms, 109–114
minimal or no evidence of active
infection, 108–109
no detectable, 105–108
data sources, 3
immune dysregulation, 6
microglia, mechanism, 100–101
mononuclear phagocyte, 63, 64
replication, 5–6
reverse transcriptase, 5
viral glycoprotein, 4–5
Human immunodeficiency virus type
1 macrophage tropism, 56–64
env-mediated cell tropism,
mechanism, 58
phenotypic association, 58–59
syncytium induction, 58–59
V3 sequence analysis, 58–59
viral determinants, 57–58
Human immunodeficiency virus type
1 neurotropism
biologic basis, 47–66
genetic basis, 47–66
in vivo correlates, 65
Human immunodeficiency virus type
1 protein, human
immunodeficiency virus-related
neuronal injury, 189–190

I

Immunomodulatory therapy, 34
Immunosuppression, development,
6–7

Transforming growth factor beta 1,
human immunodeficiency virus
neuropathogenesis, 207–212,
216–218
Tricyclic antidepressant, depression,
232–233
Tumor necrosis factor alpha, 73–74
AIDS dementia complex, 78
central nervous system, 77–78
glial cell
biological effects, 77
expression, 77–78
human immunodeficiency virus
neuropathogenesis, 214–218

U
Unmyelinated nerve fiber,
predominantly sensory
neuropathy of AIDS, 173, 174

V
V3
amino acid sequences, 60
antibody neutralization, 62
V3 sequence analysis, human
immunodeficiency virus type 1
macrophage tropism, 58–59
Vacuolar myelopathy, 16–18,
105–107, 108

Vascular endothelium
AIDS dementia complex, 32
central nervous system human
immunodeficiency virus type 1
infection, 32
vif gene, 54
Viral glycoprotein, human
immunodeficiency virus type 1
infection, 4–5
vpr gene, 54
vpu gene, 54–55
vpx gene, 55

W
White matter
gliosis, 16–18
pallor, 16–18
pediatric human immunodeficiency
virus type 1-associated central
nervous system disease,
301–302
simian immunodeficiency virus,
136, 138

Z
Zidovudine, human immunodeficiency
virus dementia, 267–268